Acquired Language Disorders
A CASE-BASED APPROACH

Second Edition

Acquired Language Disorders
A CASE-BASED APPROACH

Second Edition

James M. Mancinelli, MS, CCC-SLP
Evelyn R. Klein, PhD, CCC-SLP, BCS-CL

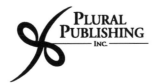

PLURAL
PUBLISHING
INC.

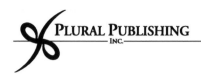

5521 Ruffin Road
San Diego, CA 92123

e-mail: info@pluralpublishing.com
Website: http://www.pluralpublishing.com

Typeset in 10½/13 Garamond Book by Flanagan's Publishing Services, Inc.
Printed in the United States of America by McNaughton & Gunn, Inc.
20 19 18 17   2 3 4 5

Library of Congress Cataloging-in-Publication Data

Klein, Evelyn R., author.
  Acquired language disorders : a case-based approach / James M. Mancinelli, Evelyn R. Klein.—Second
edition.
      p. ; cm.
  Author's names reversed on the first edition.
  Includes bibliographical references and index.
  ISBN-13: 978-1-59756-571-4 (alk. paper)
  ISBN-10: 1-59756-571-7 (alk. paper)
  I. Mancinelli, James M., author. II. Title.
  [DNLM: 1. Language Disorders—diagnosis—Problems and Exercises. 2. Aphasia—diagnosis—Problems
and Exercises. 3. Aphasia—therapy—Problems and Exercises. 4. Language Disorders—therapy—
Problems and Exercises. 5. Language Therapy—Problems and Exercises. WL 18.2]
  RC423
  616.85'5—dc23
                                                                          2013035349

Contents

Accompanying PowerPoint slides and CD include lecture material for:
    Review of Neuroanatomy
    The Target Model
    Assessment in Acquired Language Disorders (ALD)
    Nonfluent Aphasia
    Fluent Aphasia

Preface

Introduction

New and experienced clinicians may find it challenging when attempting to integrate theoretical knowledge and research into clinical practice. As professors teaching the graduate courses in acquired language disorders and clinical practicum, we realize that it isn't until the clinician actually encounters a person with a specific disorder that academic knowledge and practice coincide. Given our years of experience as both teachers and practitioners, it is our intention to bridge the gap between theory and practice by providing the reader with a case-based approach to understanding acquired language disorders (ALD). To further our goal in making ALD come to life for the reader, we have developed a model that depicts the individual's language and cognition following a cerebrovascular accident or other neurologic event. We refer to this as the Acquired Language Disorders Target Model, and each of the 14 cases that we discuss has a corresponding diagram within the chapter.

In our experience as professors at the graduate level, the student benefits from the graphic features of the ALD Target Model because it facilitates a concrete understanding of the linguistic and cognitive characteristics of each case. This model combined with features of the various disorders, case analyses, and treatment considerations connects theoretical knowledge with practical application. In our opinion, this case-based approach matches the needs of speech-language pathologists practicing in health care today.

How the Book Is Organized

Each chapter includes a fictional person based upon an actual case that was treated in a health care setting, private practice, or home health environment to exemplify a specific acquired language disorder. These case scenarios were developed based on actual patients who the authors or their colleagues have evaluated and treated. This brings to life each communication impairment for the learner, who can better conceptualize the specific characteristics of the disorder in the context of a real person. For purposes of anonymity and confidentiality, the patients' names and identifying information have been changed.

As practicing speech-language pathologists, we believe it is essential to understand not only the basic pathophysiology of a disease process associated with an acquired language disorder, but also the functional effects it may have on a person's life. The fundamentals presented here allow the reader to participate in discussions with other professionals and family members. The student or practitioner can then use this information to build a foundation for assessment and therapeutic approaches, which are found in Appendix D.

Special Features

The 14 cases in this book provide a comprehensive overview of the assessment process, major aphasic syndromes, right hemisphere disorder, traumatic brain injury, dementia, encephalopathy, and other etiologies affecting the ability to communicate. The final chapter provides detailed information about past, present, and future considerations in treating individuals with ALD. We discuss therapeutic approaches currently in use and include new trends in treatment.

Each chapter is based on a case study and includes eight sections:

- **Characteristics** of the disorder including neurologic correlates.
- **Case Scenario** providing a brief overview of the case history.

- **Diagnostic Profile** including language expression, speech production, auditory comprehension, reading, written expression, cognition, and behavioral symptoms of the case.
- The **ALD Target Model** presents a visual representation that captures the type and degree of language impairment as well as any areas of cognition that may be affected.
- **Functional Analysis** consists of a narrative that succinctly summarizes the case and helps the clinician understand the impact of the disability on daily life.
- **Critical Thinking/Learning Activity** poses questions designed to help the student or clinician develop problem-solving and practical skills necessary to maximize the patient's progress.
- **Treatment Considerations** provide areas to consider for rehabilitation based on the patient's strengths and weaknesses, individualized to his/her psychosocial context. General therapeutic objectives are also provided.
- **Therapeutic Options** include possible treatment considerations pertinent to the case, most of which are further described in Appendix D.

The Acquired Language Disorders Target Model

We developed the Acquired Language Disorders Target Model™ (ALD Target Model™) from an *embedded language framework*. This model is shown in Figure 1 and reflects the influence that cognition plays in normal communication and, by extension, in the rehabilitation of people with acquired language disorders. The physical appearance of the model depicts a schematic relationship between language and cognition as well as the relationship among functional language modalities.

There are five primary domains of the ALD Target Model: Language, Attention, Memory, Executive Functions, and Visual Spatial skills. The Language domain includes four areas: expression, comprehension, reading, and writing. Expression (E) and com-

Normal Communication Embedded within Normal Cognitive Functions

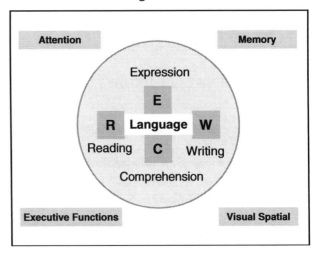

Figure 1. The Acquired Language Disorders Target Model.

prehension (C) involve the verbal modality; whereas reading (R) and writing (W) involve the visual modality. Although as speech-language pathologists we are clinically oriented to the Language domain, we must not neglect the other four cognitive areas of functioning because they are integral to functional communication.

For an individual who has normal communicative functions, the lettered squares (E, C, R, and W) remain attached to the rectangle containing the word *Language*. For an individual with an acquired language disorder, the lettered squares move further away from the Language rectangle to reflect greater impairment. For each type of acquired language disorder, the pattern is different. For example, in a person with an expressive nonfluent aphasia (Broca's), the E square and the W square are placed outside the circular border to indicate a severe degree of impairment. Depending on the acquired language disorder, any or all of these language modalities may be impaired at varying degrees. This ranges from normal, to mild-moderate, to moderate-severe, to severe-profound. Impairment level is depicted in Figure 2.

The ALD Target Model reflects our agreement with Helm-Estabrooks and Albert (2004): assessing the cognitive domains of attention, memory, visuo-

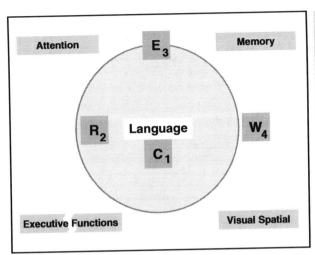

Figure 2. The key to understanding the Acquired Language Disorders Target Model.

spatial skills, and executive functions in aphasia should be a component of the standard evaluation for treatment planning. The reader will notice a fractured line through any of the four cognitive domains that are impaired in each specific case presented For example, in an individual with a severely impaired memory, the box labeled *Memory* has a fractured line going through the word.

How to Use This Book

For the Student and the Practitioner

- A graphic image of the ALD Target Model representing each disorder enhances the student's or practitioner's understanding of cognitive-linguistic changes pertinent to that specific case.
- The value of the case-based approach to ALD is that it facilitates comparisons among types of patients. This optimizes more accurate decision-making for planning treatment. As a learning tool, this approach helps the student or practicer attach clinical information to a case that is represented with a physical image
- The ALD Target Model combined with the Functional Analysis can be very useful for

clinical practice in a health care setting. This permits the student or practitioner to integrate the neurologic, cognitive, linguistic, and functional aspects of each patient to formulate a holistic picture for treatment.

- PowerPoint slides supporting lectures are provided for the topical chapters in the book.
- Critical thinking questions are provided for each case to facilitate clinical decision-making skills, and Appendix G provides a case-based exam to "test your knowledge."
- Many current treatment approaches (23) are provided to assist the practitioner in planning a program for each patient.
- Each case has a one-page diagnostic profile that describes each patient's language expression, speech, auditory comprehension, reading, written expression, cognition, and behavioral symptoms.

For the Instructor

- An overview of basic neuroanatomy for acquired language disorders is provided.
- This book offers a detailed summary of many formal and informal assessments

and treatment programs for those with ALD.

■ There are 14 case-based acquired language disorders, each with assessment and treatment considerations, to facilitate class discussion and clinical problem solving.

■ There is a section on past, present, and future considerations with a historical overview of efficacy and evidence in treating those with ALD.

■ PowerPoint slides correspond to the text and offer important lecture material, diagrams, illustrations, and online links for teaching.

■ Charts, tables, and figures including the ALD Target Model help categorize and concretize the various acquired language disorders.

■ Functional treatment can be easily planned using the Functional Communication Connections Worksheet with samples provided.

■ A Test Your Knowledge examination is also provided using seven case-based examples.

Reference

Helm-Estabrooks, N., & Albert, M. L. (2004). *Manual of aphasia and aphasia therapy* (2nd ed.). Austin, TX: Pro-Ed.

Acknowledgments

We were delighted when Plural Publishing asked us to prepare the second edition of *Acquired Language Disorders: A Case-Based Approach*. As a professor and a director of clinical education, we have many responsibilities, but writing a book for students and clinicians to benefit their patients is a high priority. We couldn't have completed this task without the support of our Speech-Language-Hearing Science Program Director, Barbara Amster, PhD, CCC-SLP, and our Dean of the School of Nursing and Health Sciences, Brain Goldstein, PhD, CCC-SLP. They provided steadfast support and are remarkable colleagues. We are also grateful for the guidance and input we received at Plural Publishing from our Executive Editor, Valerie Johns, our Project Editor, Milgem Rabanera, and our Production Editor, Megan Carter, with whom we consulted on a regular basis. We are honored they saw the repeated value in this text to produce a second edition.

Jim Mancinelli would like to thank his colleague and coauthor, Evelyn Klein for participating in this second edition. She is a generous individual with a calming spirit and fine intellect. It was an honor and a pleasure to work with her on this book. Of course, my love and gratitude goes out to SB, who listens and comforts at just the right times.

Evelyn Klein would like to thank her colleague and coauthor, James Mancinelli, for taking the lead on the second edition of this text. His ideas in the formation of this text continue to make it valuable to the profession. Working with Jim on this edition was a pleasure, and I am very grateful that he signed on for the second edition. A special thank you also goes to DF for always being there and providing daily support.

*Jim Mancinelli dedicates this book to his partner
Dave—for all the things you are.*

*Evelyn Klein dedicates this book to her husband
Dietrich—for his constant support and gentle spirit.*

Chapter 1

AN OVERVIEW OF NEUROANATOMY AND NEUROPHYSIOLOGY RELATED TO ACQUIRED LANGUAGE DISORDERS (ALD)

The Neuron

The brain has more than 100 billion neurons, or nerve cells. These structures comprise the building blocks of the nervous system and are its functional work horses. Each neuron is composed of a body, referred to as the soma; filamental extensions called dendrites; and longer fibers called axons. Each neuron has one axonal fiber that can measure from micrometers to meters in length. The axon functions as a conductor of electrical impulses. Dendrites receive stimuli or input from other neurons, and axons send stimuli to other neurons, glands, or muscles (Webb & Adler, 2008). These neurons communicate with each other electrochemically via neurotransmitters (a discussion of neurotransmitters appears in this chapter; Figure 1–1).

The nervous system has sensory neurons (receptors) and motor neurons (effectors). Sensory neurons are sensitive to light, sound, touch, temperature, smell, and chemical input, and transmit sensory information from the environment via the nervous system. Motor neurons receive excitation from other cells and send impulses to the muscles instructing them to contract and to the endocrine glands to regulate hormonal secretions. Input from sensory neurons can be transmitted to motor neurons, for example, a sensory neuron may detect a dangerous stimulus and respond by alerting interneurons in the spinal cord to notify the motor neurons to remove that body part in danger. At the endpoint or terminal of the nerve cell, neurotransmitters are released into the synaptic space between the cells. Neurotransmitters are biochemical compounds that help neurons communicate, acting as messengers between them (Figures 1–2 and 1–3).

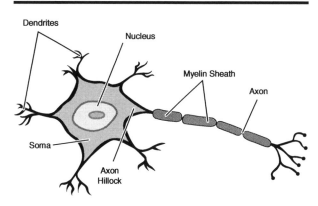

Figure 1–1. Neuron.

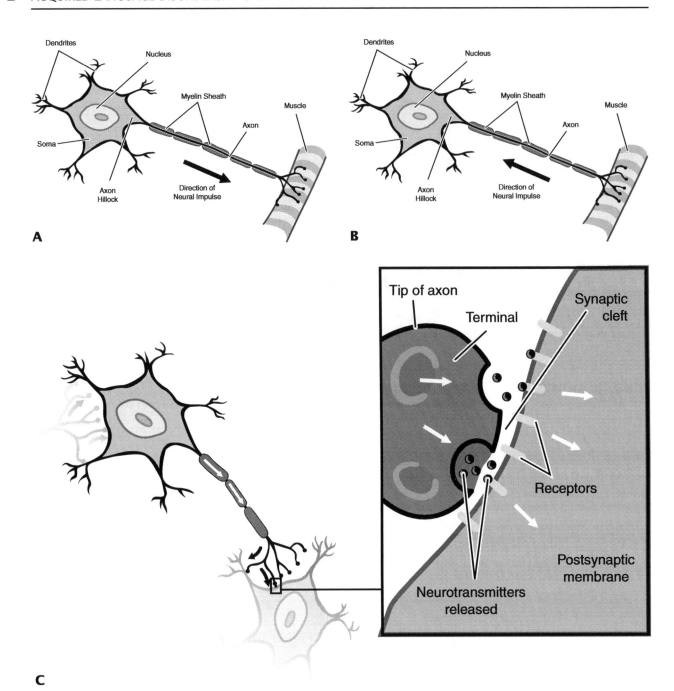

Figure 1–2. A. Motor neuron. **B.** Sensory neuron. **C.** Events at synapse.

Neurotransmitters

Neurotransmitters are chemicals that assist in the regulation of the brain's ability to control metabolic activity, speech and language, motivation, personal-

ity, mood states, and cognition including attention and memory (Bhatnagar, 2002). Each neuron releases neurotransmitters at the synapse, which is where the bulb of the axon makes contact with the dendrites. The neurotransmitter passes across the synaptic cleft and bonds with the receptor site on the postsynaptic

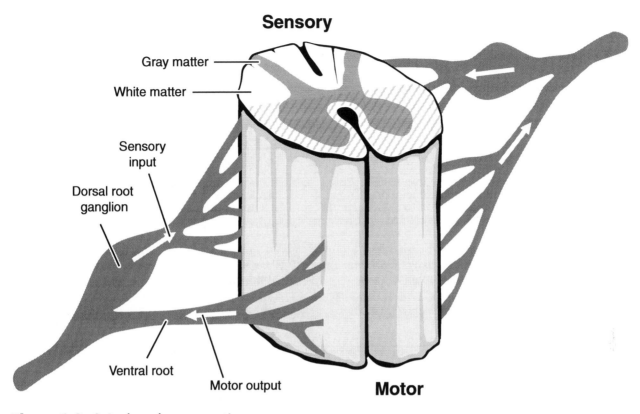

Figure 1–3. Spinal cord cross-section.

membrane. This results in a change in the electrical current across the cell membrane and the nerve fibers. The change in the electrical valence of the cell is referred to as the action potential. An excess or depletion of neurotransmitters can have significant effects on functioning. For example, excess dopamine interacting with other factors has been linked to schizophrenia, and a depletion of dopamine concentration contributes to Parkinson's disease.

There are two main types of neurotransmitters: the small molecules and the large molecules, also known as neuropeptides. The small molecule transmitters include acetylcholine, serotonin, dopamine, norepinephrine, glutamate, histamine, and gamma aminobutyric acid (GABA). In this group, GABA is primarily inhibitory whereas glutamate is excitatory. Yet in many cases, neurotransmitters can be either excitatory or inhibitory depending on the receptor site. Dopamine can act in this way. The large molecule neuropeptides include vasopressin, somatostatin, neurotensin, enkephalin, and endorphins. These neuroactive substances are hormone-mediated and affect the body's metabolic functioning. A pituitary peptide such as endorphin is opioid-like and functions in pain management. Neuroactive peptides may be specific to particular organs and have multiple roles in the body. Both groups of neurotransmitters are crucial to a person's feelings of pleasure, pain, stress, cravings, the promotion of sleep and rest, and emotional attachment, as well as basic metabolic functioning (Schwartz, 1991; Webb & Adler, 2008; Table 1–1).

The Brain: A Brief Review of Structure and Function

The central nervous system consists of the brain and spinal cord. Each segment of the spinal cord has both sensory and motor nerves that innervate our skin, organs, and muscles. During brain development in

Table 1–1. Selected Neurotransmitters

Neurotransmitter	Distribution	Proposed Impact
Acetylcholine	It is the primary neurotransmitter of the peripheral nervous system (PNS) and important to the central nervous system (CNS) as well. It is concentrated in the basal forebrain, striatum, and reticular formation. It is also concentrated within regions of the brainstem involved with cognition and memory.	Involved in voluntary movement of skeletal muscles and viscera including spinal and cranial nerves. Drugs that affect cholinergic activity within the body impact heart rate, bladder function, digestion, and may cause dry mouth. This neurotransmitter is also important to sleep-wake cycles. Decreased cholinergic projections on muscle cells are found in myasthenia gravis. Decreased projections in the hippocampus and orbitofrontal cortex are related to Alzheimer's disease.
Dopamine	Concentrated in neuronal groups in the basal ganglia. Dopaminergic projections originate in the substantia nigra and have terminals in the cortex, amygdala, and nucleus accumbens.	Decreased dopamine in the brain is linked to Parkinson's disease. An increase of dopamine in the forebrain is linked to schizophrenia. Dopamine is involved in cognition and motivation and is related to wanting pleasure associated with love and addiction.
Norepinephrine	Norepinephrine neurons are found in the pons and medulla. Most are in the reticular formation and locus ceruleus.	Important to maintaining attention and focus. It increases excitation in the brain and is involved in wakefulness and arousal. It is also associated with the sympathetic nervous system and feelings of panic, fight, or flight.
Serotonin	Synthesized from the amino acid tryptophan and found in blood platelets and the gastrointestinal tract. Terminals are localized in nerve pathways from the nuclei at the center of the reticular formation.	Controls mood, regulates sleep, involved in perception of pain, body temperature, blood pressure, and hormonal functioning. Low levels are associated with depression. It is also involved in memory and emotion.
GABA	A major neurotransmitter with cells found in the cerebral cortex, cerebellum, and hippocampus. GABA projections are inhibitory from the striatum to the globus pallidus and substantia nigra to the thalamus.	Loss of GABA in the striatum is linked to a degenerative disease that causes involuntary abnormal movements (Huntington's chorea). It is associated with the inhibition of motor neurons.

childhood, neurons create new connections with other neurons. At birth, the brain weighs about 350 grams (12 ounces) and is about 1,000 grams (2.2 pounds) at 1 year old. As an adult, the brain weighs approximately 1,200 to 1,400 grams (2.6 to 3.1 pounds) and does not have the ability to create new connections with other neurons, as most neurons cannot be replaced. This section discusses the brain's covering, the ventricles, and the following major structures of the central nervous system: the cerebral cortex, brainstem, subcortical structures, cerebellum, and the neural pathways.

The Coverings of the Brain, Ventricles, and Cerebrospinal Fluid

There are three layers of tissues, the meninges, that protect the brain. They include the dura mater, arachnoid membrane, and pia mater. Between the arachnoid membrane and pia mater is the subarachnoid space. This space contains blood vessels and cerebrospinal fluid (CSF).

The CSF protects the brain. It is a clear and colorless fluid that circulates throughout the brain and the spinal cord cushioning and protecting them from injury. There are four ventricles within the brain: two lateral ventricles, the third ventricle, and the fourth ventricle. Each ventricle contains the choroid plexus, which is the structure that produces the CSF. The CSF flows from one ventricle to the next and finally into the subarachnoid space. It is reabsorbed back into the blood. The lateral ventricles are connected to the third ventricle, and the third ventricle is connected to the fourth. Blockage in any of the spaces can cause CSF to back up, leading to a number of serious medical conditions including hydrocephalus, which increases pressure on the brain (http://www.sickkids.ca/childphysiology/cpwp/brain/csf.htm; Figures 1–4 and 1–5).

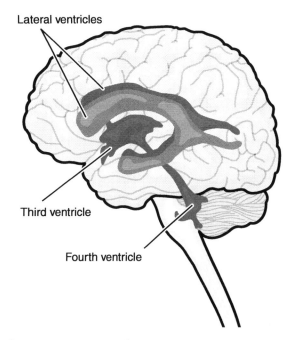

Figure 1–4. Ventricles.

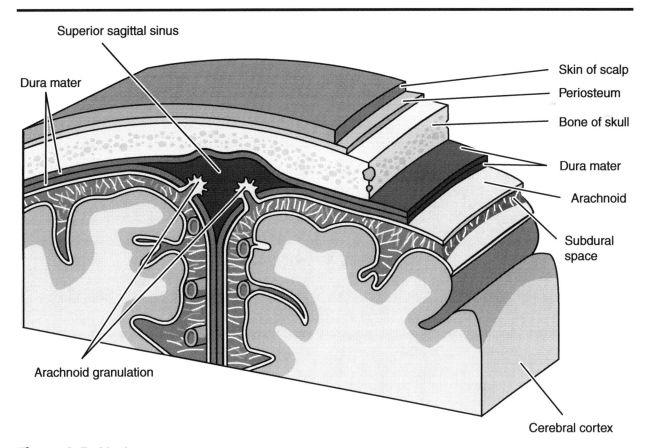

Figure 1–5. Meninges.

Cerebral Cortex

The cerebral cortex is also referred to as the cerebrum and it composes the largest part of the brain. It is involved in complex thought and executive functions learning, personality, movement, touch, and vision, and is divided into two hemispheres: right and left. The outer surface of each hemisphere is composed of gray matter that contains nerve cell bodies (more than 6 billion), glial cells, capillaries, axons, and dendrites. The gray matter directs sensory or motor stimuli to the interneurons of the central nervous system for responsiveness via synaptic activation. White matter consists of axons that travel throughout the cortex. These structures are referred to as *white matter* because of the color of the myelinated sheaths that wrap each axon. The color reflects the fact that they consist primarily of lipids, or fatty material. As noted in the section on neurons, the axon is responsible for carrying information away from the brain to the periphery. These axons form tracts, and the tracts take the information to their intended destination. Two neurologic diseases that manifest white matter changes are multiple sclerosis, which destroys the myelin shield surrounding the axons and Alzheimer's disease. In Alzheimer's disease, these white matter changes produce amyloid plaques.

The two hemispheres of the brain primarily receive sensory information from the contralateral side of the body and affect movement on the contralateral side of the body. The two hemispheres are separated by a longitudinal fissure but communicate by two large bundles of axons, the corpus callosum composed of cortical association fibers and subcortical connections. The proper and efficient functioning of the corpus callosum is critical to the transmission of information between the left and right hemispheres. The left hemisphere typically is best for processing speech and language and is involved in verbal memory. The right hemisphere has been known to process paralinguistic information and pragmatics as well as providing skills with nonlinguistic information that is visual, spatial, emotional, and musical.

The cerebral cortex integrates sensory and motor signals in order to execute the primary sensory, motor, and association area functions.

The sensory areas of the cortex receive input from the environment such as touch, taste, smell, vision, and hearing. The motor areas are responsible for muscular activity throughout the body. The association areas of the cortex connect the sensory and motor systems and give humans the ability to integrate the sensory (afferent) and the motor (efferent) information, permitting normal function.

The following website provides an overview of midsagittal brain structures and functions (Figure 1–6): http://web.psych.ualberta.ca/~iwinship/studyguide/brain_study.htm

Lobes of the Brain

Each hemisphere is composed of four lobes: the frontal, temporal, parietal, and occipital (Figure 1–7). The left side of the brain generally controls the right side of the body, and the right hemisphere controls the left side of the body. Damage to either hemisphere can result in paralysis or lost sensation. Weakness on one side of the body is referred to as hemiparesis, and paralysis on one side of the body is referred to as hemiplegia. Thus, if a person has a left hemispheric stroke with a paralysis on the right side of the body, that person has a right hemiplegia. If the right side is only weak, it is then a right hemiparesis.

The following website provides an overview of the lobes of the brain and their associated functions: http://www.stanford.edu/group/hopes/basics/braintut/ab4.html. The lateral views provide further detail of the structural landmarks and functional association areas of a cerebral hemisphere (Figures 1–8A and 1–8B).

The Frontal Lobes. The frontal lobes are at the most anterior part of the brain. The anterior limit of the frontal lobe is dorsal and posterior to the bony case of the eyes. The posterior limit of the frontal lobes is the precentral gyrus. The posterior portion of the frontal lobe is specialized for control of movement. In humans, the frontal lobe is critical for language production. The prefrontal area is important for planning and initiation, judgment and reasoning, concentration, emotional range, disinhibition of behaviors, and adaptation to change. Functions of the frontal lobes are essential to con-

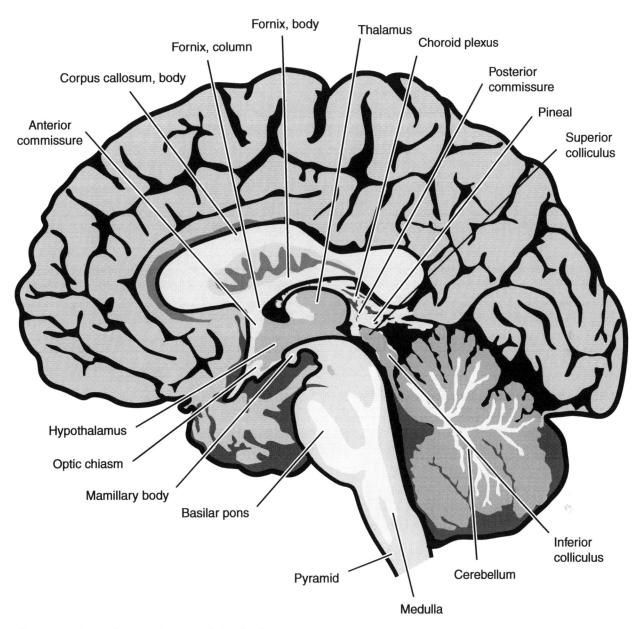

Figure 1–6. Midsagittal view of the brain.

sciousness and let us appropriately judge what we are doing in the environment and how we initiate and respond to life's events. Proper functioning assists with our emotional response and expressive language choices. Essentially, the frontal lobes make us aware of our conscious actions, and our emotional responses, memory for habits, motor activities, and expressive language are all mediated by the frontal lobe.

People who have frontal lobe damage may demonstrate the following impairments:

- Loss of simple movement (paralysis)
- Loss of spontaneously interacting with others
- Loss of flexible thinking
- Persistence on a single thought (perseveration)

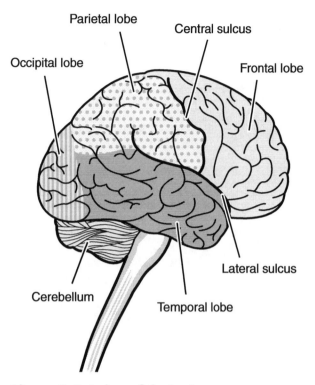

Figure 1–7. Lobes of the brain.

- Inability to focus on a task
- Mood changes that are frequent and inappropriate (emotional lability)
- Changes in personality and social behavior
- Difficulty problem solving
- Inability to express language (Broca's nonfluent aphasia)
- Inability to sequence complex movements.

The Temporal Lobes. The temporal lobes are located laterally in the cerebral hemispheres, approximately at the level of the ears. They house the primary and secondary auditory cortex, and are involved in auditory sensation and perception. Wernicke's area is located in the posterior part of the superior temporal gyrus and important to auditory comprehension of language. It is in this area that auditory stimuli are transformed for comprehension. However, many associations connect auditory input with other systems including memory needed for the auditory comprehension of language. Hearing ability, some visual perceptions, and categorization

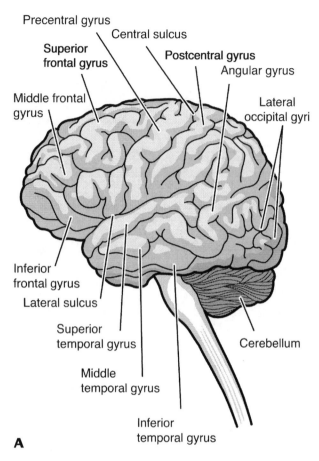

A

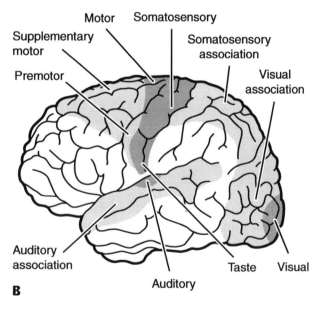

B

Figure 1–8. A. Lateral view of the brain with structural landmarks. **B.** Lateral view of the brain with primary functions and secondary association areas.

skills are dependent, in part, on the temporal lobe. The left temporal lobe contains Wernicke's area, which is critical to language comprehension. Damage to the temporal association cortex may lead to difficulty identifying and categorizing auditory stimuli. The main functions of the temporal lobe include hearing ability, memory acquisition, visual perceptions, and categorization of objects. Individuals who have lesions in this area may demonstrate the following deficits:

- Difficulty in recognizing faces (prosopagnosia)
- Difficulty understanding spoken words (Wernicke's aphasia)
- Difficulty identifying and verbalizing about objects
- Disturbance with selective attention to what is seen and heard
- Short-term memory loss
- Interference with long-term memory
- Increased or decreased interest in sexual behavior
- Inability to categorize objects
- Right lobe damage can result in persistent talking
- Increased aggressive behavior
- Poor selective attention to what is seen or heard.

The ability to understand written and spoken language occurs primarily in Wernicke's area, and the ability to produce speech movement occurs primarily in the frontal lobe (Broca's area). These two areas communicate with each other constantly via bundles of neurons that are subcortical white matter pathways known as the arcuate fasciculus and superior longitudinal fasciculus. These pathways also pass through gyri at the rim of the sylvian fissure (angular gyrus and supramarginal gyrus), which are also very important areas for the language modalities.

The Parietal Lobes. The parietal lobes are located between the occipital lobe and the central sulcus. The most anterior part is the postcentral gyrus where the axons carrying sensory information for sensation terminate. The parietal lobe receives and evaluates most sensory information including touch,

pressure, pain, temperature, and taste. Sensations from the body are represented at various parts of the postcentral gyrus. A person with parietal lobe damage may demonstrate the following deficits:

- Inability to attend to more than one object at a point in time
- Inability to name an object (anomia)
- Problems with reading (alexia)
- Inability to write words (agraphia)
- Word blindness (inability to recognize words)
- Difficulty with math (dyscalculia)
- Difficulty drawing objects
- Difficulty knowing left from right
- Lack of awareness of specific body parts
- Inability to focus visual attention
- Difficulties with eye-hand coordination
- Impaired perception of touch
- Unilateral neglect
- Inability to manipulate objects.

The Occipital Lobes. The occipital lobes are located at the posterior part of the brain. It is the primary target for projections from the thalamus, and it receives sensory information from fibers in the eyes. The retina gets visual input in the form of light flashes, shapes, and shading. This input is then transmitted through the optic nerve to the thalamus and then to the primary visual cortex in the occipital lobe. If the visual cortex is damaged, blindness or a partial visual field cut can ensue. For example, damage to the left hemisphere often impairs vision in the right visual field. A small focal area of damage or lesion can lead to a small blind area or scotoma. Although the neural information is initially meaningless, the association areas of the cortex transmit stimuli to other parts of the brain for analysis. The medial and lateral surfaces of the occipital lobe help with such visual associations. This secondary area of the occipital lobe is important to visual processing for recognizing objects and visually discriminating.

Damage to the occipital lobe may include, but are not limited to the following:

- Defects in vision such as visual field cuts
- Difficulty locating objects in the environment

- Difficulty recognizing drawn objects
- Inability to recognize movement of an object
- Difficulty identifying colors
- Visual illusions or inaccurately seeing objects
- Word blindness or inability to recognize words
- Difficulties with reading and writing.

The Insula. This portion of the cerebrum is sometimes referred to as the fifth lobe. It is not as easily visualized like the other four lobes since it is in underneath the parietal, temporal, and frontal lobes, deep within the lateral fissure. The insula is consid-

ered a critical area for both sensory and motor functions, and has been found to be related to speech and language skills. The connections and functions of the insula have not been fully described in the literature and await further investigation.

The Brainstem

The brainstem consists of the medulla oblongata, pons, and the midbrain (Figure 1–9). These structures are also referred to as the mesencephalon. The cerebellum may also be considered as part of the brainstem as it is located rostral to the spinal cord. However, it is discussed separately in this text.

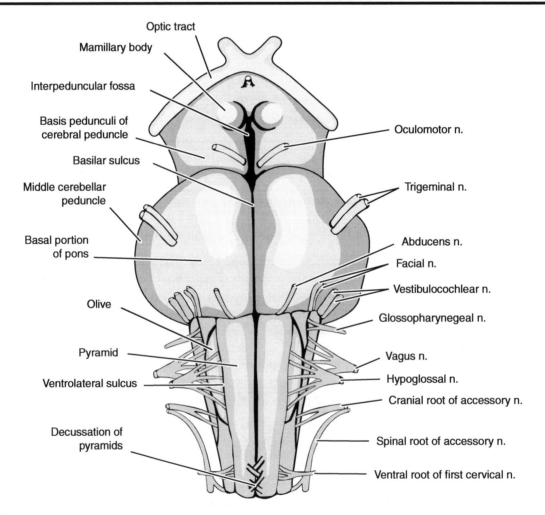

Figure 1–9. Brainstem.

The brainstem connects the brain to the spinal cord and regulates primary life functions such as respiration, swallowing, blood pressure, eye movements, and heart rate. It also mediates functions such as vomiting, salivation, sneezing, coughing, and gagging. Sensations from the skin, joints of the head, face, and neck including hearing, balance, and taste are all under the control of the brainstem. Control of the trunk and limbs for both sensation and motor control is mediated by the spinal cord (Kelly & Dodd, 2000).

The medulla actually is an enlargement of the top of the spinal cord and occasionally is referred to as the bulb. This structure is extremely important for speech motor control. It contains both ascending and descending nerve tracts as well as the nuclei of the cranial nerves controlling phonation, articulation, velopharyngeal closure, and swallowing. The medulla contains cells of the reticular activating formation that is crucial for overall arousal and important for sleep.

The pons is located superiorly to the medulla and inferior to the midbrain. It contains the nuclei for the trigeminal, abducens, facial, and vestibulocochlear nerves. It is the bridge to the cerebellum. The pons also helps control breathing and sleep, and contains part of the reticular activating system, which is important for alertness and arousal functioning.

The midbrain contains most of the brainstem and connects it to the forebrain. It contains the superior colliculus for vision and inferior colliculus for hearing. It also houses the nuclei for the oculomotor and trochlear cranial nerves, important for eye movement and sensation. The substantia nigra is also housed in the midbrain. The substantia nigra produces the neurotransmitter dopamine and plays an important role in the reward center. It is responsible for controlling sensory processes such as vision and movement. A common disorder affecting this region (specifically the substantia nigra) is Parkinson's disease.

The 12 Cranial Nerves

There are 12 pairs of cranial nerves. With the exception of cranial nerve I (olfactory) and II (optic), the cranial nerves emanate from the brainstem. They serve functions that are motor (efferent), sensory (afferent), or both. Motor nerves send impulses from the cortex via neural pathways to the spinal cord. Once there, they synapse with the cell bodies in the spinal cord. The nerve impulses are then sent to the targeted muscles, glands, or organs via the peripheral nervous system. The motor nerves include the oculomotor (III), trochlear, (IV), abducens (VI), spinal accessory (XI), and the hypoglossal (XII). Sensory nerves receive input from the periphery and send nerve impulses from the sensory organs to the brain. The sensory portions of the cranial nerves have their origin outside the brain in ganglia that divide into two branches: one that extends into the postcentral gyrus (the sensory cortex) and one that connects to the sensory organ itself. The sensory nerves include the olfactory (I), optic (II), and the vestibulocochlear (VIII). Mixed nerves have more than one originating nucleus and include the trigeminal nerve (V), the facial nerve (VII), the glossopharygeal (IX), and the vagus nerve (X; Table 1–2).

Subcortical Structures

Subcortical structures are found above the midbrain and contain the hypothalamus and thalamus, also referred to as the diencephalon. The thalamus is an oval structure that acts as the gatekeeper to relay sensory input to other areas of the brain. It is located in the center of the forebrain. Most sensory information is processed first in the thalamus and then is relayed to the cerebral cortex. Thalamic lesions may affect contralateral somatic sensations and create a lower threshold for pain. The hypothalamus is a small area located ventral to the thalamus with widespread connections to the thalamus, reticular formation, cerebral cortex, limbic system, olfactory bulb, and midbrain. Its many nuclei help regulate endocrine functions. Damage to one of the hypothalamic nuclei often leads to difficulty with feeding, drinking, temperature regulation, sexual behavior, sleep, wakefulness, activity level, and/ or fighting. The hypothalamus also exerts a major influence on regulating the body's hormonal system and can impact emotional expression, food intake, metabolism, and cycles of sleep and wakefulness as well. Attached to the base of the hypothalamus

Table 1–2. Cranial Nerves

I. Olfactory (smell)
II. Optic (vision)
III. Oculomotor (eye movement and pupil constriction)
IV. Trochlear (eye movement)
V. Trigeminal (sensations of touch, pain, and temperature from the face and head; chewing and swallowing)
VI. Abducens (eye movement)
VII. Facial (taste for anterior 2/3 of tongue, somatosensory information from ear, facial expression, and controls muscles for facial expression)
VIII. Acoustic/Vestibulocochlear (hearing and balance)
IX. Glossopharyngeal (taste for posterior half of tongue and somatosensory information from tongue, tonsils, and pharynx, and controls some muscles for swallowing)
X. Vagus (sensory, motor, and autonomic visceral functions: heart rate, glands, digestion)
XI. (Spinal) Accessory (controls muscles used in head movement)
XII. Hypoglossal (controls muscles of tongue)

The following website provides an overview of the cranial nerves with their associated locations: http://faculty.washington.edu/chudler/cranial.html

is the pituitary gland. It releases hormones into the bloodstream and to other organs. It is considered the master gland of the body, controlling secretions from the thyroid, adrenal gland, ovaries, and testes.

The hippocampus is another subcortical structure located between the thalamus and cerebral cortex, and is important for recent working memory. It is also crucial for inhibiting a habitually unsuccessful action. The amygdala also plays a role in memory. The amygdala's primary role is in forming and storing memories associated with emotional events. The hippocampus and the amygdala work as a whole system to regulate motivation and emotions (Figure 1–10).

The Cerebellum

The cerebellum is inferior to the occipital lobes and posterior to the brainstem. The cerebellum has two hemispheres and is divided into three lobes each. The white matter within the cerebellum connects it to other parts of the central nervous system. The gray matter analyzes body movement and compares it with what is needed to accomplish a specific motor task. It is crucial for maintaining balance in space and executing coordinated movements. A very critical function of this structure for speech and swallowing is the integration of sensory input from regions of the brain, allowing it to coordinate muscle groups. The cerebellum also modifies muscle tone, speed, and range of motion, allowing movements to be executed smoothly.

The cerebellum helps to make sequenced motor skills automatic. Because the cerebellum is important for motor control, it receives input from muscle spindles and tendons via the spinal cord. It also gets input from vision, hearing, touch, and the vestibular system for balance. A critical distinction between the cerebellum and the cortical structures is that the

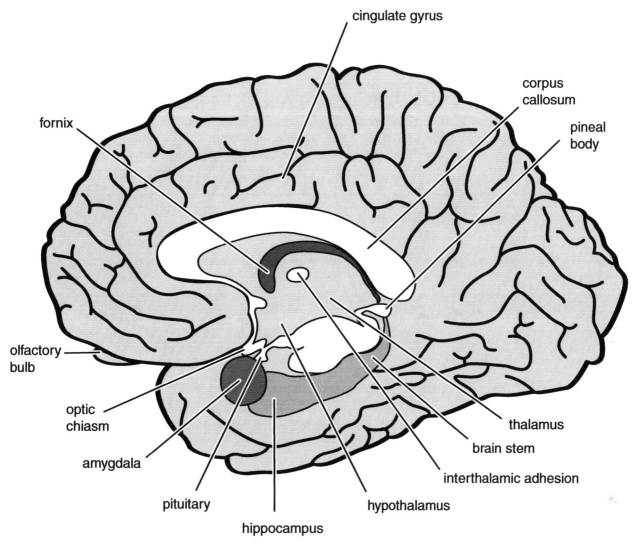

Figure 1–10. Subcortical structures of the brain.

cerebellum can only control and perform online correction of planned movements. It does not initiate motor activity (Figure 1–11).

Neural Pathways

To the left and right of the thalamus is the basal ganglia, which includes the caudate nucleus, putamen, and globus pallidus. These structures are involved in motor control and integration. They form part of the extrapyramidal system, which are neural pathways whose function is the coordination of involuntary movement. The anatomy of the extrapyramidal system remains unclear. It primarily connects the cortex with the basal ganglia, but it also has indirect influence on the lower motor neuron in the spinal cord. This system is polysynaptic, that is, it makes many connections through interneurons before its impulses reach the spinal cord. These tracts affect reflexes, locomotion, posture, and complex movement. Any degradation of the extrapyramidal system

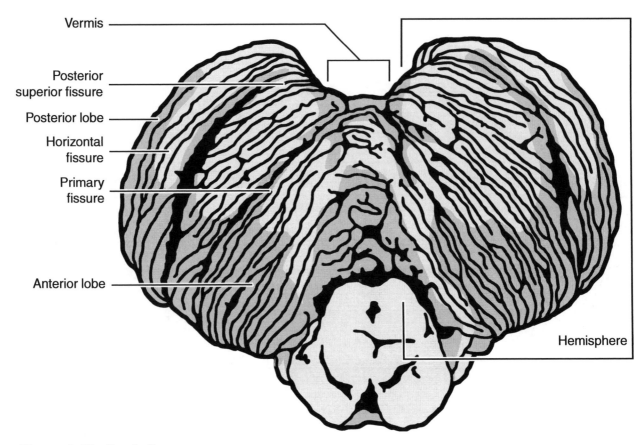

Vermis

Posterior superior fissure

Posterior lobe

Horizontal fissure

Primary fissure

Anterior lobe

Hemisphere

Figure 1–11. Cerebellum.

due to stroke or other neurological processes causes difficulties with motor control. People with extrapyramidal disorders have varied clinical presentations. They may have difficulty initiating movement (akinesia) or inability to remain still or motionless (akathisia). Tardive dyskinesia, commonly seen as a side effect from prolonged use of some psychotropic drugs, is manifested as involuntary and irregular muscle movement. Cerebral palsy of the athetoid type is another example of an extrapyramidal disorder. Huntington's chorea and Parkinson's disease are the best known examples of extrapyramidal disorders, and many speech-language pathologists who practice in an acute-care setting will encounter these patients. The extrapyramidal system plays a significant role in speech production and swallowing function, and every speech and language clinician must be aware of its structure and functions.

The pyramidal system consists of upper motor neurons in the primary motor cortex whose axons synapse with the lower motor neurons in the anterior horn of the spinal cord. The lower motor neuron axon, also referred to as the final common pathway or the alpha-neuron, begins in the spinal cord and extends to the muscles for movement of the arms and legs. The pyramidal system is a monosynaptic system and controls all voluntary movement. It is made up of three nerve tracts: the corticospinal, the corticobulbar, and the corticopontine. The corticospinal tract controls the movements of the limbs and digits. Eighty to ninety percent of corticospinal tract axons cross over to the other side in the medulla. This crossover is referred to as the point of pyramidal decussation. Injuries to upper motor neurons in the cortex at the point before they enter the pyramidal decussation will lead to spastic paralysis on the opposite side of the body. If an injury occurs to the pyramidal tract below the point of decussation, or to the lower motor neurons in the spinal cord, paralysis on the same side of the body will result. The axons of the corticobulbar tract synapse with the cranial nerves and, therefore, affect the movement of the speech musculature. The corticopontine tract connects the nuclei in the pons to the cerebellum. After receiving information from sensory input, it is the pyramidal system that activates muscles so that various body parts can move as needed (Figure 1–12).

Cerebral Blood Flow

The brain is only 2% of the average adult body weight. However, it receives 15% of the total cardiac output and uses 25% of the total body glucose. It also consumes almost 20% of available oxygen within the entire body.

There are two broad arterial systems: the carotid and the vertebrobasilar (Figure 1–13). The carotid arterial system has a left and right branch, and divides into the internal and external carotid arteries. The internal carotids supply the blood to the anterior part of the brain and subdivide into the anterior cerebral artery (ACA), middle cerebral artery (MCA), and the posterior cerebral artery (PCA). The external carotid artery supplies blood to the face, the tongue, and parts of the head.

The Circle of Willis is a critical structure because it allows blood to flow through both hemispheres of the brain and acts as a safety valve if blood flow on one side of the brain is blocked. Because of its construction, if blood flow is blocked on the left, blood from the right can reach the unnourished area (Love & Webb, 1992). Branching off from the Circle of Willis are two arterial systems that supply the forebrain and cortical areas pertinent to speech and language production: the ACA and the MCA. The posterior cortex, the midbrain, and the brainstem are all supplied by the PCA, the basilar artery, and the vertebral artery.

The ACA supplies blood to the medial surfaces of the frontal and parietal cortex. The MCA supplies

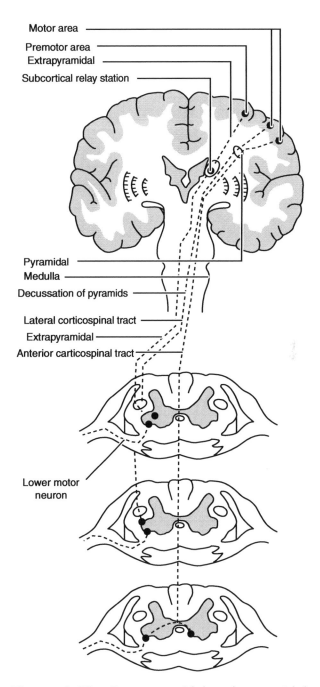

Figure 1–12. Extrapyramidal and pyramidal systems.

most of the lateral cortex of both cerebral hemispheres, including portions of the temporal lobes and frontal lobes. It provides blood flow to both Broca's and Wernicke's areas. It also has smaller

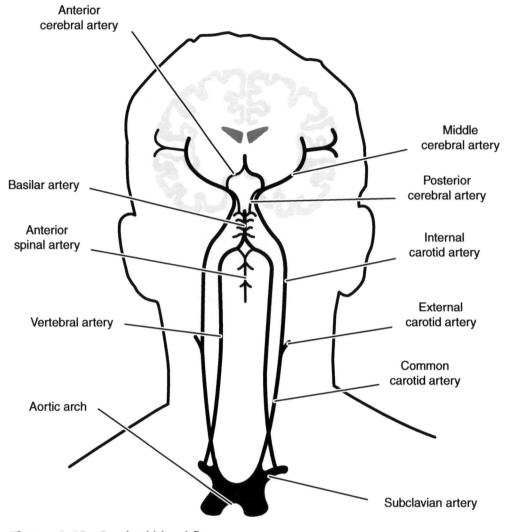

Figure 1–13. Cerebral blood flow.

branches that supply blood to the basal ganglia and internal capsule. The posterior cerebral history supplies medial and inferior surfaces of occipital and temporal lobes. The vertebrobasilar arterial system supplies the occipital lobes, medial aspects of the temporal lobes, and brainstem.

Cerebrovascular Accidents

Cerebrovascular accident (CVA), commonly known as stroke, refers to a lack of blood flow to any area of the brain, including the brainstem. As the brain is not able to store oxygen or glucose, any interruption of blood flow affects its ability to function properly. The cerebral arteries supply oxygen and blood to parts of the brain. The cerebral arteries arise from the internal carotid and vertebral arteries. At the base of the brain, the arteries form the Circle of Willis. It is there that branches of the internal carotid arteries and branches of the basilar arteries communicate. The MCA is the largest of the cerebral arteries (compared with the ACA and the PCA). The MCA is most often related to a CVA as it supplies blood and oxygen to most of the outer surface of the brain, the basal ganglia, and anterior and posterior internal capsules (Slater, 2006). Cerebral infarcts that disrupt blood flow and oxygen to the brain may arise from hemorrhagic or ischemic events in any of the arteries.

In the United States, there are 700,000 strokes annually. It is the third leading cause of death in the country and the leading cause of long-term disability (National Institute of Neurological Disorders and Stroke, 2008). Both the ischemic and hemorrhagic types of stroke are considered cerebral vascular accidents and can cause aphasia. There are approximately 100,000 cases of aphasia annually in the United States due to stroke alone (Helm-Estabrooks & Albert, 2004).

Hemorrhagic Events

The hemorrhagic stroke typifies approximately 20% of all strokes. However, the mortality rate of hemorrhagic strokes is 50% in the United States. These strokes can be due to massive edema, brain herniation, or the use of illicit drugs, especially cocaine. Other etiologies include aneurysm, clotting deficiencies, leukemia, brain tumors, and occasionally traumatic brain injury. A majority of hemorrhagic strokes are due to the rupture of a congenital berry aneurysm. In the United States, approximately one-fourth of people who suffer a stroke will die. About one half will live with long-term disabilities, and another one fourth will recover most all functions (National Institutes of Health, 2008; Figure 1–14A).

Ischemic Events

There are two types of ischemic stroke, thrombotic and embolic. The thrombotic type is due to a blood clot that forms in a vessel and remains there. Fat and blood from the diseased artery block the vessel going to the brain, and the artery narrows at the site of the thrombosis. The embolic type is caused by a blood clot that travels from the site where it was formed to a cerebral artery. The detached mass within the blood vessel is carried along with the blood flow, preventing nutrients such as oxygen and glucose from nourishing the cortical tissue. Approximately 80% of all strokes are of this type (National Institute of Neurological Disorders and Stroke, 2008). Lacunar infarcts are a type of ischemic stroke. This results from constriction of the small vessels that penetrate the brain, usually caused by hypertension. Finally, lacunar disease also can be caused by transient ischemic attacks (TIA), which

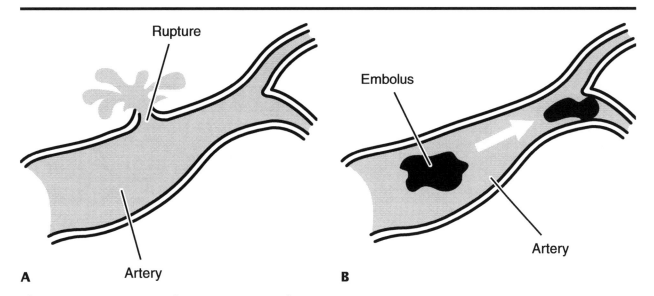

Figure 1–14. A. Hemorrhagic event. **B.** Ischemic event.

are brief events, lasting less than 24 hours. They typically last only 2 to 15 minutes without evidence of brain damage (Figure 1–14B).

Potential Sequellae to ACA Stroke

From the internal carotid artery, the ACA extends both forward and upward. It supplies blood to the frontal lobes. This part of the brain impacts personality, logical thought, and voluntary movement, particularly in the legs. Damage to this area due to stroke may result in weakness of the opposite leg; however, damage to both anterior cerebral territories may produce an akinetic form of mutism (DeFelice, 2005; Stroke Center at Washington University, 2008).

Damage to the ACA (Figure 1–15) may result in:

- Confusion
- Loss of coordination
- Impaired sensory functions
- Personality changes
- Contralateral paresis or paralysis.

Potential Sequellae to MCA Stroke

The MCA provides blood to much of the temporal lobe, anterolateral frontal lobe, and parietal lobe. Damage to this area may result in a homonymous hemianopsia, which is commonly expressed in ipsilateral head or eye deviation. Contralateral hemiplegia concerning the face, arm, and to a less significant extent, the leg, is also noted. Typically, the blockage is embolic although thrombotic blockage is frequently seen in the carotid (DeFelice, 2005; Slater, 2006).

Damage to the MCA (Figure 1–16) may result in:

- Aphasic syndromes
- Motor speech disorders
- Visual field cuts
- Contralateral paresis or paralysis.

Potential Sequellae to PCA Stroke

The PCA provides blood to the occipital lobe and the inferior section of the temporal lobe, originating from the basilar artery. When this area is damaged, problems with vision, memory, smell, and emotion may arise in conjunction with functions associated with the midbrain and thalamus (DeFelice, 2005).

Damage to the PCA (Figure 1–17) may result in:

- Visual field cut
- Sensory impairment
- Alexia
- Cortical blindness
- Color blindness
- Locked-in syndrome
- Agnosias.

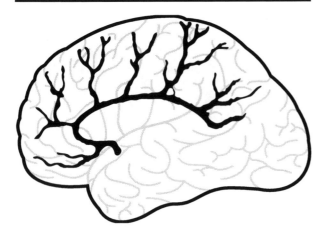

Figure 1–15. ACA (for anterior cerebral arteries).

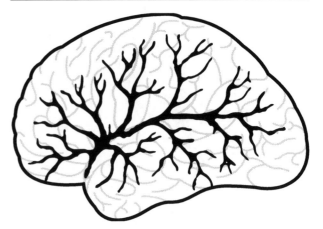

Figure 1–16. MCA (for middle cerebral arteries).

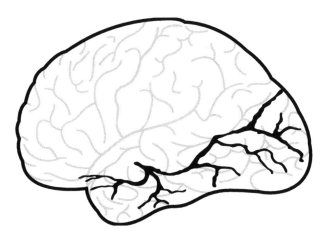

Figure 1–17. PCA (for posterior cerebral arteries).

Brain Imaging and Selected Medical Tests for Acquired Language Disorders

The medical diagnosis of stroke includes imaging studies, that is, tests that provide static or dynamic images of the damaged areas of the brain to supplement the clinical findings. Some of these tests image blood flow and metabolic activity, and some image structure. Some use radioactive materials and some do not. The most frequently used imaging studies used in the diagnosis of stroke include: computerized axial tomography (CAT or CT) scan, magnetic resonance imaging (MRI), functional magnetic resonance imaging (fMRI), positron emission tomography (PET) and single photon emission computerized tomography (SPECT) scan, and the latest technique called arterial spin labeling (ASL; Detre, Wong, Wang, & Rao, 2009).

The traditional use of imaging in aphasia and acquired language disorders has primarily focused on identifying the lesion site for diagnostic purposes, and less for therapeutic interventions. Ramage, Kiran, and Robin (2008) discuss the role of imaging in treatment and treatment planning for people with aphasia. They report some potential problems with using imaging for identifying neural regions activated during the scanning of a patient engaged in a language task. For instance, a region that is activated during a task does not necessarily indicate that it is the area responsible for processing that task. It may actually be a *residual language region* activated to perform the task secondary to the lesion. Also, scanning after treatment and substantial recovery does not necessarily indicate the mechanisms underlying that recovery. The authors suggest that the patient is scanned in the early, middle, and late stages of recovery. This more refined methodology may be more accurate for delineating the actual area of function by documenting the changes over time. Finally, the authors state that one must consider the nature of the task and level of task difficulty because these two factors can confound the analysis of imaging results.

In addition to imaging studies, the major cerebral arteries and blood flow may be tested via Doppler ultrasound, carotid phonoangiography, endocardiography, or angiography. Several brain imaging studies are outlined below.

CAT Scan or CT Scan

- This test takes 10 to 20 minutes to conduct.
- A three-dimensional picture is created from different angles in slices, linked to x-rays to detect hemorrhages, lesions, and tumors.
- Must be done to detect if a stroke is hemorrhagic or ischemic (important to know prior to giving tissue plasminogen activator or tPA).
- This is not a good test for soft tissue lesions.
- This is a good test for pinpointing the site of the lesion.

MRI

- Testing time is typically 30 to 45 minutes.
- A magnetic field is used to show fine details in the brain and spinal cord.
- MRI shows:
- soft tissues
- large blood vessels
- location and size of arteriovenous malformations

- tumors
- blood clots
- ischemic stroke

fMRI

- fMRI is a nonradioactive, noninvasive procedure that shows the use of glucose and oxygen feeding areas of the working brain.
- Movement of the patient during the procedure can adversely affect readings.
- fMRI can be used:
  - to map critical areas in patients prior to brain surgery
  - to directly measure blood flow indicating functional brain activity
  - to investigate the role of specific brain regions in human activity

PET Scan

This test is radioactive and provides imaging of metabolic activity in the brain:

- The radioactive markers assess the brain's metabolism for oxygen and glucose and blood flow.
- This test reveals how the brain is using blood flow to function.
- This test is expensive and not done routinely as a diagnostic tool but more often for research purposes in clinical settings.

SPECT Scan

- This test evaluates the amount of blood flowing through the brain's regions.
- It can identify areas of reduced or absent blood flow (known as regional cerebral blood flow or rCBF).
- This test assesses cerebral metabolism of glucose and oxygen.
- It typically is not done as an inpatient procedure due to its high expense.
- SPECT is more commonly used for research purposes.

ASL

- This test is used with structural MRI, not fMRI.
- The blood water that is proximal to the tissue of interest is magnetically labeled, and the patient is then scanned with traditional MRI technology.
- This is most useful for imaging the neural correlates of functional behavior, including speech and language.

Examination of the Carotids: Doppler Ultrasound or Auscultation of the Carotids

- Doppler examination of the carotids use an ultrasound technique with high-frequency sound waves.
- This is a noninvasive procedure that examines the blood flow in the major arteries and veins of the neck and brain.
- This examination detects bruits that are turbulent sounds within an artery and indicate extracranial carotid occlusive disease.
- Audio measurements *bear* the blood flow and produce a visual image of the carotid arteries.
- This procedure is used in patients with vascular disease to identify partial or complete occlusion of a vessel.
- Auscultation with a stethoscope also provides evidence of carotid artery disease through the detection of the turbulent sounds associated with bruits.

Endocardiography

- This procedure uses ultrasound to take images of the heart and can detect blood clots that have the potential to travel to the brain.
- Endocardiography can detect:
  - a hole in the atrium of the heart
  - a clot in a ventricle

- an infected valve of the heart
- an enlarged heart that is a risk factor for stroke (often due to chronic hypertension)

Angiography

- CT Type
  - A trace element is injected intravenously with contrast dye to detect blood flow.
  - Ischemic areas or a subaracnoid aneurysm can be detected.
  - This test delineates areas where there is a deprivation of blood flow.
- MR Type (also known as MRA)
  - This test is similar to an MRI but is conducted with contrast dye that is injected to depict blood flow to the brain.
- Cerebral Angiography
  - This is an invasive test using dye that is injected intravenously into an artery.
  - A catheter is surgically inserted into a blood vessel around the groin, which is guided through the circulatory system to an artery leading to the brain.
  - X-rays are taken to track blood flow.
  - Abnormalities that can cause stroke (aneurysm, narrowing vessels, embolus, atherosclerosis, arteriovenous malformations, etc.) can be detected.
  - There is a risk to this procedure. If a clot is present in the artery prior to the procedure, introducing the catheter into the artery can dislodge the clot, thereby increasing the probability of an embolic stroke.

References

Bhatnagar, S. C. (2002). *Neuroscience for the study of communicative disorders* (2nd ed.). Philadelphia, PA: Lippincott Williams & Wilkins.

DeFelice, E. A. (2005). *Prevention of cardiovascular disease: Atherosclerosis, carotid artery disease, cerebral artery disease/stroke, coronary artery disease, peripheral artery disease and hypertension.* Lincoln, NE: iUniverse.

Detre, J. A., Wong, J., Wang, Z., & Rao, H. (2009). Arterial spin-labeled perfusion MRI in basic and clinical neuroscience. *Current Opinion in Neurology, 22,* 348–355.

Helm-Estabrooks, N., & Albert, M. L. (2004). *Manual of aphasia and aphasia therapy* (2nd ed.). Austin, TX: Pro-Ed.

Kelly, J. P., & Dodd, J. (2000). Anatomical organization of the nervous system. In E. R. Kandel, J. H. Schwartz, & T. M. Jessell (Eds.), *Principles of neural science* (4th ed.). Columbus, OH: McGraw-Hill.

Love, R. J., & Webb, W. G. (1992). *Neurology for the speech-language pathologist* (2nd ed.). Stoneham, MA: Butterworth- Heinemann.

National Institute of Neurological Disorders and Stroke. (2008). *What you need to know about stroke.* Retrieved from http://www.ninds.nih.gov/disorders/stroke/stroke_needtoknow.htm

National Institutes of Health. (2008). *Medline plus outlook on stroke.* Retrieved from http://www.nlm.nih.gov/medlineplus/ency/article/000.htm#Expectations%20(prognosis)

Ramage, A. E., Kiran, S., & Robin, D. A. (2008). Has imaging advanced the science in aphasiology? A critical review of neuroimaging research in acquired adult language disorders. In R. Ingham (Ed.), *Neuroimaging in communication sciences and disorders* (pp. 155–193). San Diego, CA: Plural.

Schwartz, J. H. (1991). Chemical messengers: Small molecules and peptides. In E. R. Kandel, J. H. Schwartz, & T. M. Jessell (Eds.), *Principles of neural science* (4th ed.). Norwalk, CT: Appleton and Lange.

Slater, D. I. (2006). *Middle cerebral artery stroke.* Retrieved from http://www.emedicine.com/pmr/TOPIC77.htm

Stroke Center at Washington University. (2008). *Blood vessels of the brain.* Retrieved from http://www.strokecenter.org/education/ais_vessels/ais049a.html

Webb, W., & Adler, R. K. (2008). *Neurology for the speech-language pathologist* (5th ed.). St. Louis, MO: Mosby-Elsevier.

Chapter 2

ELEMENTS OF ASSESSMENT IN ACQUIRED LANGUAGE DISORDERS

Assessment

It is important to attempt to read the patient's and family's signals upon the first meeting, prior to testing. We urge the speech-language pathologist (SLP) to go slowly during the initial phases of testing. Remember, the patient has undergone a significant medical event and may be suffering in a number of ways when you receive the consult. Whether a bedside evaluation or a formal test battery is to be used, it is important to show the patient and his or her family members that you are genuinely concerned. You want to inform them that you intend to gather accurate information about the patient's communication abilities in order to plan and deliver the most appropriate treatment. Although this seems logical, it is crucial that patients know your intention to gather information to assist their recovery. One cannot assume the patient understands this without taking the necessary time to gain rapport. Don't rush into testing prior to knowing the patient is ready to try and work with you.

The purpose of the initial evaluation is to determine if the person has an acquired language disorder, and to classify it by type and severity, and to provide a functional prognosis. Throughout the therapeutic course, functional communication is emphasized and the SLP gauges the patient's recovery by charting changes in the areas of impairment. The SLP obtains important information about the patient and family during the initial interview process, which informs the development of a functional and meaningful treatment plan. A case history is obtained from the medical chart or during the interview and typically includes the following information:

- Chief complaints and admitting diagnosis
- Past medical history (PMH)
- Past surgical history
- Family history
- Psychosocial history
- Work and educational history.

If the clinician sees the patient in an inpatient setting, it is always best practice to contact family members or caregivers to confirm the information that the patient provided as well as to obtain another perspective on the patient and his or her history. Information about the patient's communication style and communicative needs in the home environment should be obtained. It is said that the eyes and ears of a clinician are sometimes the best diagnostic tools available. Consequently, informal observational findings supplement and complement the formal diagnostic testing. Using both informal and formal methods of assessment further help the SLP in the development of a proper plan of treatment. Areas of speech and language to evaluate are:

- Discourse ability (conversations and questions)
- Auditory comprehension (following commands)
- Naming skills (clothing, accessories, money, etc.)

- Repetition skills (words, sentences with increasing syllables)
- Reading and writing (read printed words and write names of objects)
- Ability to sing ("Happy Birthday")
- Praxis (waving, hammering, blowing out candles, etc.).

In addition to the case history and speech-language findings, the clinician needs to be alert to more global elements of the patient's condition and integrate that information into the clinical picture of the patient. This includes:

- Behavior
- Gait and posture
- Appearance
- Gross functioning of skin, head, neck, and spine
- Noted impairment in cranial nerves
- Reflexes
- Stereognosis (identify object felt in hand without visual help)

Aspects of the motor system should also be noted:

- Muscle tone and strength
- Muscle wasting
- Physical symmetry
- Coordination (balance, walking, sitting)
- Involuntary movements (shaking, twitching, tremors)

This information can be obtained from the medical chart, specifically in the nursing notes and the consults from other services in the hospital who are also involved in the patient's care. See the Speech-Language Pathology Case History Form provided (Appendix A). For a comprehensive overview of the characteristics of the acquired language disorders covered in this book, see Appendix 2–A.

Areas of Language Function

Six major areas of language functioning are generally considered when assessing aphasia. These areas are noted below, as well as the most common lesion sites producing the aphasic symptoms.

1. The first area is the patient's *speech fluency*. Fluency involves the length of the utterance that an individual expresses in connected words. Fluent speech generally includes phrases and sentences that are at least four words in length. Fluent aphasias involve a more posterior lesion (around the temporoparietal junction) in the cerebral cortex whereas nonfluent aphasias generally result from a more anterior lesion (the perisylvian gyrus) in the brain.

2. The second area of assessment involves *comprehension of language*. Patients with more posterior lesions typically have more comprehension difficulties than those with anterior lesions. Comprehension is a broad term and can involve understanding words, phrases, sentences, paragraphs, stories, and conversation.

3. The third area of assessment involves the ability to use *automatic speech*. Automatic speech refers to commonly used sequences of language. For example, days of the week and months of the year are considered automatic. This type of language tends to be easier to produce as it becomes rote over time.

4. The fourth area of assessment is *repetition* or *imitative speech*. The ability to repeat what one hears is a diagnostic feature. Individuals with certain types of aphasia (such as conduction aphasia) have difficulty with repetition of speech.

5. The fifth area of assessment is *naming*. Struggle, circumlocutions, recurrent utterances, paraphasias, jargon, and confrontation naming difficulty can be observed in patients with naming problems.

6. The sixth area of assessment is *grammatical use*. Agrammatism, which is typical for anterior lesions, is characterized by fragmented, incomplete use of sentences and includes omissions and substitutions of inflections and function words (prepositions, articles, conjunctions, etc.). Speech may sound telegraphic. Agrammatism is often prevalent in those with a nonfluent type of aphasia. Paragrammatism indicates a reduced syntactic complexity with substitution of function words and inflections. This tends to

coincide with paraphasic errors often seen in fluent types of aphasia and is more consistent with a posterior lesion.

Characteristics of Major Aphasic Syndromes

Each of the major aphasic syndromes have both shared and unique characteristics. In reality, very few of them are pure, and people with aphasia often have overlapping features. The primary characteristics (Figure 2–1) are used to assist in the differential diagnosis of the syndromes. In our discussion, we assume that the left hemisphere is dominant for speech and language functions.

Just as the aphasic syndromes commonly seen in the clinical setting have both shared and unique characteristics, each syndrome can have more than one name. For example, Broca's aphasia is also known as an *anterior aphasia, motor aphasia, nonfluent aphasia,* and sometimes, *expressive aphasia.* Wernicke's aphasia is sometimes referred to as a *posterior aphasia, fluent aphasia, sensory aphasia,* or *receptive aphasia.* The interchangeability of these terms reflects the culture of the medical setting and not a nosological difference.

The major aphasic syndromes are generally due to cortical lesions. However, it is also possible to see aphasia secondary to a subcortical lesion. There are two major types of subcortical aphasia. One is due to a lesion in the basal ganglia and adjacent regions of the internal capsule. The other is due to a lesion in the left thalamus. These are discussed in detail in the chapter on subcortical aphasia (Chapter 5).

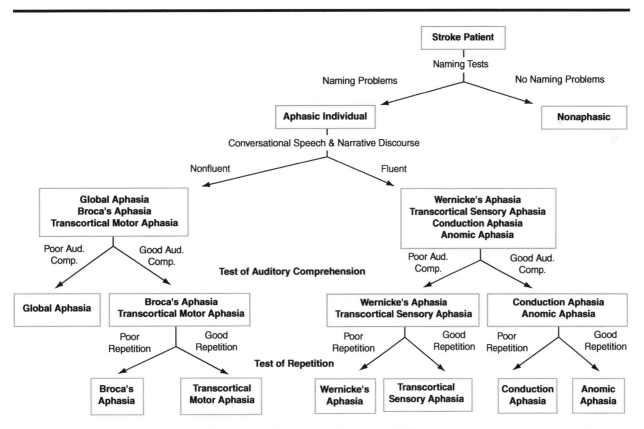

Figure 2–1. Characteristics of major aphasic syndromes. Skills Assessment Inventory. (Source: Helm-Estabrooks, N., & Albert, M. L. (2004). *Manual of aphasia and aphasia therapy* (2nd ed.). Austin, TX: Pro-ed. Copyright 2007 by Pro-Ed, Inc. Reprinted with permission.)

Definitions of the Clinical Characteristics of the Major Aphasic Syndromes

Fluency. Fluency refers to the ability to produce an uninterrupted, phrase-length utterance, typically more than four words in length.

Prosody. Prosody involves the ability to vary intonation patterns, stress, and rhythm in connected speech.

Auditory Comprehension. Auditory comprehension involves the ability to listen to and process information presented verbally. This ranges in levels from the ability to comprehend at the word level to the conversational level.

Automatic Speech. Automatic speech involves the ability to produce rote sequences such as counting, naming the days of the week, the months of the year, and so forth.

Verbal Repetition. Verbal repetition requires the ability to repeat what the examiner said. This skill is initially assessed from the monosyllabic level to sentence imitation.

Word Recall. Word recall refers to the ability to name objects and pictures during structured confrontation naming as well as at the conversational level. This can also be referred to as *lexical retrieval* or *word finding*.

Syntax. Syntactic ability involves organization of words and sentences into a logical structure based on the rules of syntax for a particular language. *Agrammatism* occurs in individuals with nonfluent aphasia and is characterized by the absence of function words, thereby creating sentences that include primarily nouns and verbs. The speech is telegraphic, and there can be omissions of grammatical morphemes. *Paragrammatism* occurs in fluent aphasia and is characterized by inaccurate syntactic rule application, for example, subject-verb agreement or incorrect tense markers, and inappropriate use of pronouns.

Perseveration. Perseveration is defined as the inappropriate repetition of a previous response that continues after the task requirements have changed and the response is no longer needed. There are three primary types of perseveration: *stuck-in-set*, *continuous*, and *recurrent*. Table 2–1 provides a definition and an example of each of these types of perseveration.

Table 2–1. Primary Types of Perseveration

Type	Definition	Example
Stuck-in-Set Perseveration Lesion: More frontal	Inappropriate maintenance of a category or framework after a new task is introduced and a new response expected.	Working on naming within a food category. When the task is changed to clothing, the patient continues to assign food names to the items of clothing.
Continuous Perseveration Lesion: Right hemispheric, subcortical, and cortical aphasias	Inappropriate prolongation of a behavior that should stop; inability to inhibit the continuation of the response.	Erasing an incorrect response as directed, but continuing until the paper is torn.
Recurrent Perseveration Lesion: Left temporal and parietal region	Inappropriate recurrence of a previous response after a new stimulus is given and a new response expected.	There can be a carryover of whole words (perseverates on *slipper* for all stimuli in the semantic category of "footwear"); or carryover of phonemic structure (perseverates on /k/ in initial position for all words subsequent to the first presentation of /k/).

Ideational perseveration also may be observed in some patients. In this type, the patient perseverates on a concept or idea despite a topic shift or change in communicative context. For example, continuing to talk about the breakfast meal, even though the topic has switched to daily activities that occur after eating breakfast. Studies indicate that 63% to 87% of aphasics have some degree of perseveration. Many people with aphasia have recurrent perseveration. There appears to be no difference in the rates of perseveration between fluent and nonfluent patients with aphasia (Helm-Estabrooks & Albert, 2004).

One must also be attentive during diagnostic testing because some errors that appear perseverative may actually be showing the therapist that the patient may have understood the task. For example, the patient may point to his head then his toe in response to your directive to point to the ceiling then the floor. However, earlier, you were asking him to point to body parts. In this case, the patient understood the directionality of the directive, but perseverated on body parts.

Clinical observations of patients with perseverative behavior have shown that certain tasks or contexts will increase the likelihood of its occurrence. This is a very important fact for a treating therapist to understand because the reduction and/or elimination of perseveration is a crucial factor for successful functional communication.

The following tasks are likely to increase the likelihood of perseveration:

- Tasks that involve non-automatic speech will increase perseveration. For example, naming tasks will increase perseveration versus counting to 10 or reciting the days of the week.
- Tasks that involve naming items, pictures, or objects that are in similar semantic fields will increase perseveration. For example, having a patient name fruits and then switch the task to naming vegetables will increase the likelihood that they will continue to name fruits (recurrent perseveration).
- Tasks that require the patient to respond more rapidly between trials will increase perseveration.

- Tasks that require the use of lexical items that occur less frequently in the language will increase perseveration. For example, this may include asking the patient to name geometric shapes such as hexagon, rectangle, and octagon.
- Tasks that use words that are close in semantic and/or phonemic properties can cause increased perseveration. For example, requiring a patient to name the following pictures: *dog, doctor, door, cat, nurse, window* may present a challenge. The semantic proximity of the words *doctor* and *nurse,* and *cat* and *dog*; the phonemic proximity of the words, *door, doctor, dog* can also increase perseveration. Consequently, the word *window* may not be produced successfully.

It is possible to decrease perseveration although it can be quite intractable. Helm-Estabrooks, Emery and Albert (1987) developed the Treatment of Aphasic Perseveration (TAP) program. In this program, the therapist writes the word that the patient is repeating on a piece of paper. One technique is to cross out the word in an attempt to extinguish the perseveration, while the patient watches. The therapist tells that patient that he or she no longer needs to say this word. Other techniques to control or reduce perseveration include:

- Establish new rules for new tasks: "Now we are going to stop talking about animals. We will now talk about clothing."
- Give the patient a break by using a distracting comment: "Do you think it will rain today?"
- Raise the patient's level of awareness about his or her perseveration: "You are repeating the same word over again, John. Do you hear yourself?"
- Do not allow the patient to see any written work that he or she has done earlier in the session, which can be a perseverative stimulus.

Paraphasia. Aphasic speech can be characterized by paraphasic errors, although not all patients demonstrate this particular characteristic. These errors reflect a disruption at the lexical level, for semantic paraphasias, or the phonological level, for the phonemic paraphasias. For more information see Kohn (1989, 1993) and Caplan (1987). There are three general types of paraphasias: phonemic, semantic, and neologistic (often referred to as a *neologism*). A *phonemic paraphasia* is characterized by a similar word substitution, where at least 50% of the word overlaps phonologically with the intended word. Examples include saying "octagon" for "octopus," or "ship" for "shirt." Phonemic paraphasias may also take the phonological shape of a non-word, for example, "ocoput" for "octopus." This is referred to as a *nonword phonemic paraphasia*. A *semantic paraphasia* is a verbal paraphasia related to the target word, for example, "jellyfish" for "octopus." This is referred to as a *related semantic paraphasia* because it is in the same class as the intended word. The *unrelated semantic paraphasia* is a real word, but not in the same class, for example, "chicken" for "octopus." Semantic paraphasias are also known as *verbal paraphasias*. A neologism is not a real word phonologically or semantically, for example, the neologism "ertig" may be said for "octopus." Notice, however, that the neologism follows the phonological rules of English, yet it is not a real word. Figure 2–2 maps the relationships of the three primary types of paraphasias.

Error Recognition. This involves the ability to recognize a phonemic (literal), semantic (verbal), or neologistic self-generated error. For individuals with error recognition problems, they are not aware that their speech contains the wrong sound, the wrong word, or a non-word.

Extralinguistic and Paralinguistic Considerations in Assessment

Assessment of right hemisphere disorders (RHD) typically involves tasks that are important for functional communication but not specific to the basic language systems (phonology, syntax, and semantics). Because the right hemisphere is more involved with complex processing of language, it is essential to nonverbal and paralinguistic aspects of communication. According to Brookshire (2003), when there is right hemisphere impairment, specific deficits typically involve the following primary categories: (1) attention, (2) perception, (3) affect, (4) communication, and (5) cognition. Within these areas, patients with RHD may experience visual neglect, difficulty recognizing faces, impulsivity, denial of deficits, lack of motivation, difficulty recognizing emotions, impaired comprehension and word retrieval, difficulty with pragmatics, impaired prosody of speech, disorientation, memory difficulties, and poor information integration, to name several. The speech-language pathologist must be cognizant of these potential deficits when conducting an evaluation, whether formal or informal in nature.

Types of Assessment

Functional Assessment

Functional testing is important to helping patients function most successfully in the world. A breakdown of visually mediated and verbally mediated

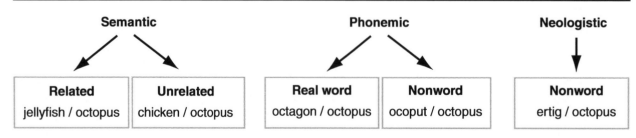

Figure 2–2. A mapping of the relationships of the three primary types of paraphasias.

functions of receptive and expressive language is delineated in Appendix 2–B. There are many measures such as *Focus on Function* (Klein & Hahn, 2007) that provide numerous functional activities for patients in therapy. Primary areas include:

- Basic communication, including expressing ideas and starting conversations
- Using the phone, including making appointments and taking messages
- Managing and understanding time, including designing a schedule and using a calendar
- Managing and understanding finances, including check-writing and using an ATM
- Shopping, including working with money and using coupons
- Meals and cooking, including planning menus, writing shopping lists, and cooking
- Getting around, including reading and understanding signs, symbols, and maps
- Activities around the house, including ordering, reading directions, writing letters
- Social participation, including social exchanges and discussing feelings and emotions
- Leisure activities, including using the Internet and communicating via e-mail
- Work-related tasks, including resume-writing and completing applications.

Appendix B (Skills Assessment Inventory) provides a checklist of functional topics that adults typically engage in during activities of daily living (ADLs).

The American Speech-Language-Hearing Association's (Frattali, Thompson, Holland, Wohl, & Ferketic, 1995) Functional Assessment of Communication Skills for Adults (ASHA FACS) is designed for assessing functional skills of adults in the rehabilitative process. The ASHA FACS provides a conceptual framework and measurement tool to assess four domains: (1) social communication, (2) communication of basic needs, (3) reading, writing, number concepts, and (4) daily planning. Within each domain is a list of behaviors to consider when evaluating

an individual's level of functioning and planning a functional treatment approach. The measure also considers qualitative dimensions of functioning. These include: adequacy (frequency with which the client understands the message); appropriateness (frequency with which the client communicates relevant information); promptness (frequency with which the client responds without delay); and communication sharing (extent to which the client's communication is a burden to the communicative partner).

- This measure was standardized on 185 adults with aphasia or cognitive impairment from 12 geographic regions of the United States.
- The scale is scored from 1 to 7 for communication independence. The scores range from 1 (does not perform even with maximal assistance or prompting) to 4 (does with moderate assistance) to 7 (does with no assistance or prompting).
- A second scale is scored from 1 to 5 for qualitative dimensions. These include ratings for adequacy, appropriateness, promptness, and communication sharing.
- Using the observational rating scale takes approximately 20 minutes.
- A communication independence score is derived.
- Test results are comprehensive and provide meaningful information to the family and help guide rehabilitation services.

ASHA developed the Functional Communication Measure (FCM) for adults and children in order to obtain outcome data. Another benefit is that it allows the clinician to track a patient's progress throughout the course of treatment in the speech and language domains. The value of this measure is two-fold: (1) it focuses on the functional aspects of communication in each domain; and (2) it provides a scoring hierarchy to monitor progress over time across domains. The FCMs range from Level 0 (Unable to Test) to Level 7 (Normal in All Situations). Table 2–2 presents the FCMs typically pertinent to ALD in adults.

Table 2–2. FCMs Pertinent to ALD in Adults

- Comprehension of Spoken Language
- Production of Spoken Language
- Recognition of Nonspoken Language
- Comprehension of Written Language
- Production of Written Language
- Cognitive Communication

For a complete review, see Kreb, R. A. (Ed.). (1996). *A practical guide to applying treatment outcomes and efficacy resources.* Rockville, MD: American Speech-Language-Hearing Association.

Bedside Assessment

Early in the assessment process, a bedside evaluation may be administered. The Western Aphasia Battery–Revised (WAB-R; Kertesz, 2006) provides a bedside evaluation component that takes approximately 15 minutes to administer. The Bedside Evaluation Screening Test (West, Sands, & Ross-Swain, 1998) may help the speech-language pathologist to secure essential language information in a shorter time than other standardized tests. Helm-Estabrooks and Albert (2004) also provide a brief informal exam that may be administered at bedside with the inclusion of several common objects. Areas to assess include: a discourse sample, auditory comprehension skills, naming common objects and coins, repetition of words and sentences, reading printed words, writing names of objects, praxis for individuals who are verbally restricted, and singing a familiar song. Table 2–3 presents sample items for a brief, comprehensive bedside screening tool for aphasia.

Cognition, Aphasia, and the ALD Target Model™

The person with aphasia has a primary disorder in the area of language; however, we cannot assume that their cognitive functions are normal or conversely, disordered after the stroke. Cognitive ability plays an important part in daily functioning. Non-brain-injured individuals must engage the world regularly using attention, memory, visuospatial skills, and executive functions combined with language. For example, it is possible that a person who is status post traumatic brain injury (TBI) may be unable to recall information over a brief time span in the presence of normal receptive and expressive language.

Helm-Estabrooks and Albert (2004) indicate that it is faulty to assume that cognition is not affected by a stroke that has produced aphasia. Furthermore, they assert that aphasia may not be "an isolated language disorder." Helm-Estabrooks, Bayles, Ramage, and Bryant (1995) have found that the level of severity of the aphasia is not significantly correlated with the severity of nonverbal cognitive skills. This suggests that cognitive impairment and language impairment after stroke are unique entities that influence one another. Just as attention impacts memory because a person must attend in order to remember information, so do memory skills impact language. The general principle is that the cognitive functions listed above interact and influence reading, writing, listening, and speaking, depending on the task. In normal-functioning individuals, it is difficult to imagine a person holding a meaningful conversation without the ability to attend and use information stored in memory. Professionals working with people with aphasia would be remiss if they did not consider a patient's ability to attend to tasks, use memory functions, perceive visuospatial details, and engage their executive functions. We suggest that clinicians screen these areas of cognitive ability using nonverbal measures such as the Cognitive Linguistic Quick Test (CLQT; Helm-Estabrooks, 2001) or the Cognitive Linguistic Evaluation (Appendix C).

In patients with cognitive deficits, the clinician must address those therapeutically before or in conjunction with language therapy (Helm-Estabrooks & Albert, 2004). Consider the task of trail making. In this activity, the client must attend to circles and triangles interspersed randomly on a page. Specifically, the task is to draw a line from a circle to a triangle keeping that pattern until all the shapes are connected. Such a nonverbal task requires general attentional skills, sequential memory, and visuospatial ability. Once the clinician has obtained the results, a therapy plan for the patient must incorporate this information. For instance, if the clinician

Table 2–3. Sample Items for a Brief, Comprehensive Bedside Screening Tool for Aphasia

Language Functions	Sample Tasks (Ex = Example)
Basic Auditory Comprehension *Directions*: The clinician gives five commands.	The patient will follow directions and/or manipulate objects from the environment based on clinician instruction: Ex: "Hand me your comb." Ex: "Point to the door."
Complex Auditory Comprehension *Directions*: The clinician will ask five questions about a narrative or story.	The patient will demonstrate the ability to understand a short narrative presented verbally: Ex: "Tell me what happened to X."
Naming *Directions*: The clinician asks the patient to name five common objects within the patient's field of vision.	The patient will name objects in the room: Ex: "What is this?"
Writing and Functional Word Retrieval *Directions:* The clinician will give the patient paper and pen in order to execute the task.	The patient will write the names of family/friends: Ex: "Write the names of your closest family members/friends."
Reading *Directions:* The clinician will locate functional reading material within the patient's room.	The patient will read greeting cards, menus, and newspapers available in the room: Ex: "Read this greeting card to me."
Expressive Language *Directions:* The clinician asks leading questions to facilitate expressive language.	The patient will describe a room of his or her house: Ex: "Describe your bedroom at home for me."
Repetition *Directions:* The clinician asks the client to repeat words, phrases, and sentences of increasing length.	The patient will repeat a word/phrase/sentence: Ex: "Repeat after each word or phrase: *book, my big book, I want my big book.*"
Verbal Memory *Directions:* Upon entering the room and greeting the patient, the clinician will offer his or her name.	The patient will remember the clinician's name once introduced: Ex: "I gave you my name three minutes ago. What is my name?"
Reasoning/Judgment *Directions:* The clinician can choose to develop the question from any home-based safety scenarios.	The patient will respond to a home-based scenario: Ex: "What would you do if you ran out of a very important medicine?"
Speech/Voice *Directions:* The clinician will monitor the patient's voice for quality, pitch, resonance, respiration and loudness, articulatory accuracy, and speech intelligibility.	The patient will produce an automatic speech sequence: Ex: "Name the days of the week."

Directions for Use: Use this beside screening instrument to delineate deficit areas. The clinician can then determine the most appropriate diagnostic instrument to administer in order to provide further clinical insights into the patient's communication profile. This would optimize treatment planning and goal selection.

plans to use a therapy program such as Melodic Intonation Therapy (MIT) (Helm-Estabrooks & Albert, 2004, p. 221) or the Sentence Production Program for Aphasia (SPPA) (Helm-Estabrooks & Albert, 2004, p. 235), which requires attention to black and white line drawings, it is necessary to consider information about their visuospatial skills. This will impact the patient's success and may require the clinician to select other stimuli. Without a cognitive screening and/or evaluation, the clinician may miss vital details to support the patient's success.

The Target Model and Cognitive Assessment in Acquired Language Disorders

According to Donovan, Kendall, Heaton, Kwon, Velozo, and Duncan (2008), up to 65% of people who sustain a stroke, experience cognitive impairments that affect their ADLs, that is, planning activities for the day. Table 2–4, lists the 10 domains of functional cognition recommended by an advisory panel of experts referenced in the above study.

The ALD Target Model includes all of these domains except for Limb Praxis, which is not within the scope of practice for speech-language pathologists. The ALD Target Model separates memory, executive function, attention, and visuosaptial functions, as does the model above. However, our model includes all areas of language functions (reading and writing, numeric/calculation, and social use of language) within the ALD Language area (expression, comprehension, reading, and writing). The domain of Emotion Function is not covered in the ALD Target Model in the same manner as in Donovan et al. (2008). However, the specific areas of anosagnosia and behavioral changes due to stroke are developed within each case study presented, because people with stroke can manifest both of these aspects status post CVA. Emotional and/or behavioral changes due to stroke will certainly affect communicative abilities, and clinicians should address this through counseling and education of patients and caregivers as well as more directly in therapy as needed.

As noted above, cognitive ability plays an important part in daily functioning. For people who have cognitive-linguistic deficits, operating within the world is challenging due to their impaired language, attention, memory, executive functions, and/or visuospatial abilities. Once the clinician has obtained a thorough case history of the person with aphasia, we believe that the most important aspects of cognition to be addressed are:

- Attention
- Memory
- Language
- Executive functions
- Visuospatial skills

Attention

The ability to pay attention has important therapeutic implications, that is, attending to tasks within the therapy session. In addition, attention is of primary importance if one is to be safe and interactive in the environment. Therefore, we suggest that the clinician determine if the patient demonstrates *vigilance,* which is the ability to maintain attention over time. The underlying abilities necessary for vigilance are obviously being awake and alert. The patient must also be able to shift attention as needed, that is, demonstrate *selective attention.* This is an important cognitive skill that is necessary for success in therapy as well as for the individual to participate in social life and in their environment. The clinician must also evaluate the patient's ability to plan and multitask. In order to live independently or with minimal supervision, a patient must be able to plan their daily activities and manage information and situations that may happen simultaneously, typically an everyday occurrence. Two very simple methods of testing attention are using symbol cancellation tasks and trail-making tasks. Both require the patient to maintain attention (vigilance), shift attention continuously (selective attention), and plan their next move (executive attention). Many cognitive workbooks include these types of tasks, and clinicians can devise their own.

Memory

In general, there are three types of cognitive memory (memory requiring thought). They are called episodic, working, and semantic memory. *Episodic*

Table 2–4. Domains of Functional Cognition Supported by the World Health Organization (WHO)

Language	Ability to understand and/or produce spoken language.
Reading and Writing	Ability to read printed material and write words and numbers.
Numeric/Calculation	Ability to process numerical information and/or perform mathematical calculations.
Limb Praxis	Ability to perform skilled purposeful limb movements in the presence of motor function.
Visuospatial Function Ability	To perceive and process visual information in one's environment.
Social Use of Language Ability	To use language to interact with others, including use of appropriate content, expression or comprehension of pitch, loudness or rate that conveys the speaker's emotional intent (prosody), management of a conversational topics (cohesion), and interplay between speakers (turn-taking).
Emotional Function	Awareness of emotional state of oneself and others, and the ability to manage those emotions in terms of both personal emotional management and the management of emotions in interpersonal interactions. Also encompasses self-awareness of deficits and abilities (anosagnosia), and the presence of emotional dysfunction (i.e., depression).
Attention	A variety of functions that include: selectivity, focusing, sustaining concentration or vigilance, switching, and modulating the intensity of attention.
Executive Function	The group of cognitive processes responsible for guiding, directing, and managing cognitive, emotional, and behavioral functions, during novel tasks such as organizing thoughts and activities, prioritizing tasks, managing time efficiently, and decision making.
Memory	The capacity to retain a variety of information, for varying durations, and use it for adaptive purposes.

memory is used when we are remembering our own past experiences and events that we have participated in throughout the day. Evaluating this aspect of cognitive memory can help the clinician with a differential diagnosis (e.g., raising questions about one's ability to recall events, which is important to know in assessing for dementia). For example, the patient may benefit from a memory book to assist with planning and keeping appointments. *Working memory* is necessary for normal conversation. An individual must have the ability to retrieve words to express their thoughts and retain the content of the other speaker's information in order to respond appropriately. People with aphasia may lack the working memory necessary to engage in discourse. The ability to sequence information and hold it in

memory for processing and manipulation is a complex task requiring several systems to work simultaneously. *Semantic memory* is the storehouse for our conceptual knowledge of the world and for factual information that we have learned. It is obvious that a patient with an impaired semantic memory will be at a severe disadvantage due to their inability to retrieve facts and concepts pertinent to activities of daily living.

In addition to the more cognitive domains of memory, *procedural memory* is used during execution of automatic tasks that were previously learned by the patient. This would include activities such as typing, dressing, gardening, and cooking to name a few. In the aphasic patient, the clinician must determine if procedural memory has been affected by the neurologic event in case the clinician wants to use any of those previously learned tasks in therapy. Consulting with the occupational therapist (OT) is recommended during an evaluation in order to eventually cotreat the patient optimally. The OT can assess and treat the patient's functional capabilities for activities of daily living, giving the SLP insight into the patient's procedural memory for those tasks. This can help the SLP with functional goal formulation.

Language

The relationship between language and cognition is intricate and well-established. Any comprehensive diagnostic language instrument designed to evaluate the person with aphasia should include the following linguistic areas for assessment:

- Semantics
- Syntax
- Morphology
- Pragmatics
- Phonology

Cognition is dealt with in more detail in the following chapters on the aphasic syndromes. However, we believe that the ability to compensate for one's language deficits must take into account one's cognitive skills. The extent of damage to the patient's cognition will influence therapeutic considerations. Areas assessed in a comprehensive cognitive-linguistic evaluation typically include the following:

- Perception
- Discrimination
- Orientation/awareness
- Organization of thoughts
- Memory (immediate/recent/long-term)
- Reasoning/problem-solving/inference
- Auditory processing and comprehension
- Calculation
- Reading and visual processing
- Writing
- Pragmatics and affect

Executive Functions

Executive functions refer to the highest level of human cognitive ability. It is very possible to sustain significant language impairment secondary to stroke and still have intact executive functions. The patient may simply not be able to demonstrate this to the clinician verbally. Therefore, assessing executive functions nonverbally must be considered in the person with aphasia. Executive functions include tasks such as *planning, sequencing, accomplishing goal-directed behavior, maintaining flexibility, problem-solving, reasoning,* and *judgment.* These skills are needed in order to function independently in the world. Evaluating these skills will help the clinician in post-discharge planning by informing other team members of cognitive assessment outcomes. Furthermore, the status of a patient's executive functioning will impact selection of language goals. Some tests that the SLP can use to evaluate this area include the Wisconsin Card Sorting Test (Psychological Assessment Resources, 2003), Tower of Hanoi, and/or the Maze Solving subtest from the CLQT.

Visuospatial Skills

Visuospatial skills must be assessed in order to know if any confrontation naming deficits, writing, and/or reading problems are affected by this type of impairment. The clinician must evaluate the patient's visual fields to rule out visual inattention, visual neglect, or a visual field cut due to hemianopsia. The occupational therapist will also be invaluable for consultation in this area. *Visual perception* encompasses the ability to discriminate, analyze, recognize, and interpret visual stimuli. Visual perception is an extremely important skill when working with the aphasic patient as the SLP tends to use visual stimuli to facilitate language production. Another visuospatial skill necessary for language therapy is *visual construction.* This is defined as the ability to combine visual perception with a motor response. This skill is critical for writing, printing, and drawing, which in some cases remains the only functional communication modality in people with aphasia. Both the Rey Complex Figure Test (Meyers & Meyers, 1995) and the Boston Assessment of Severe Aphasia (BASA; Helm-Estabrooks, Ramsberger, & Nichols, 1989) assess some of these skills.

Integrating Tasks: Clock Drawing. The clock drawing task has been used for many years as a quick but very effective tool in the assessment of cognition in the person with aphasia. Why? Here is the instruction:

> Draw a clock, put in all the numbers, and set the clock to 10 minutes after 11.

In order to complete this task, the patient must possess the *language skills* to process the directions and write the numbers in the correct place on a clock. The patient must have the *memory* to store and later retrieve the time setting. He or she must have the *visuospatial skills* to represent the clock correctly. He or she must possess *visuoperceptual attention* and motor skills to execute the mental image. Finally, he or she must have the *executive functions* that are needed to plan the task and make adjustments if necessary. In short, clock drawing enables the speech-language pathologist to get a glimpse of the patient's cognitive skills to plan therapeutically.

Modifications to Standard Approaches to Assessment

It is important for SLPs to know if the tasks on the assessment tool could be influencing a patient's performance on the test, for example, sentence comprehension may be influenced by the nature of the assessment task. It is conceivable that a patient may be more or less successful depending on the materials used to assess a particular language function. In a study by Salis and Edwards (2009), 10 aphasic speakers (3 fluent and 7 nonfluent) were given three different comprehension tasks. Task 1 included sentence-picture matching using a field of four pictures. Task 2 included sentence-picture matching using a field of two pictures plus an enactment piece that involved hearing a sentence that in turn had to be acted out by manipulating animal figures (i.e., "it is the gorilla that kicks the hippo"). Task 3 (a no-picture condition) included a truth-value judgment involving the figures. For that task, the experimenter acted out a scenario using the toy figures, and then made a statement that either matched or did not match the scenario. The person

with aphasia was required to judge if the sentence and scenario matched.

Outcomes of the study revealed that enactment tasks were effective for identifying syntactic deficits and in fact identified more comprehension deficits than the sentence-picture matching tasks. Using toy figures proved to be a good way to evaluate syntactic comprehension. This included figure identification, parsing of the sentence, and the lexical processing necessary to plan, mentally represent, and use the figures to execute the sentence. On a truth-value judgment task, people with aphasia took longer to verify false sentences relating to the figures' actions, compared with true ones. They also had more difficulty comprehending noncanonical sentences (passives such as "the girl is chased by the boy" and object relatives such as "there's a woman who the dog is chasing") than canonical sentences (actives such as "the cat is chasing the mouse" and subject relatives such as "there's the boy who is chasing the cat").

Salis and Edwards (2009) concluded that by using different modes of testing, the speech-language pathologist can develop a hierarchy of difficulty for training various sentence types because syntactic comprehension appears sensitive to the assessment conditions imposed by the SLP.

Assessment of expressive language in people with aphasia should include functionally relevant speech production. Although daily conversations have ecological validity, that is, real-world applicability, Lind, Kristofferson, Moen, and Simonsen (2009) argue that a more controlled monologue may be easier to acquire and analyze. Verbal descriptions and/or narratives of pictures such as the "Cookie Theft" (Goodglass, Kaplan, & Barresi, 2001) can be effective methods to obtain these samples. Picture descriptions and story retells may offer an alternative that promotes semispontaneous discourse and valuable intra- and interindividual comparisons. Using picture stimuli like the "Cookie Theft" (Figure 2–3) as well as structured tasks, clinicians may be better able to identify anomia, a general problem found in various aphasic syndromes (Laine & Martin, 2006). In their study, the data confirmed the need to assess different lexical categories separately and not assess overarching groupings such as *function words* and *content words*. Laine and Martin

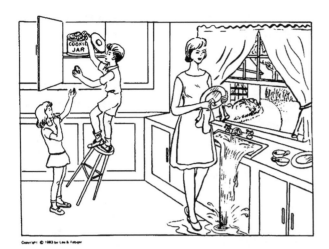

Figure 2–3. "Cookie Theft." (Source: Goodglass, H., Kaplan, E., & Barresi, B. (2001). *Boston Diagnostic Aphasia Examination: Stimulus Cards, Short Form* (3rd ed.). Philadelphia, PA: Lippincott Williams & Wilkins.)

(2006) suggest the following types of analyses of aphasic discourse:

- Proportion of nouns and verbs
- Type-token ration (TTR) of nouns and verbs (lexical diversity)
- Proportion of nouns and verbs used only once (lexical richness)
- Proportion of high-frequency nouns and verbs
- Proportion of nouns and verbs with a general meaning.

Conversational Analysis as a Component to the Evaluation of People with Aphasia

The analysis of the spontaneous speech production in daily life of people with aphasia is typically not part of the standard evaluation. This is understandable when one considers: (1) the time it takes to obtain a valid sample and to analyze that sample using standard conversational analysis techniques; and (2) the fact that payers, for example, the Centers for Medicare and Medicaid Services (CMS), and pri-

vate insurances, prefer quantified results because it is easier to monitor change and functional outcomes by comparing scores on tests and percentages in progress notes. Despite these practical limitations, there is great value in examining the spontaneous speech of aphasic speakers.

Prins and Bastiaanse (2004) conducted a review of the methodology for obtaining these types of speech samples. They distinguish among four types of samples:

a. Semispontaneous speech based on picture stimulation or a story retell.
b. Semispontaneous speech elicited in role-playing scenarios.
c. Spontaneous speech elicited in a conversation or a dialogue with someone familiar with the patient, for example, a spouse or therapist.
d. Spontaneous speech elicited in an interview format, with open-ended questions.

The sample can be part of the more objective standard battery of testing. Wright and Capiluto (2009) found that spontaneous speech elicited by a question such as, "Tell me what you see in this picture" is impoverished when compared with a narrative elicited by the question, "Look at the picture and then tell me a story that has a beginning, middle, and end." This suggests that clinicians must consider the type of stimulus question so that it will elicit a speech sample pertinent to their needs as evaluators. Prins and Bastiaanse (2004) point out that conversational analysis of aphasic speech, which is part of a "communicative/pragmatic analysis," is helpful because it provides the clinician with a better picture of the patient's communicative behaviors in real-life situations and settings. There are assessment instruments used with people with aphasia that do take spontaneous samples into consideration. These include:

a. Functional Communication Profile (FCP; Sarno, 1969)
b. Communicative Abilities in Daily Living (CADL; Holland, 1980).
c. Pragmatic Protocol (PP; Prutting & Kirchner, 1987)
d. ASHA FACS (Frattali et al., 1995)

Unfortunately, their review raised the question of the reliability and validity of these standardized aphasia measures for analyzing the samples that they provide, with the exception of the Communication Activities of Daily Living, Second Edition (CADL-2; Holland, Frattali, & Fromm, 1999). This problem is complicated by the fact that the *qualitative* nature of conversation does not lend itself to *quantification,* which they believe is essential because "aphasia is a linguistic disorder and not a pragmatic one." They suggest that measuring "collaborative repair" is one way to quantify the conversational output between an aphasic speaker and a nonaphasic conversation partner. Collaborative repair is operating when the nonaphasic partner initiates repairs to the aphasic speaker's output, correcting the errors. These can be measured over the course of treatment by the number of turns per repair sequence, and the average length of each repair. Thus, therapeutic success, that is, improvement to functional communication, can be measured with a more objective method.

Conversational analysis, discourse analysis, and/ or narrative analysis can provide the clinician with important insights into the everyday talk of people with aphasia (PWA). Furthermore, these types of analyses fit nicely within the International Classification of Functioning (ICF) framework in that one can obtain information not only on the impairment (language), but also on social participation, the patient's psychosocial adjustment to their aphasia, and the barriers that prevent effective and meaningful communication (Papathanasiou, Coppens, & Potagas, 2013). Adding an analysis of everyday talk to the assessment battery will give the clinician a glimpse of the way that people with aphasia convey meanings. Whereas, the more traditional psycholinguistic, cognitive, and neuropsychological model of assessment focuses primarily on the impairment within the ICF framework, leaving the social factors and adjustment issues outside the scope of the evaluation process.

Use of Standardized Tests for Individuals with Cognitive-Communication Disorders

It is a challenge to assess individuals with cognitive-communication disorders. The Academy of Neurologic Communication Disorders and Sciences (ANCDS) has written on the topic of use of standardized, norm-referenced tests for individuals with cognitive-communication disorders (Turkstra, Coelho, & Ylvisaker, 2005). A committee analyzed the use of performance measures and questionnaires regarding strengths and limitations. Reliability and validity were also important factors in consideration of appropriate tests. Four key questions for test evaluation included: (1) Does the person have a problem?, (2) If there is a cognitive-communication disorder, what are the characteristics?, (3) What are the implications of the test results beyond the test session?, and (4) Where should I begin with treatment? For a complete list of the standardized tests that were reviewed, see Turkstra et al. (2005). Of the 32 assessment measures reviewed, the following eight tests met most of the criteria for standardized assessment of individuals with cognitive-communication disorders:

- ASHA FACS (Frattali et al., 1995)
- Behavior Rating Inventory of Executive Function (BRIEF) (Gioia, Isquith, Guy, & Kenworthy, 2000)
- CADL-2 (Holland, Frattali, & Fromm, 1999)
- Functional Independence Measure (FIM, 1996; Uniform Data System for Medical Rehabilitation, 1996)
- Global Deterioration Scale (GDS; Reisberg, Ferris, De Leon, & Crook, 1982)
- Repeatable Battery for the Assessment of Neuropsychological Status (RBANS) (Randolph, 2001)
- Test of Language Competence-Extended (TLC-E) (Wiig & Secord, 1989)
- Western Aphasia Battery (WAB) (Kertesz, 1982), updated to the WAB-R (Kertesz, 2006)

Commonly Used Assessments for Acquired Language Disorders: Key Concepts and Information

The assessment measures listed below are frequently used to assess individuals with aphasia and cognitive-communication disorders. Details regarding testing purpose, appropriateness for patient types, standardization information, and administration factors are included.

Arizona Battery for Communication Disorders of Dementia (ABCD)

The Arizona Battery for Communication Disorders of Dementia (ABCD; Bayles & Tomoeda, 1993) is designed for patients with neurologic disorders including dementia and head injury.

- It assesses:
  - Linguistic expression
  - Linguistic comprehension
  - Verbal episodic memory
  - Visuospatial construction
  - Mental status
- The ABCD was designed to identify and describe information about nonlinguistic and linguistic communication deficits in dementia.
- The ABCD was standardized on patients with Alzheimer's and Parkinson's disease, as well as young and older healthy individuals.
- The ABCD allows clinicians to have an understanding of the patient's mental status and their ability to read, name, describe, define, repeat, answer questions, follow directions, retell a story, recall, and recognize words, copy figures, and draw.
- There are 14 primary subtests in the ABCD. These include:
  Mental status, story retelling, following commands, comparative questions, word learning (free recall, total recall, recognition), repetition, object description, reading comprehension (word and sentence levels), generative naming, confrontation naming, concept definition, generative drawing, figure copying, and story retelling (delayed).
- The test is easy to administer and score. Single subtests can be used.
- Test responses can aid clinicians in planning intervention strategies.

- Testing the full battery takes from 45 to 90 minutes.
- Test results help determine how coherent the patient is to the environment and how well he or she is able to follow directions, compare information to make judgments, and recognize and identify uses for objects that are common in the home.

Addenbrooke's Cognitive Examination (ACE)

The Addenbrooke's Cognitive Examination (ACE; 2012) is designed for assessing mental status in individuals suspected of experiencing cognitive decline:

- Attention
- Memory
- Verbal Fluency
- Language
- Visuospatial abilities

Results from a national dementia research register indicated that ACE is highly correlated with the Mini-Mental State Examination (MMSE) and has better estimates of cognitive ability over the MMSE by 16% (Gray & Starr, 2013). The ACE has been found to be a useful measure in detecting and tracking dementia (Leyton, Hornberger, Mioshi, & Hodges, 2010).

Using the ACE with 63 individuals with semantic dementia (SD) and 45 individuals with progressive nonfluent aphasia (PNFA), a cutoff score of 88 points (out of a possible 100) detected 95% of those with both types of dementia. Results also showed an average annual decline of 10 points with no significant group differences. Regarding prognosis, change over 12 or 24 months was considered average for these disorders.

Leyton et al. (2010) identified the ACE as a global cognitive bedside assessment useful in detecting early stages of dementia. The ACE has been able to reliability distinguish between frontotemporal dementia (FTD) and Alzheimer's disease as well as other affective disorders (Davies Dawson, Mioshi, Erzinclioglu & Hodges, 2008). It has also been identified as having fewer ceiling effects and includes more language tasks that have a broader diagnostic utility. Using the upper cut-off of 88 points on the ACE, very few cases of SD or PNFA would be missed.

The newest version of the ACE (2012) can be found at http://neura.edu.au/sites/neura.edu.au/files/page-downloads/ACE-III%20Administration%20(UK).pdf, and scoring guidelines can be found at http://neura.edu.au/sites/neura.edu.au/files/page-downloads/ACE-III%20Scoring%20(UK)_0.pdf

Assessment of Language-Related Functional Activities (ALFA)

The Assessment of Language-Related Functional Activities (ALFA; Baines, Martin, & McMartin Heeringa, 1999) test assesses language-related functional activities in 30 to 90 minutes, and it requires that the patient perform each of these tasks. In order for the patient to perform on these functionally-based subtests, they must have supportive auditory comprehension, express themselves verbally, read, and write, as well as use cognitive and motor skills. While a client performs each activity, the examiner records an objective, quantitative score. This test can be used in any health care service delivery sector. The 10 tasks are:

1. Telling time
2. Counting money
3. Addressing an envelope
4. Solving daily math problems
5. Writing a check/balancing a checkbook
6. Understanding medicine labels
7. Using a calendar
8. Reading instructions
9. Using the telephone
10. Writing a phone message

The value of this test lies in its utility for assessing the patient's abilities to perform their activities of daily living and can be used with patients 16 years and older.

Mini Mental State Exam (MMSE)

The MMSE is the most commonly used assessment tool for evaluating the person with memory impair-

ment and is used to help diagnose dementia in cognitively impaired patients. The MMSE broadly assess the following areas:

- Orientation to time and place
- Immediate and delayed memory
- Naming common objects
- Repetition of phrases
- Reading
- Following written and oral directions
- Writing a sentence
- Copying a design.

Scoring the MMSE is very simple. It is based on a 30-point scale. Point ranges correlate with the level of severity. A score of 16 to 24 points correlates with an early stage dementia; a score of 8 to 15 correlates with a middle stage dementia; and a score 0–9 is indicative of a late stage dementia. The MMSE is also useful as a screening tool and/or part of an assessment battery for newly admitted patients to a rehabilitation facility, long-term care facility, sub-acute facility, or acute rehabilitation facility. This tool can also be used to monitor a patient's progress over the treatment period. Below is a link to the MMSE.

http://www.health.gov.bc.ca/pharmacare/adti/clinician/pdf/ADTI%20SMMSE-GDS%20Reference%20Card.pdf

Global Deterioration Scale (GDS)

The GDS (Reisberg et al., 1982) considers cognitive, functional, and behavioral impairments in dementia. The test was designed to evaluate the stages of Alzheimer's disease, from normal to late dementia; however, we believe that its use can be expanded to other forms of dementia due to its content. It has a seven-stage rating scale that can be correlated with the MMSE (Eisdorfer et al., 1992) and is described below:

- Stage 1 Objectively normal
- Stage 2 Independent; mild memory loss; subjective complaints (MMSE score 26–30)
- Stage 3 Mild cognitive impairment; declining work performance; denial (MMSE score 21–25)

■ Stage 4   Early dementia; problems with complex tasks; assistance may be necessary; denial is common; withdraw from challenging situations (MMSE score 17–20)

■ Stage 5   Moderate dementia; need assistance for ADLs; cannot live independently; disorientation; cannot recall address and phone; general memory impairment (MMSE score 11–16)

■ Stage 6   Moderately-severe dementia; usually in long-term care facilities; family becomes unfamiliar; need assistance with basic ADLs; incontinent; delusions; repetitive behaviors; agitation (MMSE score 1–10)

■ Stage 7   Severe dementia; loss of language; incontinent of bowel and bladder; nonambulatory (MMSE score 0)

Boston Diagnostic Aphasia Examination-3 (BDAE-3)

The Boston Diagnostic Aphasia Examination-3 (BDAE-3; Goodglass, Kaplan, & Barresi, 2001) is designed for assessing patients with aphasia. It assesses the following aspects of speech and language function in the person with aphasia:

■ Auditory comprehension
■ Articulation
■ Fluency
■ Word finding
■ Repetition
■ Serial speech
■ Grammar and syntax
■ Paraphasia

■ The BDAE-3 is a diagnostic test to diagnose the presence and type of aphasic syndrome, to measure performance of a wide range of abilities, and to provide a comprehensive assessment of the patient's

strengths and weaknesses in language areas to guide treatment.
■ The test has both long and short forms and also includes the Boston Naming Test to assess lexical retrieval abilities.
■ The test assesses five areas of functioning: conversational and expository speech, auditory comprehension, oral expression, reading, and writing.

Testing of conversational and expository speech includes simple social responses, free conversation, picture description, and narrative discourse. It provides a severity rating and speech output characteristics profile. Auditory comprehension testing assesses word comprehension, following commands of increasing complexity, understanding complex ideational material, and syntactic processing with comprehension of embedded sentences. Oral expression is assessed for oral agility, automatic sequences, recitation, melody and rhythm, repetition abilities, and naming. Reading is assessed for basic symbol recognition, word identification, phonics, derivational and grammatical morphology, and oral reading with comprehension of words, sentences, and paragraphs. Writing assessment includes mechanics, writing to dictation, oral spelling, written picture naming, grammar, and narrative writing. Praxis is also tested for limb and hand, as well as for buccofacial and respiratory abilities.

■ Using the rating scale profile form, the type of aphasic syndrome can be identified with a degree of validity.
■ The test was standardized on 85 aphasic subjects from inpatient, outpatient, and private practice sources with a range of severity ratings and 15 normal elderly volunteers.

Burns Brief Inventory of Communication and Cognition

The Burns Brief Inventory of Communication and Cognition (Burns, 1997) is designed for adults with neurologic impairment. It can be used effectively with individuals with left hemispheric lesions, right hemispheric lesions, and patients with other complex neuropathologies. Listed below are the features of this measure:

- Assess specific skills a patient has and their level of functioning.
- Determine if individuals with left hemisphere lesions have language deficits consistent with aphasia.
- Determine if individuals with right hemisphere lesions have patterns of aprosodia (lack of speech prosody) or visuospatial cognitive deficits consistent with right hemisphere syndrome.
- Determine if individuals with head injury or early dementing diseases have attention and memory problems consistent with these disease processes.
- Its scoring is set up to help determine what areas to treat first (scored areas falling within the shaded zones are optimal for initial treatment).
- It is standardized on individuals from 18 to 80 years and is to be administered by speech-language pathologists.
- Reliability and validity studies have been completed with adequate results found.
- It is easy to administer and score—each inventory (3 total) takes about 30 minutes.
- Differential scoring is considered for repetition, self-correction, cueing, or delayed responses.

Cognitive Linguistic Evaluation

The Cognitive Linguistic Evaluation (Shipley & McAfee, 2004) (see Appendix C) is an informal tool that is comprehensive in its range of content and provides an overview of cognitive-linguistic skills of adults and teens.

- It assesses:
  - Perception
  - Discrimination
  - Orientation/awareness
  - Organization of thoughts
  - Memory (immediate/recent/long-term)

- Reasoning/problem-solving/inference
- Auditory processing and comprehension
- Calculation
- Reading and visual processing
- Writing
- Pragmatics and affect

The area of cognitive-linguistics developed from the field of linguistics with an understanding that language development and language use are best explained in reference to human cognition. In the area of cognitive linguistic study, there are three primary premises: (1) there is no autonomous linguistic faculty in one's mind, (2) grammar is a conceptualization, and (3) knowledge of language comes from language use (Croft & Cruse, 2004). Cognitive-linguistic evaluations typically include knowledge that addresses the following types of items:

- Orientation to the date, time, season, where someone lives and for how long, one's name, profession, and additional items as pertinent to the individual.
- Memory for recall of numbers and words, retelling a story, indicating food eaten during the day, activities of the day, where born, birth date, family members' names, and additional facts.
- Auditory processing and comprehension involving yes-no questions for basic information including one's name and residence, answering yes/no questions for factual and abstract information.
- Problem-solving for questions given situations, logic and reasoning, inferential knowledge for correcting illogical statements, providing meanings for common expressions and proverbs, naming items given a series of clues, and indicating categories for similar items.
- Thought organization for providing definitions of words, steps taken to accomplish tasks, and planning strategies in addition to higher level tasks pertinent to the individual.
- Calculation for numerical word problems involving quantities, money, and time.

■ Reading and visual processing for reading words and determining ones that do not belong in the group, following a series of written directions, reading sentences aloud and answering questions about a paragraph, telling time from clock drawings, and attending to specific shapes on a page.

■ Writing one's name and date, writing a short description of activities accomplished during the day, and other written work pertinent to the individual.

■ Pragmatic behaviors of language including appropriateness of physical proximity, eye contact and facial expression, use of gestures, prosody, topic maintenance, turn taking, initiation, attention, organization, and ability to limit distractibility.

Cognitive Linguistic Quick Test (CLQT)

The CLQT (Helm-Estabrooks, 2001) is a criterion-referenced test for English and Spanish-speaking adults with acquired neurologic dysfunction.

■ It assesses individuals with deficits affecting:
  ■ Attention
  ■ Memory
  ■ Language
  ■ Visuospatial skills
  ■ Executive dysfunction
■ Assesses strengths and weaknesses of the five cognitive domains: attention, memory, language, visuospatial skills, and executive functions.
■ Used to identify cognitive strengths and weaknesses.
■ It is not considered a comprehensive tool for differential diagnosis.
■ Patients must be able to use a pen and give verbal responses to take this test.
■ More abstract items may require a professional with experience for interpretation and application.
■ It provides a performance review of cognitive abilities affecting functioning.

■ The test takes approximately 30 minutes to administer.

Coma Recovery Scale–Revised (CRS-R)

The Coma Recovery Scale–Revised (CRS-R; Giacino & Kalmar, 2004) measure is useful with any patient who has been in a coma. The purpose of this scale is to assist with differential diagnosis and treatment planning for patients who exhibit varied levels of consciousness. The items within each scale are hierarchically arranged so that a higher number reflects a higher skill level and better prognosis. The CRS-R is particularly useful for tracking progress along the six functional scales. The six scales are listed below:

■ Auditory Function Scale
  Consistent movement to command = 4
  Reproducible movement to command = 3
  Localization to sound = 2
  Auditory startle = 1
  None = 0

■ Visual Function Scale
  Object recognition = 5
  Object localization/reaching = 4
  Visual pursuit = 3
  Fixation = 2
  Visual startle = 1
  None = 0

■ Motor Function Scale
  Functional object use = 6
  Automatic motor response = 5
  Object manipulation = 4
  Localization to noxious stimulation = 3
  Flexion withdrawal = 2
  Abnormal posturing = 1
  None/flaccid = 0

■ Oromotor/Verbal Function Scale
  Intelligible verbalization = 3
  Vocalization/oral movement = 2
  Oral reflexive movement = 1
  None = 0

- Communication Scale
  Functional/accurate = 2
  Nonfunctional/intentional = 1
  None = 0

- Arousal Scale
  Attention = 3
  Eye opening without stimulation = 2
  Eye opening with stimulation = 1
  Unarousable = 0

The CRS-R also includes a Brain Stem Reflex Grid, an Arousal Facilitation Protocol, a supplementary Assessment of Contingent Behavior to assess vocalizations, gestures, and affective responses, and charts to track and score progress. This measure is available online at http://www.coma.ulg.ac.be/images/crs_r.pdf

Comprehensive Aphasia Test (CAT)

The Comprehensive Aphasia Test (CAT; Swinburn, Porter, & Howard, 2005) was the first new aphasia assessment tool to appear in English for 20 years. The CAT is intended to assess language, screen for cognitive deficits, monitor changes in aphasia over time, and consider the effects of aphasia on the individual's life. The authors state that the CAT, a short standardized aphasia battery, assists in providing a prognosis and designing therapy. The CAT has three parts.

1. The Cognitive Screen
2. The Language Battery
3. The Disability Questionnaire

- The Language Battery assesses auditory comprehension at varying levels of complexity, written comprehension, oral reading, verbal expression, written expression, and repetition, all at varying levels with a variety of tasks using real words, nonwords, sentences, and digits.
- The Cognitive Screen screens for cognitive deficits that can influence language performance and includes subtests to assess visual neglect, memory problems, acalculia, and ideational apraxia.

- The Disability Questionnaire has a disability self-rating scale and assessments of self-image and emotional support.
- The CAT does not assign people with aphasia to syndromes. According to some investigators (Gordon, 1998; and Feyereisen, Pillon, & de Partz, 1991), assigning an aphasic syndrome on the basis of spontaneous speech characteristics can be unreliable.
- The CAT compares degree of impairment across different tests (language comprehension, repetition, spoken output, reading aloud, and writing) to assess the level of performance across subtests.
- It can also differentiate between those who have aphasia and those with normal language as well as predict relative outcome (12 months post-onset) for those tested during the first few months after the onset of aphasia.

Communication Activities of Daily Living, Second Edition (CADL-2)

The CADL-2 (Holland et al., 1999) is designed for adults with neurogenic disorders.

- It assesses functional communication skills of:
  - Reading
  - Writing
  - Using numbers
  - Social interaction
  - Context utilization
  - Role-playing
  - Sequential relationships
  - Divergences
  - Nonverbal communication
- This test was standardized on 175 individuals 20 to 96 years old with neurologically based communication disorders across 17 states in the United States.
- The test provides information about the patient's communication strategies, pragmatic skills, and interaction abilities that are functional in nature.

- Areas assessed include greetings, answering questions, and performing activities of daily living such as ordering from a menu, reading a bus schedule, determining what to do next in a given situation, completing forms, matching symbols with pictures, making plans and scheduling, to name several.
- It can also be used for individuals with mental retardation, dementia, traumatic brain injury, and right hemisphere syndrome.
- It contains 50 items and is generally administered in 30 to 50 minutes by a licensed, certified speech-language pathologist.
- Patients can ask for repetition of items.
- Video-recording is encouraged for assessing nonverbal as well as verbal behaviors.
- Differential scoring is provided for adequacy of responses.
- Results can pinpoint strengths in communication and determine what the patient is functionally able to communicate.

The Kentucky Aphasia Test (KAT)

The Kentucky Aphasia Test (KAT; Marshall & Wright, 2007) is an objective test of language functioning for aphasia. It is considered a clinician-friendly measure that helps determine language functioning at the early post-onset phase following a stroke. This clinician-friendly test is one that can be given in its entirety in a brief amount of time. It is also applicable to people with various degrees of language impairment and is convenient to administer in a variety of health care settings. It incorporates a multidimensional scoring system and permits response features such as self-corrections and delays. A variety of response modes (gesture, drawing, pointing, and writing) are considered in the scoring module.

This measure includes both orientation and picture description tasks. The subtests include picture naming, repetition span, defining words, following commands, answering yes/no questions, and word-to-picture matching. It is considered to be sensitive for accurately differentiating people with aphasia from normally functioning adults.

The reader can find the entire measure in Marshall and Wright (2007). Appendices A through D within the journal article include the subtests of the KAT in its early developmental stages.

Psycholinguistic Assessments of Language Processing in Aphasia (PALPA)

The Psycholinguistic Assessments of Language Processing in Aphasia (PALPA; Kay, Lesser, & Coltheart, 1992) is designed for patients with acquired brain damage and aphasia.

- It assesses language processing and evaluates:
  - Recognition
  - Comprehension
  - Production of spoken words and sentences
  - Production of written words and sentences
- The PALPA consists of 60 assessments to help diagnose language processing difficulties in people with acquired brain damage.
- Subtest areas are selected according to the patient's individualized needs.
- The battery is divided into four primary areas: (1) auditory processing, (2) reading and spelling, (3) picture and word semantics, and (4) sentence comprehension. Modules include recognizing printed words, understanding printed words, reading aloud, recognizing objects and pictures, recognizing and repeating speech, spelling, writing, sentence processing, and more.
- Data was obtained on 25 subjects with aphasia and 32 nonbrain-damaged subjects, matched for age, education, and social variables. Descriptive statistical analyses (means and standard deviations)

are provided as a gauge for abnormal performance.

- The materials provided may also be used for a variety of procedures and tasks.
- This lengthy test has studies reporting on its use.

Reading Comprehension Battery for Aphasia (RCBA-2)

The Reading Comprehension Battery for Aphasia, Second Edition (RCBA-2; LaPointe & Horner, 1998) evaluates reading impairments in people with brain injury, for example, stroke, TBI, encephalopathies. This test is suitable for anyone with an acquired reading disability, who was premorbidly literate. The RCBA-2 is also valuable for treatment planning. The new, supplemental material in this second edition includes seven additional subtests that measure the different varieties of acquired dyslexia. This new material measures oral-reading comprehension, as well as silent reading comprehension. The subtests can be used at the examiner's discretion, that is, all subtests can be administered or just selected subtests. All, or just one, subtest can be administered, based upon an individual's need. These cover a diverse range of activities including:

- Single-word comprehension for visual confusions
- Auditory confusions and semantic confusions
- Functional reading
- Synonyms
- Sentence comprehension
- Short paragraph comprehension
- Paragraphs
- Morpho-syntactic reading with lexical controls
- Allows for entirely nonverbal responses
- Covers a wide range of difficulty, from single words through complex paragraphs
- Numerous aspects of reading are assessed, including:
  - Word order
  - Factual versus inferential reading
  - Synonym recognition

Ross Information Processing Assessment-2 (RIPA-2)

The Ross Information Processing Assessment-2 (RIPA-2; Ross-Swain, 1996) is designed for individuals 15 to 90 years old with neurogenic disorders.

- It assesses:
  - Memory
  - Orientation
  - Organization
  - Reasoning
  - Auditory processing
- The RIPA-2 was developed as an efficient, standardized test that quantifies and qualifies cognitive-linguistic deficits.
- The subtests assess aspects of memory, orientation, recall of information, problem solving, abstract reasoning, organizational ability, auditory processing, and retention.
- Scoring is based on a three-point system that considers intelligibility, perseveration, confabulation, and tangential information as errors.
- The test requires minimal materials and is easy to administer.
- Scoring requires use of different diacritical markers.
- Reliability and validity studies have been performed on individuals with TBI.

The Scales of Cognitive and Communicative Ability for Neurorehabilitiation (SCCAN)

The Scales of Cognitive and Communicative Ability for Neurorehabilitiation (SCCAN; Milman & Holland, 2012) was developed to assess impairment and activity limitations across eight cognitive domains. These include: speech comprehension, oral expression, reading, writing, orientation, attention, memory, and problem solving. The SCCAN also considers the effect that the patient's condition has on their daily functioning. The measure incorporates less items than traditional batteries to determine the patient's abilities, which is more expedient during administration. It has been found to accurately identify individuals with neurological disorders. The measure, intended to be brief, takes an average of 34 minutes to administer and has good reliability. The SCCAN accurately classified 98% (50/51) of neurologically impaired individuals and 95% (38/40) of the healthy control subjects. The measure accurately identified and differentiated individuals diagnosed with left-hemisphere pathology, right-hemisphere pathology, and probable Alzheimer's disease. It is considered a reliable and valid measure for assessing adult cognitive-communicative disorders.

Subtests are as follows:

- Speech Comprehension
  Single Word
  Connected Speech
- Oral Expression
  Repetition
  Naming
  Connected Speech
- Reading
  Single Words
  Connected Text
- Writing
  Single Words
  Connected Text
- Orientation
- Attention
  Verbal
  Visuospatial
- Memory
  Verbal
  Visuospatial
- Problem Solving
  Verbal
  Visuospatial
  Numeric

Scales of Cognitive Ability for Traumatic Brain Injury (SCATBI)

The Scales of Cognitive Ability for Traumatic Brain Injury (SCATBI; Adamonovich and Henderson, 1992) is designed for patients with acquired brain damage.

- It assesses cognitive deficits associated with TBI including:

- Perception and discrimination (including attention)
- Orientation
- Organization
- Recall
- Reasoning

- This measure assesses cognitive-linguistic status during recovery from head injury and measures the extent of change during a program of rehabilitation.
- The test was standardized on head-injured patients throughout the United States and Canada. The subjects ranged from 15 years to 88 years old.
- The SCATBI provides a systematic method to assess cognitive deficits.
- Test items are arranged with increasing difficulty.
- Administration takes approximately 2 hours with each section taking from 10 to 45 minutes, ranging from lower to higher difficulty levels.
- The five scales of the SCATBI are: perception/discrimination, orientation, organization, recall, and reasoning. Items include: Initiating, sustaining, and shifting attention, discriminating between shapes and sounds, knowing time, place, and setting, grouping and sequencing based on rules, recalling information from semantic memory and episodic memory with immediate, delayed, and long-term memory stores, and inductive and deductive reasoning.
- Within each section, there are tests to determine the patient's cognitive abilities. These comprise 40 testlets.
- Minimal materials are needed to administer the test, and the testlets can be given separately.
- The instructions are clear. Stimulus cards and the manual must be used simultaneously.
- A severity score is determined from the patient's overall performance. Scores can reflect an initial level and patient progress with readministering throughout the patient's recovery.

Western Aphasia Battery-Revised (WAB-R)

The WAB-R (Kertesz, 2006) is designed for differential diagnosis of English-speaking adults and teens with neurologic disorders.

- It assesses individuals with: stroke, head injury, and dementia.
- It contains a bedside evaluation as a screening tool that takes 15 minutes.
- It contains a comprehensive evaluation composed of eight subtests with oral/verbal sections taking 30 to 45 minutes and reading sections taking 45 to 60 minutes.
- It provides diagnostic information about linguistic and key nonlinguistic skills most frequently affected by aphasia.
- It provides an Aphasia Quotient, Cortical Quotient, Auditory Comprehension Quotient, Oral Expression Quotient, Reading Quotient, Writing Quotient, and bedside WAB-R scores based on 32 short tasks.
- Areas tested include: content, fluency, auditory comprehension, repetition, naming, word finding, reading, writing, drawing, block design, calculation, and praxis.
- It contains statistical research with evidence of reliability and validity along with information about its use for people with head injury and dementia.
- The WAB-R is considered a good predictor of patients' vocational outcomes.
- The test can be administered in sections, and it gives a comprehensive aphasia classification (Global, Broca's, Isolation, Transcortical Motor, Wernicke's, Transcortical Sensory, Conduction, and Anomic).
- It has been standardized on 150 patients with aphasia and 59 control subjects.
- The test booklet provides an outline for each section and provides details linking scores with aphasia types.

Selected Assessments for Aphasia by Category

Comprehensive Language Batteries:

- Examining for Aphasia (EFA-4; LaPointe & Eisenson, 2008)
- Comprehensive Aphasia Test (CAT; Swinburn et al., 2005)
- Minnesota Test for Differential Diagnosis of Aphasia (MTDDA; Schuell, Jenkins, & Jimenez-Pabon, 1964)
- Boston Diagnostic Aphasia Examination (BDAE-3; Goodglass, Kaplan, and Barresi, 2001)
- Western Aphasia Battery–Revised (WAB-R; Kertesz, 1982, 2006)
- The Porch Index of Communicative Ability (PICA; Porch, 1971)
- Aachen Aphasia Test (AAT; Huber, Poeck, & Willmes, 1984)
- Multilingual Aphasia Examination (Benton & Hamsher, 1978)
- Bilingual Aphasia Test (Paradis & Libben, 1987)

Functional Tests of Communication

- Functional Communication Profile (Sarno, 1969)
- Communication Activities of Daily Living, Second Edition (CADL-2; Holland, Frattali & Fromm, 1999)
- Pragmatics Profile of Communication Skills in Adults (Dewart & Summers, 1996)
- ASHA FACS (Frattali et al., 1995)

Tests Based on a Cognitive Neuropsychological Model

- Psycholinguistic Assessments of Language Processing in Aphasia (PALPA; Kay et al., 1992)

Tests Examining Specific Areas of Language Performance

- Boston Naming Test (Kaplan, Goodglass, & Weintraub, 1976)
- Reading Comprehension Battery for Aphasia (LaPointe & Horner, 1979)
- Discourse Comprehension Test (Brookshire & Nicholas, 1997)

Screening Tests of Aphasia

- Frenchay Aphasia Screening Test (FAST; Enderby, 1987)
- Bedside Evaluation Screening Test (BEST-2; Fitch West, Sands, & Ross-Swain, 1998)

We refer the reader to Appendix C (Cognitive Linguistic Evaluation) for specific information regarding the Cognitive-Linguistic Evaluation.

Treatment and Goal Setting

Suggested functional activities are listed in Appendix 2–B. This partial list of activities further illustrates the many reading-writing-listening-speaking connections individuals engage in during activities of daily living. Both verbal (listening and speaking) and visual (reading and writing) modalities must be considered when planning functional treatments for patients. It is important not to frustrate the patient by exceeding his or her skill level, yet we want to provide them with meaningful tasks to enhance their quality of life. Furthermore, and most important, all goals must be measurable and transparent, that is, easily understood by any reader. In an acute care setting, the SOAP note tends to be very succinct in order to avoid lengthy and wordy reporting. However, the SLP may keep more detailed information in their own soft chart.

Working with patients within a rehabilitation framework requires the SLP to consider the patient's individual needs and desires while simultaneously considering their level of impairments and functional abilities. Family members, friends, and significant others are excellent resources in establishing appropriate goals. The goals of treatment in therapy should always meet the following criteria:

- Promote function.
- Promote an effective communicative environment.
- Provide compensatory strategies to communicate if a return to the patient's premorbid communication status is not possible or feasible.
- Provide education and counseling for adjustment of the patient and family.
- Reduce interfering behaviors.
- Provide a relevant home program to the patient and family.

Documentation of Progress

It is essential to continually record progress regarding the patient's performance of therapeutic tasks. In the acute care setting, the SOAP note is the preferred form of documentation for patient progress. The note is divided into four sections:

- Subjective—general impressions of the client during the session (feelings and statements about the client from the client and/or the family are given, information about the client's behavior during the session may be written, and factors that may have affected the client's progress or lack of progress may be included in this section).
- Objective—measurable information about the treatment, indicating the behavioral objectives (data that is quantitative and/or qualitative, behavioral objective(s) and current data are written in this section).
- Assessment—an analysis of the session with objective findings, interpretation of results of the session reflecting if the client is making progress (indicate if the client is making progress in therapy, provide a cohesive statement, indicate if performance has improved, declined, or

remained the same with factors that may be contributing).

- Plan—the course of treatment and plans are provided in this section. Provide a logical follow-up to the previous section on assessment, indicating your next steps for the upcoming session.

Each section of the note reflects an important aspect of the session. The Subjective section reflects the status of the patient. The Objective section describes the goals and procedures of therapy for that session and the results, indicating the patient's performance. Please note that if the patient does *not* achieve the criterion set for a particular goal, the clinician must then intervene, that is, implement a technique to improve the patient's performance. In essence, this *is* the therapy for that session. The clinician is using a technique to improve performance, to scaffold the patient to the next level of success. In the Assessment section of the note, the clinician summarizes the session for the reader, without reporting the numbers and percentages from the Objective section. Finally, in the Plan section of the note, the clinician states the goals for the next session, based on the patient's performance during the session being reported. Below is a sample SOAP note:

Speech-Language Pathology
Date: 11/08/12
Time: 1300–1400

S: Pt. seen bedside; alert/cooperative; sitting in bedside chair; motivated; inappropriate laughter noted when session began; wife present; wife educated re: emotional lability; pt. redirected.

O: The patient will execute one-step commands with common objects with 60% accuracy independently.

- One-step commands: 40% accuracy × 5 trials; increased to 60%, with visual cues, and repetition.

The patient will identify his paraphasias on 50% of occurrences at the sentence level, after a verbal prompt.

- Self-identified neologism on 40% of occurrences × 10 opportunities; no change noted after a binary choice, for example, "Is it a *cup* or a *teptee?*"

The patient will write single words to dictation with 80% accuracy independently.

- Writing single functional words: *eat, drink, help, pain, bathroom, wife*
  - 60% accuracy × 5 trials per word; increased to 80% imitatively.

The patient will read the words denoting common objects with 80% accuracy, independently.

- Reading words was 60% accurate; increased to 80% with articulatory cue.

A: Pt. increased in one-step accuracy compared with baseline; pt. beginning to self-correct neologistic output with verbal cues compared with baseline; improvement in reading and writing compared with baseline; session pace good for patient skill level.

P: (1) Increase one-steps to 70% via repetition, visuals, slower presentation—note on data sheet as reminder.
(2) Decrease neologistic paraphasias to 50% of trials via verbal and self-corrective cues.
(3) Review reading and writing targets before next session; if performance continues to be low, consider other targets/activities.
(4) Provide counseling and education to family regarding stroke and aphasia.

Signature: _____

Service Delivery to People with Acquired Language Disorders

The SLP will typically encounter the patient with an acquired language disorder in five different settings: acute care settings, rehabilitation settings (free-standing rehabs or acute rehabs), home care settings, outpatient settings, and long-term care settings. The continuum of care for these patients has an expected course if the patient's medical status is supportive, that is, acute care to rehabilitation to outpatient. However, understandably this is not always the case. This section discusses the models of service delivery appropriate to each setting, without referring to any specific disorder as that is addressed separately within each chapter of the book.

The Acute Care Setting

In the acute care setting, information and assessment are the focus of service delivery. Miller and Groher (1990) state that acute care is the stage of a person's medical care where the symptoms of a particular illness are severe, but immediate illness is of a short duration; however, this is not always the case. For example, if the patient is admitted with a stroke, or pneumonia, the immediate goal is to stabilize the patient so that treatment can proceed. This can be accomplished in a short period of time, if there are no other comorbidities complicating the clinical picture. It could also become a protracted stay due to unforeseen medical problems that arise. Miller and Groher's (1990) description is one that acts as a good differentiator between acute care and post-acute care settings, but in our opinion, it is too general to cover the myriad circumstances

that may arise. Nevertheless, the acute care setting does demand its own model of service delivery, and Johnson and Jacobson (2007) provide a realistic and valid one. They refer to it as the Acute Care Consultative Model (ACM; Figure 2–4).

The most salient feature of this model is that there is no direct therapeutic component to it. The SLP is situated in the center of a matrix that revolves around three critical concepts in the acute care clinical encounter: *assessment, counseling/education,* and *monitoring.* The most obvious cause of this shift in service delivery in this setting is related to reimbursement. Patients in acute care will not be in the hospital for a lengthy stay unless there are complications to an otherwise straightforward diagnosis. As a consequence, the primary role of the SLP in this setting is to *evaluate, inform,* and *monitor* trends in the patient's status, all in preparation for the next level of care. Of course, the details will change based on the disorder type.

The Rehabilitation Setting

Rehabilitation is concerned with optimization and recovery of patient function. As a consequence, there is a shift in focus once the patient reaches the rehabilitation setting from acute care, and the ACM no longer applies. However, a revision to the ACM (Figure 2–5) can be made to reflect the role and responsibilities of the clinician in that setting.

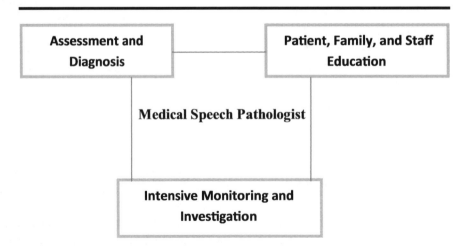

Figure 2–4. The Acute Care Consultative Model (ACM).

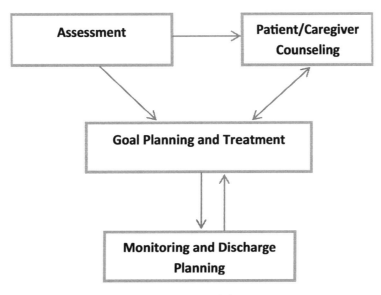

Figure 2–5. A Rehabilitation Model.

The most salient differences in the rehabilitation setting is the *bidirectional* feature to patient care and planning, indicating the importance of patient or caregiver input and ongoing monitoring of the patient's progress inherent to the rehab process. More specific, the following elements stand out: (1) the treatment component is now at the center of patient's plan; (2) the arrows indicating the flow of information reflect the importance of the caregiver in the goal planning and the treatment of the patient; and (3) monitoring continues as treatment proceeds, but discharge planning also is considered as the patient's status changes. There is great variability in the ALD population due to etiology and level of severity; therefore, these patients can have lengthy admissions to rehabilitation, at least compared with their stays in the acute care setting. Both of these factors—patient variability and level of severity—influence patient outcomes.

The Home Care Setting

The number of elderly people who choose to stay in their homes longer is likely to increase, primarily due to socioeconomic factors. This will foster a need for a general expansion in home health services. For speech-language pathologists, this will mean higher caseloads and the need for a firmer foundational understanding of service delivery in this setting. Home health care is preferable for many families and insurance companies because it is more cost-effective than outpatient treatment, and also because it enhances the quality of life of the patient. There are currently 2 million people receiving home health services in the United States (Malone & Loehr, 2013) for acute illnesses, long-term disabling processes, terminal illness, or permanent disability. Respondents to the *ASHA 2011 Health Care Survey* (American Speech-Language-Hearing Association, 2011) reported that their caseload in this setting consisted of 37% swallowing-related disorders, 20.2% aphasia, 21% cognitive-linguistic disorders including dementia and TBI, and 7.4% motor speech disorders, with the remainder dispersed among augmentative and alternative communication (AAC) and voice disorder cases.

The Home Health Model

Many patients in acute care are referred for home care upon discharge. This decision is multifactorial and can include factors such as level of acuity of the illness, reimbursement issues, lack of need for an extensive rehab admission, and/or the nature of the intended treatment—for example, a person with

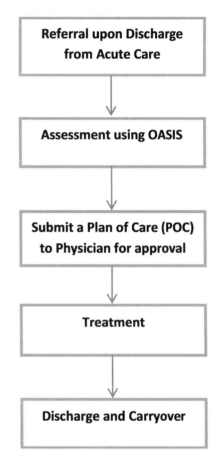

Figure 2–6. The Home Health Model.

dementia who may not need direct therapy, but the caregivers may need some instruction on the patient's communication status. The model (Figure 2–6) is more unidirectional in this case; however, because treatment is in the home, family or caregiver input influences every level of the model once the patient is discharged from acute care. Home health services are primarily reimbursed through CMS and commercial insurance companies, although reimbursement fees can vary. Under Medicare, approval is given for a 60-day period. The direct role of the physician is notable and much more directly related to treatment planning, when compared with acute care or rehabilitation settings.

Assessment in the Home Health Setting.
Optimization and recovery are the focus of service delivery in the home health setting, similar to that

in the rehab setting. Of course, in some cases, recovery is not feasible, for example, dementia; however, optimization may still apply. CMS mandates practitioners in the home health setting use the Outcome and Assessment Information Set (OASIS) for the evaluation of patients. More detailed Information about OASIS can be found at the CMS website (http://www.cms.gov/Medicare/Quality-Initiatives-Patient-Assessment-Instruments/OASIS/index.html?redirect=/oasis/). At this time, an SLP, a physical therapist, an occupational therapist, or a nurse are the only authorized providers who can complete the OASIS. The speech-language pathology section of the OASIS includes the following sections and must be provided by the SLP:

- Motor speech production
- Augmentative communication
- Swallowing
- Cognition
- Language processing
- Language expression
- Reading comprehension
- Written formulation

Plan of Care. The plan of care (POC) is based on the results of the evaluation. Long-term and short-term goals are required, and the long-term goals typically cover the 60-day reimbursement period. Goals can be patient-centered or family-centered, must be measurable and attainable, and be within the scope of practice of the SLP. CMS requires 60-day reassessments in order for treatment to continue and will only be approved if the patient is making progress. The POC also must specify the frequency and duration of visits, and there are different options available to the SLP. Malone and Loehr (2013, p.11) provide the following examples:

- Speech intervention—one visit for the first week, and two visits per week for the next 4 weeks.
- Speech intervention—one visit for the first week, two visits per week for the next 4 weeks, and then one visit per week for the last 4 weeks.
- Speech intervention—two visits per week for 9 weeks.

Therapeutic approaches in the home health setting can use formal treatment programs, for example, Promoting Aphasic Communicative Effectiveness (PACE), or use materials/activities found in the home that will increase the patient's functionality in the social setting. The SLP can be creative in this setting, but must never lose sight of the need to provide evidence-based care.

Discharge from Home Health Care. When the patient has achieved the goals established by the SLP, the clinician must submit a discipline specific discharge summary or complete an OASIS discharge assessment. The last discipline remaining on the case must complete the OASIS discharge assessment, that is, if PT, OT, and nursing have pulled out of the case, then the SLP must complete the OASIS at discharge. Maintenance of the patient's progress is an important factor in any therapeutic setting, and in a home health setting, the family can be very helpful. Training the family to implement and carry over the strategies or skills that you have given the patient can be done through videotaping your sessions, using charts and drawings, and encouraging the family to include the patient in other social settings where the new skills can be implemented. Although home health is just as highly regulated as rehabilitation, service delivery in this setting is the best option for some patients with ALD.

The Outpatient Setting

Ambulatory acute care patients with ALD who are not being admitted to rehabilitation hospitals may be candidates for outpatient (OP) SLP services. This setting is also referred to as *outpatient rehab*. The Rehabilitation Model (see Figure 2–5) can also be used to characterize this service delivery sector as well, making optimization and recovery the focus of SLP services. However, the reimbursement for outpatient treatment is different than it would be in acute rehab or for therapeutic services delivered in a free-standing rehab hospital. Both CMS and commercial insurances will reimburse for OP speech-language pathology services as long as the goals are measurable, attainable, and functionally oriented.

Also, the ICF Model of patient care is applicable to this patient population (see Appendix E).

The reimbursement issues are very complex and ever-changing, so we refer the reader to ASHA's website for the most current information on CMS, the latest Medicare Fee Schedule, and other critical funding aspects of the discipline for this service delivery sector (http://www.asha.org/practice/reimbursement/).

Although health care statistics change often, ASHA reports the following demographics for this population: 44% of the adult patients seen in the outpatient setting are people with stroke, 11% have sustained a head injury, and 7% have a type of central nervous system (CNS) disease. Based on these statistics, it is clear that the majority of the OP caseload will need a comprehensive assessment battery, because many of these patients have speech, swallowing, and language disorder secondary to neurological impairment.

Evaluations in OP settings are typically automatically covered by the insurer, and this includes patients covered by CMS. Standard evaluation procedures would apply, based on the disorder type, presenting symptoms, and so forth. Once the evaluation is complete, a commercial insurer must approve the patient for treatment. Patients are granted a specific number of visits based on their insurance plan, and all therapy goals are expected to be met by the end of that time. Some insurers will request evidence that the treatment approach you are planning to use has proven efficacy. For example, a patient may be granted 30 visits. The case manager at the insurance company will inform the clinician that the patient can be seen in many ways, for example, 30 days in a row (rare), 2 times per week for 15 weeks, and so forth. Appeals for more therapy are common, but not guaranteed. It is the responsibility of the clinician treating the patient to monitor the number of visits and to always ask the patient if they have had a change in insurance so that the appropriate company can be charged by the hospital. It is important to note that insurers reserve the right to deny reimbursement retroactively, which lends further import to the necessity of writing and planning measurable, attainable, and functional goals for your patient once the assessment is completed.

Treatment in the OP setting uses any therapeutic approach that has evidence-based efficacy and is not specific to this particular setting, that is, there are no "OP only" treatment procedures. The clinician can adapt any program or therapy technique to meet the needs of this patient type, with the understanding that unlike home health care and rehabilitation settings, the time allotted to achieve one's goals is much more limited. Family counseling and education also plays a significant role in this patient population. Family members and caregivers can be very helpful with information regarding barriers and facilitators (see ICF Model in Appendix E) to the patient's rehabilitation. Furthermore, the clinician can train the family in techniques to facilitate carryover and maintenance of the skills attained during treatment. To summarize, SLP services in the OP setting share most features with the Rehabilitation Model. The critical differences are two: reimbursement for services and the time allotted to achieve the patient's goals.

The Long-Term Care Setting

The popular view of the residents of long-term care (LTC) facilities is that they do not change, yet that is not an accurate depiction of their status. These patients *do* change, and their care plans most often reflect the fluctuations in their needs, for example, in medical status, cognitive status, and/or behavioral status. Many of these patients will have multiple acute care hospital admissions during their life at the facility, and the SLP will reassess many of these patients many times, with varying results. The SLP working in this setting will quickly learn that flexibility, interdisciplinary care, and creative problem-solving are necessary in order to provide effective service to these residents. Although recovery may not always be part of the rehabilitation equation for these patients, optimization of their current communication and swallowing functions are certainly realistic goals. Interesting, one can apply features of both the ACM and the Rehabilitation Model to these patients because some elements of each are relevant to the care of these patients (Figure 2–7).

Assessment

Upon admission, the patient is assessed by a professional in the facility (typically a nurse, but not necessarily), using the Minimum Data Set (MDS) in order to determine the patient's needs or *resource utilization*. The MDS is the mandated initial assessment according to Centers for Medicare and Medicaid Services (CMS), and the current version is the MDS 3.0 (Wisely, 2010). The form can be found at the CMS website (http://www.cms.gov/). The MDS is also used by CMS and some states' Medicaid programs to determine reimbursement rates for that patient's first 100-day stay in the facility. The patient is interviewed for personal history and preferred activities, and family involvement is encouraged by CMS throughout this initial process. If the patient is still a resident after 100 days, without an intervening acute care admission, then the patient switches to Medicare Part B reimbursement rates.

Once this initial assessment is conducted by the MDS administrator at the facility and the patient's needs are determined, the SLP may receive a consult to formally assess the patient. The SLP in the LTC setting can use any test instrument or methodology that is pertinent to the disorder type, as long as the test instrument is objective and standardized. There are three sections of the MDS that pertain to communication and swallowing, which must be completed by the MDS administrator. Wisely (2010) reports these as:

- Section B: Hearing, Speech, and Vision
  - Document the resident's ability to hear with/without assistive hearing devices.
  - Document the resident's ability to understand language.
  - Document the resident's ability to communicate with others.
  - Document any visual disturbances associated with common illnesses associated with aging.
- Section C: Cognitive Patterns
  - Document any changes to long-term and short-term memory.
  - Document evidence for clear thinking.

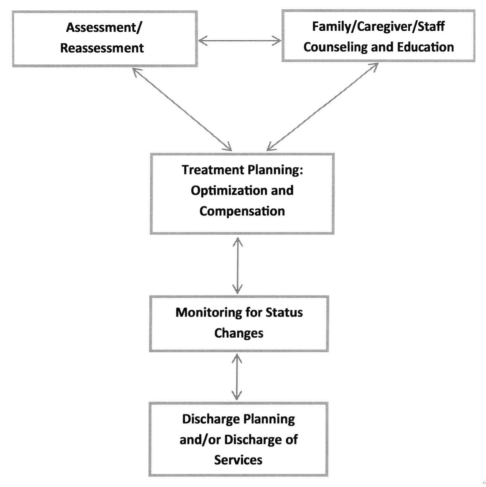

Figure 2–7. The Long-Term Care Model as a hybrid of the ACM and Rehabilitation models.

■ Section F: Preferences for Customary Routine and Activities
  ■ Document the resident's preferences for his or her daily routine and activities. CMS prefers that this information come directly from the patient; however, if that is not possible, a person familiar with the patient can supply the information.

Treatment in LTC

Treatment for Medicare Part A patients (first 100 days) in LTC is based on the results of the assessment and is included in the patient's plan of care (POC). The patient is then assigned to a RUG level—*Resource Utilization Group*—based on the patient's communication, cognitive, and/or swallowing needs. The RUG levels are low, high, and ultra-high, and are differentiated by minutes of therapy per week. For example, a patient may be assigned to an ultra-high RUG and be given 700 minutes of therapy per week. These minutes must be split by the disciplines, based on the patient's greatest need, that is, PT, OT, or SLP. The CMS website noted above offers information about RUGs and their use in LTC. It should be apparent that interdisciplinary care is very common in LTC settings because all treatment is determined by the MDS, which reflects the patient's global needs.

The SLP is an integral part of this team, so understanding the roles and responsibilities of the other disciplines prevents professional encroachment and promotes collegiality.

One of the more pressing issues in LTC for the SLP is the concept of providing specialized/individualized care. This includes restorative care, maintenance programs, and facilitative and/or inhibitory programs. The challenge is to design a care plan for this type of patient that is both reimbursable, functional, and is consistent with their own personal goals, as mandated by CMS. Therefore, any therapeutic approaches that can meet the patient's current functional needs and are based on the MDS findings and the formal assessment, are acceptable.

Monitoring Change and Continuation of Services

In the introduction to this section, the prevailing thought about patients in LTC as unchanging or unable to change was challenged. It is important that these patients be monitored for any changes during their stay in the facility, and rescreening is very common in as a result. Furthermore, patient outcomes are just as important in LTC as they are in the rehabilitation setting because the patient's quality of life is immediately dependent on those outcomes in LTC. The SLP in this setting must walk a fine line between demands for 85% to 90% productivity over the work week and providing ethical, efficacious, functional, and individualized service to the patients on the caseload. Therefore, determining the appropriate time for discharge from SLP services is a very important responsibility in this setting.

Summary

This section addressed service delivery in the ALD population in acute care, rehabilitation, outpatient, home health, and LTC settings. All of these settings are regulated by accrediting agencies along with state and government legislation whose intent is to promote quality of service and patient safety. Adult patients who are present with ALD in any of these settings can progress toward greater functionality or

regress due to a myriad of circumstances. In either scenario, the SLP is responsible for providing optimal services and "holding the welfare of the patient paramount" (American Speech-Language-Hearing Association, Code of Ethics, 2010).

References

Adamonovich, B. L. B., & Henderson, J. (1992). *Scales of cognitive ability for traumatic brain injury*. Chicago, IL: Riverside.

American Speech-Language-Hearing Association. (2010). *Code of ethics*. Retrieved from http://www.asha.org/policy

American Speech-Language-Hearing Association. (2011). *2011 SLP health care survey summary report: Number and type of responses*. Retrieved from http://www.asha.org

Baines, K. A., Martin, A. W., & McMartin Heeringa, H. (1999). *Assessment of Language-Related Functional Activities*. Austin, TX: Pro-Ed.

Bayles, K. A., & Tomoeda, C. K. (1993). *Arizona Battery of Communication Disorders of Dementia (ABCD)*. Austin, TX: Pro-Ed.

Benton, A., & Hamsher, K. (1978). *Multilingual Aphasia Examination manual*. Iowa City: University of Iowa.

Brookshire, R. H. (2003). *Introduction to neurogenic communication disorders* (6th ed.). St. Louis, MO: Mosby.

Brookshire, R., & Nicholas, L. (1997). *Discourse comprehension test*. Bloomington, MN: BRK.

Burns, M. (1997). *Burns brief inventory of communication and cognition*. San Antonio, TX: Psychological Corporation.

Caplan, D. (1987). *Neurolinguistics and linguistic aphasiology*. Cambridge, UK: Cambridge University Press.

Croft, W., & Cruse, D. A. (2004). *Cognitive linguistics*. Cambridge, UK: Cambridge University Press.

Davies, R. R., Dawson, K., Mioshi, E., Erzinclioglu, S., & Hodges, J. R. 2008). Differentiation of semantic dementia and Alzheimer's disease using the Addenbrooke's Cognitive Examination (ACE). *International Journal of Geriatric Psychiatry, 23*, 370–375.

Dewart, H., & Summers, S. (1996). *The pragmatics profile of communication skills in adults*. London, UK: Whurr.

Donovan, N. J., Kendall, D. L., Heaton, S. C., Kwon, S., Velozo, C. A., & Duncan, P. W. (2008). Conceptualizing functional cognition in stroke. *Neurorehabilitation and Neural Repair, 22*, 122–135.

Eisdorfer, C., Cohen, D., Paveza, G. J., Ashford, J. W., Luchins, D. J., Gorelick, P. B., . . . Shaw, H. A. (1992). An empirical evaluation of the Global Deterioration Scale for staging Alzheimer's Disease. *American Journal of Psychiatry, 149*, 190–194.

Enderby, P. (1987). Frenchay Aphasia Screening Test. *International Rehabilitation Medicine, 8*, 162–165.

Feyereisen, P., Pillon, A., & de Partz, M. (1991). On the measures of fluency in the assessment of spontaneous speech production by aphasic subjects. *Aphasiology, 5*(1), 1–21.

Fitch West, J., Sands, E. S., & Ross-Swain, D. (1998). *Bedside Evaluation Screening Test* (2nd ed.). Austin, TX: Pro-Ed.

Frattali, C., Thompson, C., Holland, A., Wohl, C., & Ferketic, M. (1995). *The American Speech-Language-Hearing Association Functional Assessment of Communication Skills for Adults (ASHA FACS).* Rockville, MD: American Speech-Language-Hearing Association.

Functional Independence Measure. (1996). *Uniform data set for medical rehabilitation.* Buffalo, NY: University of Buffalo.

Giacino, J., & Kalmar, K. (2004). Coma Recovery Scale-Revised. *The Center for Outcome Measurement in Brain Injury.* Retrieved from http://www.tbims.org/combi/crs

Gioia, G. A., Isquith, P. K., Guy, S. C., & Kenworthy, L. (2000). *Behavior rating inventory of executive function.* Odessa, FL: Psychological Assessment Resources.

Goodglass, H., & Kaplan, E. (1972). *The assessment of aphasia and related disorders.* Philadelphia, PA: Lea & Febiger.

Goodglass, H., & Kaplan, E. (1983). *The assessment of aphasia and related disorders* (2nd ed.). Philadelphia, PA: Lea & Febiger.

Goodglass, H., Kaplan, E., & Barresi, B. (2001). *The Boston Diagnostic Aphasia Exam* (3rd ed.) Baltimore, MD: Lippincott Williams & Wilkins.

Gordon, J. (1998). The fluency dimension in aphasia. *Aphasiology, 12*(7), 673–688.

Gray, S., & Starr, J. M. (2013). Does the Addenbrooke's Cognitive Examination–Revised add to the Mini-Mental State Examination in established Alzheimer disease? Results from a national dementia research register. *International Journal of Geriatric Psychiatry, 28*(4), 351–355.

Helm-Estabrooks, N. (2001). *Cognitive Linguistic Quick Test.* San Antonio, TX: Psychological Corporation.

Helm-Estabrooks, N., & Albert, M. L. (2004). *Manual of aphasia and aphasia therapy* (2nd ed.). Austin, TX: Pro-Ed.

Helm-Estabrooks, N., Bayles, K., Ramage, A., & Bryant, S. (1995). Relationship between cognitive performance and aphasia severity, age, and education: Females versus males. *Brain and Language, 51*(1), 139–141.

Helm-Estabrooks, N., Emery, P., & Albert, M. L. (1987). Treatment of aphasic perseveration (TAP) program. A new approach to aphasia therapy. *Archives of Neurology, 44*(12), 1253–1255.

Helm-Estabrooks, N., Ramsberger, A. R., & Nichols, M. (1989). *Boston Assessment of Severe Aphasia.* Dedham, MA: AliMed.

Holland, A., Frattali, C., & Fromm, D. (1999). *Communication activities of daily living* (2nd ed.). Austin, TX: Pro-Ed.

Huber, W., Poeck, K., & Willmes, K. (1984). The Aachen Aphasia Test. In F. C. Rose (Ed.), *Advances in neurology 42: Progress in aphasiology* (pp. 291–303). New York, NY: Raven Press.

Johnson, A. F., & Jacobson, B. H. (2007). *Medical speech-language pathology: A practioner's guide.* New York, NY: Thieme.

Kaplan, E., Goodglass, H., & Weintraub, S. (1976). *The Boston Naming Test.* Boston, MA: Veteran's Administration.

Kay, J., Lesser, R., & Coltheart, R. M. (1992). *Psycholinguistic Assessments of Language Processing in Aphasia.* Hove, UK: Lawrence Erlbaum.

Kertesz, A. (1982). *The Western Aphasia Battery.* New York, NY: Grune & Stratton.

Kertesz, A. (2006). *Western Aphasia Battery-Revised.* San Antonio, TX: Psychological Corporation.

Klein, E. R., & Hahn, S. E. (2007). *Focus on function: Gaining essential communication* (2nd ed.). Austin, TX: Pro-Ed.

Kohn, S. (1989). The nature of the phonemic string deficit in conduction aphasia. *Aphasiology, 3*, 265–285.

Kohn, S. (1993). Segmental disorders in aphasia. In G. Blanken, J. Dittmann, H. Grimm, J. Marshall, & C. W. Wallesch (Eds.), *Linguistic disorders and pathologies: An international handbook* (pp. 197–209). Berlin, Germany: Walter de Gruyter.

Kreb, R. A. (Ed.). (1996). *A practical guide to applying treatment outcomes and efficacy resources.* Rockville, MD: American Speech-Language-Hearing Association.

Laine, M., & Martin, N. (2006). *Anomia: Theoretical and clinical aspects.* Hove, UK: Psychology Press.

LaPointe, L., & Eisenson, J. (2008). *Examining for aphasia (EFA-4)* (4th ed.). Austin, TX: Pro-Ed.

LaPointe, L., & Horner, J. (1998). *Reading comprehension battery for aphasia* (2nd ed.) Austin, TX: Pro-Ed.

Leyton, C. E., Hornberger, N. M., Mioshi, E., & Hodges, J. R. (2010). Application of Addenbrooke's Cognitive Examination to diagnosis and monitoring of progressive primary aphasia. *Dementia and Geriatric Cognitive Disorders, 29*, 504–509.

Lind, M., Kristoffersen, K. E., Moen, I., & Simonsen, H. G. (2009). Semi-spontaneous oral text production: Measurements in clinical practice. *Clinical Linguistics & Phonetics, 23*(12), 872–886.

Malone, M. L., & Loehr, J. (2013). Home health care for adults: A tutorial for SLPs. *Perspectives on Gerontology, 18*(1), 7–13.

Marshall, R. C., & Wright, H. H. (2007). Developing a clinician-friendly aphasia test. *American Journal of Speech-Language Pathology, 18*, 295–315.

Meyers, J. E., & Meyers, K. R. (1995). *Rey Complex Figure Test and Trial.* San Antonio, TX: Pearson Education.

Miller, R. M., & Groher, M. E. (1990). *Medical speech-language pathology.* Rockville, MD: Aspen.

Milman, L. H., & Holland, A. (2012). *SCCAN: Scales of Cognitive and Communicative Ability for Neurorehabilitation.* Austin, TX: Pro-Ed.

Papathanasiou, I., Coppens, P., & Potagas, C. (2013). *Aphasia and related neurogenic communication disorders.* Burlington, MA: Jones & Bartlett Learning.

Paradis, M., & Libben, G. (1987). *The assessment of bilingual aphasia.* Hillsdale, NJ: Lawrence Erlbaum.

Porch, B. E. (1971). *Porch index of communicative ability.* Palo Alto, CA: Consulting Psychologists Press.

Prins, R., & Bastiaanse, R. (2004). Analysing the spontaneous speech of aphasic speakers. *Aphasiology, 18*(12), 1075–1091.

Prutting, C., & Kirchner, D. (1987). A clinical appraisal of the pragmatic aspects of language. *Journal of Speech and Hearing Disorders, 52*, 105–119.

Psychological Assessment Resources. (2003). *The Wisconsin Card Sorting Test: Computerized Version 4 (WCST).* Lutz, FL: Psychological Assessment Resources.

Randolph, C. (2001). *Repeatable battery for the assessment of neuropsychological status.* San Antonio, TX: Psychological Corporation.

Reisberg, B., Ferris, S. H., De Leon, M. J., & Crook, T. (1982). The Global Deterioration Scale for assessment of primary degenerative dementia. *American Journal of Psychiatry, 139*, 1136–1139.

Ross-Swain, D. (1996). *Ross Information Processing Assessment* (2nd ed.). Austin, TX: Pro-Ed.

Salis, C., & Edwards, S. (2009). Tests of syntactic comprehension in aphasia: An investigation of task effects. *Aphasiology, 23*(10), 1215–1230.

Sarno, M. T. (1969). *The functional communication profile.* New York, NY: Institute of Rehabilitation Medicine, New York University Medical.

Schuell, H. M., Jenkins, J. J., & Jimenez-Pabon, E. (1964). *Aphasia in adults: Diagnosis, prognosis and treatment.* New York, NY: Harper & Row.

Shipley, K. G., & McAfee, J. G. (2004). *Assessment in speech-language pathology: A resource manual* (3rd ed.). Clifton Park, NY: Delmar.

Swinburn, K., Porter, G., & Howard, D. (2005). *The Comprehensive Aphasia Test.* Hove, UK: Psychology Press.

Turkstra, L. S., Coelho, C., & Ylvisaker, M. (2005). The use of standardized tests for individuals with cognitive-communication disorders. *Seminars in Speech and Language, 26*(4), 215–222.

West, J. F., Sands, E., & Ross-Swain, D. (1998). *Bedside Evaluation Screening Test.* Austin, TX: Pro-Ed.

Wiig, E., & Secord, W. (1989). *Test of language competence—Expanded edition.* San Antonio, TX: Psychological Corporation.

Wisely, J. M. (2010). Skilled nursing facility assessment tool focuses on patient communication. *ASHA Leader.*

Wright, H. H., & Capiluto, G. J. (2009). Manipulating task instructions to change narrative discourse performance. *Aphasiology, 23*(10), 1295–1308.

APPENDIX 2–A
Quick Reference Diagnostic Chart For Acquired Language Disorders

The Major Nonfluent Aphasias

Function	Broca's	Transcortical Motor	Global
EXPRESSIVE LANGUAGE			
Automatic	Variable	WNL	Poor
Repetition	Fair	WNL	Poor
Lexical Retrieval	Variable	Poor	Poor
Conversation	Telegraphic	Paraphasic	Limited output
Pragmatics	WNL	Poor	Poor
Grammatical Structure	Agrammatic	WNL	Impaired; sparse output
AUDITORY COMPREHENSION			
Simple Yes/No Questions	WNL	Good	Fair, with perseveration noted
Executing Commands	WNL	Good	Variable
Conversation	WNL	Poor	Poor
Object Identification	WNL	Challenged by nonfluency	Poor
Object Function Identification	WNL	Challenged by nonfluency	Poor
SPEECH PRODUCTION			
Rate	Irregular due to nonfluency	Irregular due to nonfluency	Sparse output prevents valid assessment
Intelligibility	WNL	WNL	N/A
Prosody	Poor	Poor	Absent
Articulation	Impaired	WNL	Sparse output prevents valid assessment
Fluency	Nonfluent	Nonfluent	Nonfluent
ORAL READING			
Word Level	Poor	Slow with struggle	Poor
Sentence Level	Poor	Slow with struggle	Poor
Paragraph Level	Poor	Slow with struggle	Poor
READING COMPREHENSION			
Word Level	WNL	WNL	Poor
Sentence Level	WNL	WNL	Poor
Paragraph Level	Variable	Variable	Poor

continues

Function	Broca's	Transcortical Motor	Global
WRITING			
Copying Words	WNL	Poor	Poor
Copying Sentences	WNL	Poor	Poor
Writing to Dictation	Laborious with graphic paraphasias	Poor	Poor
Self-Generated Writing	Agrammatic; error-prone	Poor	Poor
SPELLING			
Oral	Variable	Paraphasic	Poor
Written	Success is length dependent	Poor	Poor
DRAWING			
Copying	WNL	Variable	Poor
Functional Use	WNL	WNL	Poor
COGNITION			
Attention to Task	WNL	Attends when engaged; distractible	Limited; requires cues
Visuospatial Skills	WNL	WNL	Poor
Memory	WNL	WNL	Functional for procedural memory
Problem Solving	WNL	WNL for ADL needs	Poor, for language-dependent problems
Safety Awareness	WNL	WNL	Patient dependent
Organizational Skills	WNL	WNL for ADL needs	WNL for ADL needs
BEHAVIOR			
Level of Alertness (LOA)	WNL	Patient dependent	Variable
Deficit Awareness	WNL	WNL	Variable
Emotional Lability	Variable	Patient dependent	Not noted
Frustration	High	Variable	Increases with task complexity
Personality Changes	Patient dependent	Apathetic, withdrawn; disinterested	Depressed; anxious

The Major Fluent Aphasias

Function	Wernicke's	Transcortical Sensory	Conduction	Anomic
EXPRESSIVE LANGUAGE				
Automatic	Poor	WNL	WNL	WNL
Repetition	Poor	Good	Poor	WNL
Lexical Retrieval	Paraphasic	Poor	Poor	Poor
Conversation	Empty speech; neologistic; logorrhea possible	Paraphasic	Circumlocutionary; literal paraphasias may be noted	Circumlocutionary; semantic paraphsaias
Pragmatics	Poor	Poor turn-taking skills	WNL	WNL
Grammatical Structure	Paragrammatic		WNL	WNL
AUDITORY COMPREHENSION				
Simple Yes/No Questions	Poor	Poor	WNL	WNL
Executing Commands	Poor	Poor	WNL	WNL
Conversation	Poor	Poor; empty; neologistic	WNL	Poor
Object Identification	Poor	Poor	Poor	Poor, due to naming difficulties
Object Function Identification	Poor	Poor	Poor	WNL
SPEECH PRODUCTION				
Rate	WNL	WNL	WNL	WNL
Intelligibility	WNL	WNL	WNL	WNL
Prosody	WNL	WNL	WNL	WNL
Articulation	WNL	WNL	WNL	WNL
Fluency	Fluent	Fluent	Variable, due to attempts at self-correction	Impacted by word-finding difficulties
ORAL READING				
Word Level	Poor	Good	Highly variable	WNL
Sentence Level	Poor	Good	Highly variable	WNL
Paragraph Level	Poor	Good	Highly variable	WNL
READING COMPREHENSION				
Word Level	Poor	Poor	Better at silent reading	WNL
Sentence Level	Poor	Poor	Better at silent reading	WNL
Paragraph Level	WNL	Poor	Better at silent reading	WNL

continues

Appendix 2–A. Quick Reference Diagnostic Chart For Acquired Language Disorders *continued*

Function	Wernicke's	Transcortical Sensory	Conduction	Anomic
WRITING				
Copying Words	Poor; paraphasic; error-prone	Parallels expressive output	Poor	WNL
Copying Sentences	Poor; paraphasic; error-prone	Parallels expressive output	Poor	WNL
Writing to Dictation	Poor; paraphasic; error-prone	Parallels expressive output	Poor	WNL
Self-Generated Writing	Poor; paraphasic; error-prone	Parallels expressive output	Poor	WNL
SPELLING				
Oral	Neologistic	Variable	Poor > 4 words	Substitutions noted
Written	Paraphasic errors	Variable	Poor	WNL
DRAWING				
Copying	Variable	WNL	WNL	WNL
Functional Use	Poor	WNL	WNL	WNL
COGNITION				
Attention to Task	Poor	Variable	WNL	WNL
Visuospatial Skills	WNL	Visual neglect possible	WNL	WNL
Memory	WNL for ADL needs	WNL for ADL needs	WNL	WNL
Problem Solving	Poor for language dependent solutions	Accurate assessment prohibited by language impairment	WNL	WNL
Safety Awareness	Poor for language dependent solutions	Accurate assessment prohibited by language impairment	WNL	WNL
Organizational Skills	WNL for ADL needs	WNL for ADL needs	WNL	WNL
BEHAVIOR				
Level of Alertness (LOA)	Patient dependent	Patient dependent	WNL	WNL
Deficit Awareness	Anosagnosia	Anosagnosia	Heightened	WNL
Emotional Lability	Patient dependent	Patient dependent	Not noted	WNL
Frustration	Variable	Variable	Heightened	Heightened
Personality Changes	Patient dependent	Patient dependent	Variable	Patient dependent

Other Aphasic Syndromes

Function	Subcortical-Thalamic	Subcortical Nonthalamic (Striatocapsular lesions)[1]	Primary Progressive Aphasia (PPA[2])
EXPRESSIVE LANGUAGE			
Automatic	WNL	WNL	Variable
Repetition	WNL	WNL	Variable
Lexical Retrieval	Poor	Impaired	Moderately impaired; typically a presenting feature
Conversation	Initially mute; semantic paraphasias may be present during recovery phase	Fluent; pauses and hesitations may be present; semantic paraphasias in some cases	Nonfluent
Pragmatics	Impaired due to lethargy	WNL	WNL
Grammatical Structure	WNL	Impaired	Agrammatic
AUDITORY COMPREHENSION			
Simple Yes/No Questions	WNL; moderate impairment for complex material	WNL; variable for complex material	Variable
Executing Commands	WNL	WNL	Variable
Conversation	WNL	Variable, depending on complexity	Variable
Object Identification	Poor	Impaired	Variable
Object Function Identification	Poor	Impaired	Variable
SPEECH PRODUCTION			
Rate	WNL	May be impaired	WNL
Intelligibility	WNL	Variable	WNL
Prosody	WNL	Impaired	WNL
Articulation	WNL	Impaired	WNL
Fluency	WNL	Fluent	WNL
ORAL READING			
Word Level	Impaired	Variable	Variable
Sentence Level	Impaired	Variable	Variable
Paragraph Level	Impaired	Variable	Variable
READING COMPREHENSION			
Word Level	Impaired	Variable	Variable
Sentence Level	Impaired	Variable	Variable
Paragraph Level	Impaired	Variable	Variable

continues

Appendix 2–A. Quick Reference Diagnostic Chart For Acquired Language Disorders *continued*

Function	Subcortical-Thalamic	Subcortical Nonthalamic (Striatocapsular lesions)[1]	Primary Progressive Aphasia (PPA[2])
WRITING			
Copying Words	Impaired	WNL	Variable
Copying Sentences	Impaired	WNL	Variable
Writing To Dictation	Impaired	WNL	Variable
Self-Generated Writing	Impaired	WNL	Variable
SPELLING			
Oral	Impaired	Variable	Variable
Written	Impaired	Variable	Variable
DRAWING			
Copying	WNL	Variable	Variable
Functional Use	WNL	Variable	Variable
COGNITION			
Attention To Task	Variable, due to low-level arousal and lethargy	Variable, due to low-level arousal and lethargy	WNL
Visuospatial Skills	WNL	Variable	WNL
Memory	Declarative memory impaired; procedural spared	Variable	WNL
Problem Solving	WNL for ADL needs	Variable	WNL
Safety Awareness	WNL for ADL needs	Variable	WNL
Organizational Skills	WNL for ADL needs	Variable	WNL
BEHAVIOR			
Level Of Alertness (LOA)	Variable, due to low-level arousal and lethargy	Variable, due to low-level arousal and lethargy	WNL
Deficit Awareness	Variable	Not typical	Present
Emotional Lability	Not typical	Not typical	Not typical
Frustration	Not typical	Variable	Present; reactive depression
Personality Changes	Lack of motivation may be observed	Lack of motivation may be observed	Not noted

[1]Subcortical aphasias can present with the symptomatology of any of the cortical aphasias. This is secondary to the fact that subcortical stroke typically involves the M-1 portion of the MCA, which also supplies the overlying cerebral cortices. Therefore, a subcortical ischemic event in that distribution territory can cause aphasic symptomatology consistent with any of the major aphasic syndromes. We have used the term *variable* in order to convey this fact in the *Quick Reference Chart*.

[2]The person with PPA can present with features of any of the aphasias, depending on the area(s) of cortical degeneration. Therefore, we have used the term *variable* to capture that variability. The symptomatology described in the Quick Reference Chart reflects PPA up to and including the second year post onset. The patient may become more cognitively impaired as the disease progresses.

Quick Reference Diagnostic Chart For Acquired Language Disorders

Function	Right Hemisphere Disorder	Dementia[3]	Cerebral Encephalopathies[4]
EXPRESSIVE LANGUAGE			
Automatic	WNL	Variable, based on stage of dementia	WNL
Repetition	WNL	WNL	WNL
Lexical Retrieval	WNL	Impaired (noted early)	WNL
Conversation	Tangential/ circumlocutionary	Deteriorates progressively	Tangential output
Pragmatics	Impaired	WNL	Poor topic maintenance and turn-taking
Grammatical Structure	WNL	WNL	WNL
AUDITORY COMPREHENSION			
Simple Yes/No Questions	WNL; could be impacted by attentional problems	WNL	WNL for concrete and personal questions
Executing Commands	WNL; could be impacted by attentional problems and distractibility	WNL for simple 1-step commands	1-steps commands— WNL; complex commands—impaired
Understanding Conversation	Tangential and circumlocutionary	WNL; progressively deteriorates	Variable depending on complexity of information
Object Identification	WNL	WNL for common objects	WNL
Object Function Identification	WNL	WNL	WNL
SPEECH PRODUCTION			
Rate	If no accompanying dysarthria: WNL	WNL	If no accompanying dysarthria: WNL
Intelligibility	If no accompanying dysarthria: WNL	WNL	If no accompanying dysarthria: WNL
Prosody	If no accompanying dysarthria: WNL	WNL	If no accompanying dysarthria: WNL
Articulation	If no accompanying dysarthria: WNL	WNL	If no accompanying dysarthria: WNL
Fluency	If no accompanying dysarthria: WNL	WNL	If no accompanying dysarthria: WNL
ORAL READING			
Word Level	WNL	WNL	WNL based on level of alertness (LOA)
Sentence Level	WNL	Variable	WNL based on level of alertness (LOA)
Paragraph Level	WNL	Variable	WNL based on level of alertness (LOA)

continues

Function	Right Hemisphere Disorder	Dementia[3]	Cerebral Encephalopathies[4]
READING COMPREHENSION			
Word Level	WNL	WNL	WNL based on level of alertness (LOA)
Sentence Level	May be affected by attentional issues and distractibility	Variable, based on type and stage	WNL based on level of alertness (LOA)
Paragraph Level	May be affected by attentional issues and distractibility	Variable, based on type and stage	WNL based on level of alertness (LOA)
WRITING			
Copying Words	WNL	WNL	WNL
Copying Sentences	WNL	WNL	WNL
Writing to Dictation	Variable	WNL	WNL up to sentence level
Self-Generated Writing	Mimics verbal expression	WNL	Variable based on level of severity
SPELLING			
Oral	WNL	More impaired for irregularly spelled words and multisyllabic words	WNL for regularly spelled words
Written	WNL	Same as above	WNL for regularly spelled words
DRAWING			
Copying	WNL; visuospatial problems may affect performance	WNL	WNL
Functional Use	WNL; visuospatial problems may affect performance	Variable	Variable
COGNITION			
Attention to Task	Impaired	Impaired	Impaired
Visuospatial Skills	Variable; neglect or left inattention may be present	Impaired	Variable
Memory	Variable	Impaired for episodic and semantic memory	Impaired
Problem Solving	Impaired	Impaired	Impaired
Safety Awareness	Impaired due to impulsivity	Impaired	Impaired
Organizational Skills	Impaired	Impaired	Impaired

Function	Right Hemisphere Disorder	Dementia[3]	Cerebral Encephalopathies[4]
BEHAVIOR			
Level of Alertness (LOA)	WNL	Agitation noted in some cases	Variable; very low in acute phase of illness; lethargy common
Deficit Awareness	Anosagnosia	Variable impairment based on stage	Impaired
Emotional Lability	Not typical	Not noted	Impaired
Frustration	Not noted	Commonly noted	Can be observed along with agitation and depression
Personality Changes	Not typically associated with this disorder	Yes	May be noted

[3]These characteristics reflect the early-middle stages of most dementias. The cognitive-linguistic characteristics of this patient type will change as the process continues to deteriorate to the end stage.

[4]Performance in many tasks depends on the patient's level of alertness and ability to focus and concentrate. Lethargy is common in these patients, especially in the acute phase of the illness.

Quick Reference Diagnostic Chart For Traumatic Brain Injury (TBI) and Post-Concussive Syndrome

Cognitive-linguistic functions in the TBI population vary based on level of functioning (see *Rancho Los Amigos Scale*). Consequently, a "Quick Reference" chart would not offer a comprehensive summary of their deficits due to the variability inherent in TBI. We suggest using the RLA paired with appropriately sensitive test instruments, and clinical observations to obtain the most reliable communicative and behavioral picture of these patients.

APPENDIX 2–B
Functional Communication Connections™

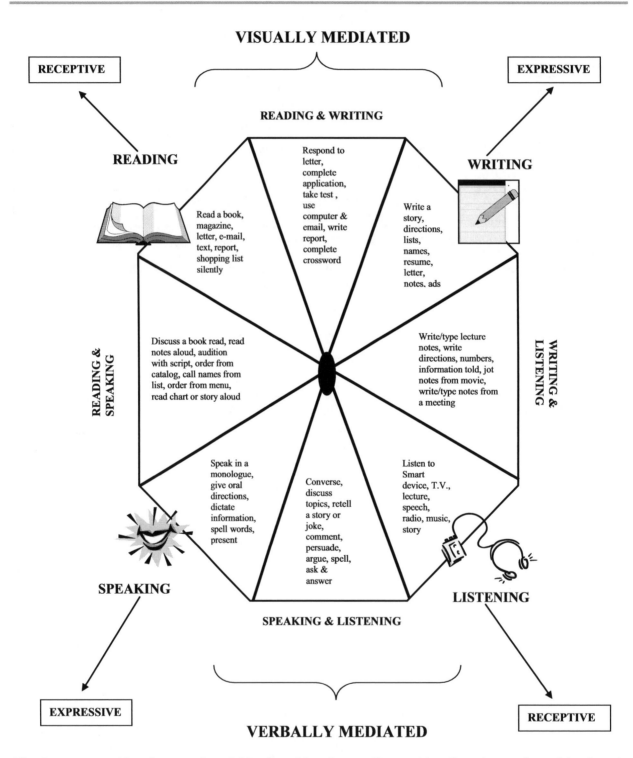

VISUALLY MEDIATED

RECEPTIVE

EXPRESSIVE

READING & WRITING

READING

WRITING

Read a book, magazine, letter, e-mail, text, report, shopping list silently

Respond to letter, complete application, take test, use computer & email, write report, complete crossword

Write a story, directions, lists, names, resume, letter, notes, ads

READING & SPEAKING

Discuss a book read, read notes aloud, audition with script, order from catalog, call names from list, order from menu, read chart or story aloud

Write/type lecture notes, write directions, numbers, information told, jot notes from movie, write/type notes from a meeting

WRITING & LISTENING

Speak in a monologue, give oral directions, dictate information, spell words, present

Converse, discuss topics, retell a story or joke, comment, persuade, argue, spell, ask & answer

Listen to Smart device, T.V., lecture, speech, radio, music, story

SPEAKING

LISTENING

SPEAKING & LISTENING

EXPRESSIVE

RECEPTIVE

VERBALLY MEDIATED

The Octagon provides therapeutic activities for addressing reading, writing, listening, and speaking impairments (see Appendix F for a reproducible blank Octagon to use with a client).

Chapter 3

THE MAJOR NONFLUENT APHASIAS

Introduction

There are numerous treatment programs and approaches for improving speech and language in individuals with nonfluent aphasia (Appendix E). One of the latest advances in treating people with nonfluent aphasias is neural stimulation (Barwood et al., 2012). There are two neural stimulation methods currently in use with people with aphasia: Repetitive Transcranial Magnetic Stimulation (rTMS) and Anodal Transcranial Direct Current Stimulation (A-tDCS), which has an excitatory effect and its counterpart Cathodal Transcranial Direct Current Stimulation (C-tDCS), which has an inhibitory effect.

Transcranial Magnetic Stimulation (TMS) is a noninvasive procedure that creates a magnetic field in a coil of wire. This is placed on the skull of the subject, over the targeted brain region. This magnetic field penetrates the skull and induces a small current that is parallel to the plane of the coil. This field depolarizes the neuronal membranes and creates action potentials in the area beneath the coil. In rTMS, a *series of pulses* are generated over a specific period of time at specific frequencies, with low frequencies having an inhibitory effect and higher frequencies acting as excitatory effect (Hamilton, Chrysikou, & Coslett, 2011). This technique has shown promise with in people with communication disorders. Pairing rTMS with behavioral therapy for the anomia can improve naming in people with aphasia (PWA), however, the findings are not always conclusive (Hamilton et al., 2011). When it is applied to the right hemisphere, it may

suppress overactivation in the right hemispheric homologue of Broca's area, increasing activation of the left hemispheric area. Winhuisen et al. (2005) did report, however, that recruiting the right hemisphere to help with a language task may not always be beneficial and in some cases unfavorable. Martin, Naeser, Ho, Doron, and Kurland (2009) conducted a study with two patients with chronic, nonfluent aphasia using rTMS in an attempt to improve naming skills. One patient was a good responder following activation and made significant gains in naming and phrase length over treatment. At 46 months post-TMS, activation continued and phrase length increased from three to six words. The other patient did not make significant gains and was only able to produce single words. This individual's lesion was frontal and extended high and near the brain vertex with deep white matter lesions near the left supplementary motor area, and showed initial activation, but effects did not persist beyond 6 months post-TMS. The authors concluded that the site of lesion may influence an individual's functional magnetic resonance imaging (fMRI) activation pattern and TMS response. From fMRI data, it is suggested that rTMS may help restore the left hemisphere language network for better naming and phrase length in good responders. This method is most often used with people who have chronic aphasia. Barwood et al. (2012), in an open-label study, applied rTMS to modulate bilateral language networks by stimulating the right hemispheric homologue to Broca's area. There were seven nonfluent aphasic participants who received 1 Hz stimulation of rTMS for 10 days. Results indicated significant improvements in auditory comprehension, picture naming, and spontaneous elicited speech. This improvement was sustained for up to 8 months post rTMS treatment. The authors concluded that rTMS appears to facilitate a positive change in receptive and expressive language in people with nonfluent aphasia. The research in this area is ongoing.

A-tDCS and C-tDCS uses fMRI guided placement of two saline-soaked electrodes—one anodal (excitatory) and one cathodal (inhibitory). Small electrical currents (1–2 mA) are passed through the anode, placed over the desired cortical region and out through the cathode, and placed on the shoulder (Fridriksson, 2011; Hamilton et al., 2011). These weak electrical currents stimulate the resting potentials of neurons. If the anode is placed on the scalp, the effect is excitatory; if the cathode is placed on the scalp, the effect is inhibitory. Fridriksson (2011) used this tDCS with 10 subjects all with an anomic aphasia. They received A-tDCS concurrently with 20 minutes of behavioral treatment for their anomia. His results showed that A-tDCS targeting the left hemisphere can improve outcomes, and those who benefited most recruited the left hemisphere for the speech task. The therapeutic effect persisted for 1 week post-stimulation. The research in this area is continuing.

Hamilton et al. (2011) do list some caveats in their review. These include the following:

1. The exact area of stimulation must be refined, that is, are the correct cortical regions being targeted by TMS and tDCS?
2. Image-guided techniques, for example, fMRI, PET, must be used concurrently during stimulation.
3. Because some results are paradoxical, intersubject variability must be considered when planning and implementing neural stimulation technologies.

Another therapeutic approach for people with nonfluent aphasia is SentenceShaper. Albright and Purves (2008) conducted a case study over a period of 4 months to support narrative speech production and everyday communication, using SentenceShaper, a sentence production software program supporting those with nonfluent aphasia. Sentence-Shaper uses recorded and saved spoken messages to help the individual communicate his or her needs and wants. After 12 weeks of using the program, the patient with nonfluent aphasia demonstrated increases in morphosyntactic complexity. However, informativeness, efficiency, and narrative structure remained the same. This suggests that although language form improved, content and use remained impaired.

Semantic Feature Analysis (SFA), which is another treatment approach designed to facilitate naming ability, has been investigated as a therapy to support individuals with nonfluent aphasia. In a study by Marcotte and Ansaldo (2010), event-related fMRI (ER-fMRI) was reported for two patients with severe nonfluent aphasia: one with primary progressive aphasia and the other with Broca's aphasia. Using ER-fMRI during oral picture naming, both patients improved in their naming performance after brief and intensive Semantic Feature Analysis (SFA) treatment. Although there were differences in their adaptive brain plasticity, both made similar gains in naming ability following treatment.

Cherney (2010) explored oral reading for improving language outcomes in individuals with chronic nonfluent aphasia using the Oral Reading for Language in Aphasia (ORLA) treatment approach (see Appendix D). This utilizes the reading modality to facilitate expressive language improvement and requires the patient to systematically read sentences aloud. To start, the clinician and patient read in unison and then independently. Cherney conducted her study with 25 patients with chronic nonfluent aphasia. These individuals received therapy over 24 sessions, one to three times weekly. Following ORLA, patients made significant improvement on Western Aphasia Battery (WAB) aphasia quotients (AQ) from pre- to posttreatment times. Medium effect sizes were found for all severity levels on reading subtests; medium effect sizes were found for the moderate aphasia group on discourse only and for those with mild to moderate aphasia on discourse and writing subtests. It was concluded that low-intensity ORLA treatment can improve language skills in people with nonfluent aphasia.

Finally, Computer Assisted Treatment (CAT) now utilizes tablet technologies (both Apple and

Android applications) therapeutically, with the clinician present and also in the home, so that patients can work more independently on their goals. Choe, Azuma, Mathy, Liss, and Edgar (2007) studied four patients with nonfluent aphasia. In an attempt to improve naming skills using a 13-week clinician-assisted treatment program, the authors found that patients who were also assigned a daily home computer component demonstrated significantly greater naming ability and were able to maintain the gains 5 weeks posttreatment than those who did not use the home computer and those in the control group.

Broca's Type Aphasia

Characteristics

Individuals who have Broca's aphasia are nonfluent. Their speech is effortful, imprecisely articulated, and their melodic line, or prosody, ranges from aprosodic to normal intonation contours in short phrases (Basso, 2003). Even though the person with a Broca's aphasia is nonfluent, they are able to repeat, although with varying difficulty (Basso, 2003). The articulation deficit is generally considered by most researchers and clinicians to be apraxia of speech (Rosenbek, Kent, & LaPointe, 1989). The person with a Broca's aphasia generally uses simplified grammar that does not include function words or morphemes, and consists mainly of nouns. This renders their output agrammatic (Basso, 2003; Davis, 2007; Thompson, 2008). In some individuals, verbal output may not extend beyond the word level. An individual with a nonfluent aphasia tends to be more fluent when producing automatic sequences, that is, counting days of the week and months of the year.

Anomia is also a predominant feature of Broca's aphasia (Basso, 2003). An interesting feature of this impairment is that the ease of word finding is proportional to verbal fluency. For example, if the individual is limited in verbal output, word finding tends to be more impaired. In addition, auditory comprehension is usually mildly or moderately impaired (Basso, 2003; Davis, 2007); however, in lengthy paragraphs or when there are multiple speakers in a conversational context, comprehension can be further compromised. People with Broca's aphasia can be effective communicators because the words they are able to produce do have semantic content, and the listener can fill in the blanks based on context (Davis, 2007).

The presence of motor speech disorders, that is, apraxia of speech and dysarthria, in a person with Broca's aphasia is common, further complicating the speaker's ability to communicate effectively. A mild dysarthria typically is observed; however, if apraxia of speech is also present, the person's speech intelligibility may be more compromised due to the interaction of these two speech disorders (LaPointe, 2005). Despite the general constellation of features common to a particular type of communication disorder, the clinician must keep in mind that patient variability is high in neurogenic impairments. As a consequence, level of severity is always a factor in the clinical presentation of a particular patient, that is, a mild dysarthria may be the general case, but a particular patient may present with more significant impairment, if even for a short time.

Broca's aphasia was historically attributed to a lesion in Broca's area. Figure 3–1 shows Brodmann's areas 44 and 45. This area is located at the foot of the inferior frontal gyrus within the third frontal convolution of the left hemisphere, which receives its blood supply from the left middle cerebral artery (LMCA) (see Figure 3–1). However, it is now recognized that damage to this area does not produce a *frank* Broca's aphasia. Instead, the observed deficits include a mild dysarthria with dysprosody and a mild agraphia, that is, difficult writing. Current imaging techniques have revealed that a *chronic* Broca's aphasia results from sizable damage to the frontal operculum and the insula. More specific, a frank Broca's aphasia results from a large lesion and includes the left lateral frontal suprasylvian, pre-Rolandic region (Johnson & Jacobson, 2007). This lesion also extends into the periventricular white matter, some tracts of the posterior internal capsule, and often includes the inferior parietal lobe (Davis, 2007). Notably, in the *acute phase* of the stroke, a much smaller infarct is needed to produce a typical Broca's aphasia.

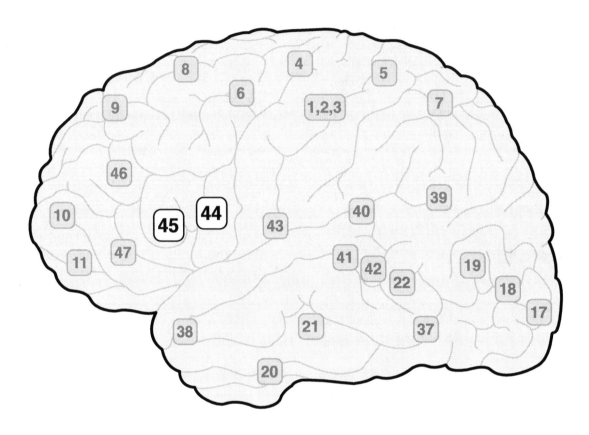

Areas 1, 2 & 3 – Primary Somatosensory Cortex

Area 4 – Primary Motor Cortex

Area 5 – Somatosensory Association Cortex

Area 6 – Premotor and Supplementary Motor Cortex

Area 7 – Somatosensory Association Cortex

Area 8 – Includes Frontal Eye Fields

Area 9 – Dorsolateral Prefrontal Cortex

Area 10 – Frontopolar Area

Area 11 – Orbitofrontal Area

Area 17 – Primary Visual Cortex (V1)

Area 18 – Visual Association Cortex (V2)

Area 19 – V3

Area 20 – Inferior Temporal Gyrus

Area 21 – Middle Temporal Gyrus

Area 22 – Superior Temporal Gyrus

Area 37 –Fusiform Gyrus

Area 38 – Temporopolar Area

Area 39 – Angular Gyrus (part of Wernicke's area)

Area 40 – Supramarginal Gyrus (part of Wernicke's area)

Areas 41 & 42 – Primary and Auditory Association Cortex

Area 43 – Subcentral Area
(between insula and post/precentral gyrus)

Area 44 – Pars Opercularis (part of Broca's area)

Area 45 – Pars Triangularis (part of Broca's area)

Area 46 – Dorsolateral Prefrontal Cortex

Area 47 – Inferior Prefrontal Gyrus

Figure 3–1. Brodmann's areas.

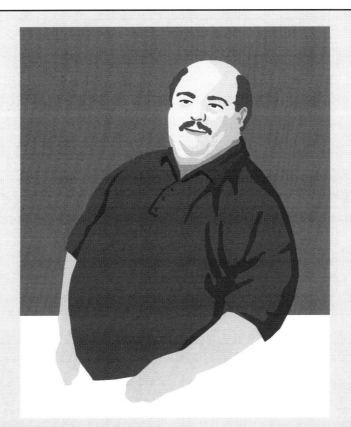

Case Scenario: Maurice

History and Physical (H & P): 48 yrs., white male, right-handed, admitted via the emergency department with stroke in progress characterized by "slurred speech" and right upper extremity weakness.

Past Medical History (PMH): Insulin-Dependent Diabetes Mellitus Type II (IDDM), hypertension (HTN), morbidly obese, carotid artery occlusion bilaterally, worse on left.

Social History: Married; two children (22 yrs. and 19 yrs.); insurance salesman; lives with wife.

Surgical History: status post (s/p) appendectomy.

A Functional Analysis of Maurice

Maurice's expressive language skills are the most significantly impaired of his language functions (see Figure 3–2 for the Diagnostic Profile for Maurice and Figure 3–3 for his ALD Target Model). Reading comprehension and auditory comprehension approximated normal; however, at more abstract paragraph levels, in both modalities, he has more difficulty comprehending than at the simple

Language Expression	**Automatic Speech:** None; attempts characterized by vowel sounds.	**Repetition Ability:** Fair at monosyllabic level.	**Lexical Retrieval-Naming:** Unable to determine secondary to sparse, nonfluent output.	**Conversational Ability:** Agrammatic; unable to converse.	**Pragmatic Skills:** Social gestures used appropriately.	**Paraphasias:** None.
Speech	**Rate:** Cannot determine due to nonfluent speech.	**Intelligibility:** Beyond monosyllables, intelligibility is poor secondary to apraxia of speech.	**Prosody:** Intonation contours observed in phrases such as oh, boy!	**Articulation:** Substitutions, omissions predominate; distortions noted secondary to unilateral upper motor neuron (UMN) dysarthria.	**Fluency:** Poor.
Auditory Comprehension	**Answering Yes/No Questions:** Very good for concrete/personal content.	**Executing Commands:** WFL	**Understanding Stories & Paragraphs:** Good at paragraph level.	**Understanding Conversational Speech:** WFL; group settings pose some difficulty.	**Identifying Objects & Their Functions:** WFL
Reading	**Word-level Comprehension:** Good.	**Sentence-level Comprehension:** Good at paragraph level with concrete information.	**Oral Reading:** Unable to assess secondary to severity of apraxia of speech.	**Oral Spelling:** Unable to spell orally.
Written Expression	**Copying:** Able to copy written words and recalls them to communicate in telegraphic writing.	**Writing to Dictation:** Unable to write numbers or letters to dictation.	**Self-generated:** Able to write numbers in sequence to 20 and names of family members and friends.	**Written Spelling:** Fair to good at the word level.	**Drawing:** Functional for communicating wants/needs.
Cognition	**Attention/Concentration:** Very good.	**Visuospatial Skills:** WFL		**Memory:** Long-term memory and working memory intact for procedural, semantic, and episodic systems.	**Executive Functions:** WFL for planning activities of daily living (ADLs).
Behavioral Symptoms	**Alertness:** Alert and cooperative.	**Deficit Awareness:** Aware of his limitations.	**Frustration:** Appropriate to social context; demonstrates anxiety as task complexity increases.	**Emotional Lability:** None.	**Current Personality Characteristics:** Pleasant and motivated; no change from premorbid state.

Figure 3–2. Diagnostic profile for Maurice.

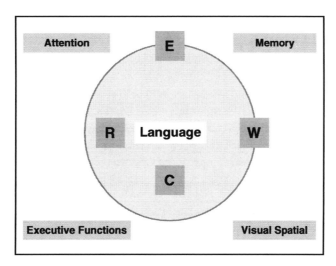

Figure 3–3. The Acquired Language Disorders Target Model for Maurice.

sentence level. Based on observation and family report, Maurice demonstrates a consistent ability to attend to therapeutic tasks when visual stimuli are provided. This is a good prognosticator for Maurice's ability to participate in therapy.

Maurice's speech production capabilities are severely limited, and this causes him great frustration, to the point of anger. His apraxia of speech combined with his dysarthria render most of his verbal output unintelligible, despite relatively spared prosody. Therefore, speech is not Maurice's strongest communication modality, but as he has intact visual motor skills, writing can be his primary communication modality.

Maurice's visuospatial skills for drawing and writing were functional, although his written letters are larger than the norm, and there are misspellings and omissions. However, it is possible that writing can be optimized for communication purposes. Also consistent with his strong visuospatial skills, Maurice is also able to follow a geographic route and has a good visual memory, which has functional value in public venues.

Maurice's executive functions were not significantly affected by his stroke. For example, his episodic memory for recent events in his daily life is preserved, and that allows him to remain connected to those around him. Maurice is able to solve simple problems necessary to complete his activities of daily living, for example, prepare food, request refills of his medications, and judge dangerous situations in the home and in the community. Although Maurice cannot communicate verbally in a functional way, his intact executive functions, functional auditory comprehension, and writing ability all serve to keep him woven into the social fabric.

Critical Thinking/Learning Activity

- What information indicates that this patient is a Broca's aphasic?
- This patient would most likely be seen in outpatient therapy. Knowing that the insurance carrier will give you a limited number of sessions, how would you prioritize this patient's functional outcomes?
- What are the family counseling and education issues in this case, and how would you address them?
- How would you include the family and/or caregivers in this patient's treatment plan?
- Write a SOAP note on this patient. Assume that you are seeing the patient for the first time after the evaluation session. Include three short-term therapeutic objectives in your note.

Treatment Considerations

Maurice was able to produce one to two-syllable words that were largely unintelligible. His repetition attempts were at the two-to-three word phrase level. He was able to comprehend language at the phrase and sentence level and 85% at the paragraph level. Therefore, treatment for Maurice must include methods that improve his expressive output.

- Use a rhythm or melodic-based approach (Melodic Intonation Therapy, MIT) to increase his MLU.
- Maurice independently began to use gestures with the non-paralyzed left hand. The Nonsymbolic Movements for Activation of Intention (NMAI) program may optimize this functional skill.
- Encourage Maurice to use monosyllabic and bisyllabic words as opposed to polysyllabic words to minimize the effects of apraxia of speech.
- Associate a drawing to represent a particular consonant's sound. For example, "bubbles" may be drawn to represent the sound /b/; a "snake" to represent the sound /s/, and so forth. Then blending these sounds together with a vowel to form a CVC syllable may facilitate coarticulation. This has the potential of minimizing the effects of the apraxia of speech.
- Develop an alternative communication system for Maurice in the form of a picture book to augment verbal communication. This book should include pictorial representations of family members, friends, and activities of daily living (ADL).

Some Therapeutic Options

- MIT (Sparks, Helm, & Albert, 1974; Sparks & Holland, 1976)
- NMAI (Richards, Singletary, Gonzalez-Rothi, & Koehler, 2002)

- Stimulation-Facilitation Approach (Schuell, Jenkins, & Jiménez-Pabón, 1964)
- Sentence Production Program for Aphasia (SPPA; Helm-Estabrooks & Nicholas, 2000)
- Promoting Aphasics' Communicative Effectiveness (PACE; Davis & Wilcox, 1981)
- Visual Action Therapy (VAT) (Helm-Estabrooks, Fitzpatrick, & Barresi, 1982)
- Response Elaboration Training (RET) (Kearns, 1985)
- MossTalk (Fink, Brecher, Montgomery, & Schwartz, 2003)
- Oral Reading for Language in Aphasia (ORLA) (Cherney, 2010)

Transcortical Motor Aphasia

Characteristics

Lichtheim (1895) referred to the aphasic disturbances due to lesions outside of the area around the sylvian fissure as *transcortical aphasias*. Transcortical motor aphasia (TMA) is a nonfluent type of aphasia. One of the distinguishing features of the transcortical aphasias, motor and sensory (which are discussed separately), is that repetition is preserved (Webb & Adler, 2008). More often, lesions are subcortical and located anterior to the frontal horn of the left lateral ventricle, part of the anterior watershed area, which prompted Benson (1979) to name them *border zone aphasias*. Other areas implicated in TMA involve the prefrontal and premotor cortices (Damasio, 2008). The lesions causing TMA are smaller than those causing Broca's aphasia, although there may be damage to the white matter below Broca's area. It is also possible that this type of lesion may interrupt communication between Broca's region and the basal ganglia and/or the thalamus, because there are areas in these regions that may have premotor capabilities. The prognosis for a person with TMA is good due to the spared linguistic features of this disorder (Alexander & Schmitt, 1980). Typically, progress occurs early after onset. There are three primary patterns typically seen with TMA:

1. Frontal lobe lesion affecting middle cerebral artery area (MCA) = motor speech deficits.
2. Frontal lobe lesion affecting anterior cerebral artery area (ACA) = lack of spontaneous speech.
3. Lesion in watershed area between MCA and ACA typically due to vascular pathology (most common).

The person with TMA manifests communication difficulties that are most obvious at the conversational level. These patients initially may present as mute due to the absence of the impulse to speak. When they do initiate, they produce syntactically correct utterances, but overall they have significantly reduced verbal output. This forces their communication partner to carry the burden of the communicative event. Their best performance is noted in short, highly structured communication scenarios, as opposed to situations characterized by many open-ended questions and free-flowing exchanges. They do best when the exchange requires few words of high predictability. For example, a person with TMA would struggle to answer the question, "What brought you to the hospital?" whereas a question such as, "How many children do you have?" would be more easily answered. The information below is from Goodglass and Kaplan (1982) and describes the common features of transcortical motor aphasia:

- Nonfluent language
- Repetition is intact compared with limited speech output
- Paraphasia is evident, especially phonemic type
- Syntax errors
- Perseveration
- Difficulty initiating conversation

- Difficulty organizing responses in conversation
- Syntactic errors
- Confrontation naming is preserved.
- Auditory comprehension is excellent
- Articulation is fair to good, although rate may be slow
- Repetition is normal

Besides stroke, the clinician may also see frontal lobe pathology in individuals who have suffered trauma, tumor, and other progressive neuropathologies (Cimino-Knight, Hollingsworth, & Gonzales-Rothi, 2005). Therefore, having a clear understanding of the relationship between lesion site and linguistic function is always very helpful when confronted with these *border zone* disturbances.

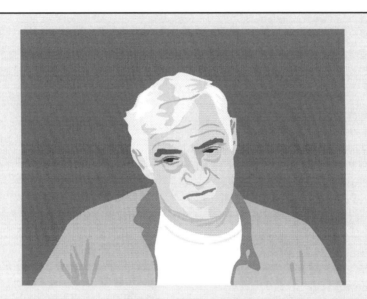

Case Scenario: Vincent

History and Physical (H & P): 75-year-old, right-handed, male Caucasian, admitted to local hospital. Right hemiparesis involving the lower extremity only was evident. On examination, he ambulated well. Family brought him to the hospital describing him as "mute." Blood pressure in the emergency department (ED) was 210/100, and heart rate was 92. He was aware of his inability to speak evidenced by his frustration and by pointing to his mouth and shaking his head in a "no" gesture.

Past Medical History(PMH): Vincent has no prior history of stroke. His PMH includes coronary artery disease, s/p angioplasty with stents; hyperlipidemia; left total knee replacement (TKR); seasonal allergies; obstructive sleep apnea (OSA). Sleep using a Klearway oral appliance to treat the OSA.

Social History: One adult daughter lives nearby. Vincent lives alone in an apartment complex that has an elevator. He has many friends and was a very active and socially engaged man prior to this stroke. He was an educator at the university level for 30 years before retirement at age 65.

Surgical History: Uvulo-palatal-pharyngoplasy (UPP) surgery for obstructive sleep apnea 10 years PTA (prior to this admission).

A Functional Analysis of Vincent

This patient has good auditory comprehension, intact word and sentence repetition, but nonfluent speech output (see Figure 3–4 for Vincent's Diagnostic Profile and Figure 3–5 for his ALD Target Model)This is complicated by his lack of volitional initiation of speech. In Vincent's case, treatment is geared toward increasing volitional initiation of speech with less phonemic paraphasias. Based on observation and family report, Vincent's speech consists mostly of immediate imitation. Although he understands what people say to him, he is continually challenged by the frustration of not being able to respond fluently and with ease. The family may consider purchasing an augmentative alternative communication device (AAC) for Vincent. For example, purchasing an iPad which is portable, reasonably priced, and supports applications for people with communication disorders, can supplement his verbal communication (see Chapter 10).

Cognitively, Vincent is able to attend to a task when his frustration level is manageable. His memory for information that is verbally or visually presented appears intact. Visuospatial skills remain good. This will help him negotiate his home and external environment safely. Furthermore, because of his intact visuospatial skills, Vincent can draw his messages if they have emotional valence. His problem-solving skills, judgment and reasoning, and safety awareness are intact for his ADL needs. For example, Vincent can be left alone at home for a limited amount of time as he knows how to access 911 via his medical alerting system; use the phone to access family members; and prepare light meals for himself. Vincent only needs minimal assistance with his morning care due to his right lower extremity weakness.

Critical Thinking/Learning Activity

1. What features of this person's aphasia indicate that the patient has TMA?
2. How do you bridge the gap between immediate repetition and delayed repetition to help the patient to build longer utterances?
3. Name three activities that you could use to facilitate speech initiation. Provide a rationale for each and give a scripted example of how that would happen in the therapy room.
4. What information would you provide to family members about TMA?
5. How would you use LPAA (life participation approach to aphasia) to facilitate functional communication in this patient?

Language Expression	**Automatic Speech:** WFL for counting, days of the week, alphabet with a verbal prompt to facilitate initiation.	**Repetition Ability:** WFL for words and sentences.	**Lexical Retrieval-Naming:** Confrontation naming compromised by initiation difficulties; better with cloze procedure.	**Conversational Ability:** Verbal output limited; syntactic complexity reduced in attempts at longer utterances.	**Pragmatic Skills:** Understands turn-taking; maintains eye contact, uses appropriate social gestures; however, nonfluent speech limits thorough evaluation of speech acts.	**Paraphasias:** Phonemic paraphasias.
Speech	**Rate:** Slow and halting.	**Intelligibility:** WFL in known and unknown contexts.	**Prosody:** Reduced intonation contours, stress pattern altered.	**Articulation:** WFL	**Fluency:** Speech output is nonfluent; struggles to produce utterances in response to open-ended questions. Speech output is fluent on repetition tasks.	
Auditory Comprehension	**Answering Yes/No Questions:** WFL	**Executing Commands:** WFL	**Understanding Stories & Paragraphs:** WFL	**Understanding Conversational Speech:** WFL at conversational level.	**Identifying Objects & Their Functions:** WFL	
Reading	**Word-level Comprehension:** WFL	**Sentence-level Comprehension:** WFL at paragraph level.	**Oral Reading:** Reading aloud is difficult to produce fluently and is slow and labored.	**Oral Spelling:** Unable to test due to nonfluent speech.		
Written Expression	**Copying:** WFL	**Writing to Dictation:** Unable to initiate writing to dictation secondary to an ideomotor apraxia.	**Self-generated:** Functional for name and address, when not prompted verbally.	**Written Spelling:** Paragraphic.	**Drawing:** If self-initiated, he is able to produce simple line drawings.	
Cognition	**Attention/Concentration:** Attends to a task when his frustration is manageable.	**Visuospatial Skills:** WFL	**Memory:** Procedural memory is WFL; semantic memory for basic information is intact; episodic memory difficult to assess due to limited expression.	**Executive Functions:** Problem solving, safety awareness, and judgment are intact for ADL needs.		
Behavioral Symptoms	**Alertness:** WFL	**Deficit Awareness:** He is aware of his communication deficits.	**Frustration:** Demonstrates intermittent frustration with his inability to "get it out."	**Emotional Lability:** None noted.	**Current Personality Characteristics:** His frustration is causing anger and social isolation.	

Figure 3–4. Diagnostic profile for Vincent.

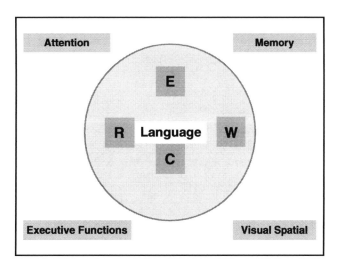

Figure 3–5. The Acquired Language Disorders Target Model for Vincent.

Treatment Considerations

Vincent's treatment will focus on:

- Optimizing initiation of speech output
- Reducing paraphasic speech output
- Increasing utterance length
- Developing appropriate intonation at the sentence level.

Vincent's good auditory comprehension and ability to repeat accurately could be used to support verbal output. For example, in the following task both of these preserved skills are called into play to promote speech initiation and fluency. The therapist can give Vincent a sentence supplemented with a visual stimulus (picture or object) to help him initiate and expand verbal output.

SLP: [Shows keys to Vincent]: I will open the door with my *keys*. What will I use to open the door? [SLP can provide a phonemic cue if needed.]

Vincent: Key.

SLP: What should I do with the key?

Vincent: Open the door.

This task allows the speech-language pathologist (SLP) to work not only on increasing verbal initiation and fluency, but can also help with intonation. For example, the SLP can ask, "Who will open the door?"

■ This question prompts Vincent to respond with lexical stress on the subject of the sentence in his response.

Some Therapeutic Options

■ MIT (Sparks et al., 1974; Sparks & Holland, 1976).
■ NMAI (Richards, Singletary, Gonzalez-Rothi, & Koehler, 2002).
■ SPPA (Helm-Estabrooks & Nicholas, 2000).
■ LPAA (Chapey, Duchan, Elman, Garcia, Kagan, Lyon, & Simmons-Mackie, 2008).

Global Aphasia

Characteristics

Global aphasia is a severe impairment of communication that involves all language modalities. Milder forms of global aphasia are often referred to as mixed aphasia. The incidence of global aphasia is noted to be as high as 10% to 40% of all strokes (Peach, 2008). The pathophysiology of global aphasia is typically described as a large perisylvian lesion greater than 6 cm, and involves damage to the frontal, temporal, and parietal lobes.

The lesions are especially noted in the posterior temporal gyrus, and the infarct is attributed to abnormalities in both branches of the middle cerebral artery (MCA), extending deep into the subadjacent white matter. Certain focal lesions within this damaged area can degrade the white matter and result in a disconnection between interacting brain regions. Possible sequellae to this disconnection are behavioral dysfunctions. According to Basso and Farabola (1997), the pathophysiology of the stroke has a bearing on the prognosis in global aphasia (Figure 3–6).

Auditory comprehension will improve more than verbal expression in these patients, and patients with global aphasia make the most gains during the first 6 months of recovery (Collins, 2004). Unfortunately, prognosis for recovery is poor, and it is dependent on lesion site, (see Figure 3–6), as well as the size of the lesion: the larger the infarcted area, the worse the prognosis. Prognosis is also related to the presenting symptoms in these patients. For example, not every patient with a global aphasia may not have an accompanying hemiparesis. If motor abilities are preserved, the prognosis for recovery is better. Similarly, if auditory comprehension and verbal expression are both severely impaired, then prognosis for recovery is poorer. Of particular importance is the patient's ability to successfully answer simple yes/no questions. The higher the accuracy of such responses, the better the prognosis is for recovery.

The most salient characteristic of global aphasia is that the patient is impaired in all areas of language. They will present with deficits in comprehension and expression for syntax, semantics, and phonology. It is inconclusive whether the deficits in verbal expression are due to a lack of knowledge for linguistic rules and operations, that is, *linguistic competence,* or due instead to an individual's language competence and performance deficits (Peach, 2008). The auditory comprehension skills of individuals with global aphasia are variable. Research shows that the individual's auditory comprehension skills likely to be preserved are familiar environmental sounds, for example, a toilet flushing, a car horn, a siren, and so forth (Spinnler & Vignolo, 1966); names of famous people (Van Lancker & Klein, 1990); auditory recognition of word categories, for example, food, clothing (McKenna & Warrington, 1978); and better comprehension for personally rel-

Type	Lesion	Outcome
I.	Large Pre-and Post-Rolandic middle cerebral artery infarcts	Very poor prognosis
II.	Pre-Rolandic	Prognosis good for recovery
III.	Subcortical	Prognosis good for recovery
IV.	Parietal	Variable; improving to Broca's or Transcortical Aphasia
V.	Double Frontal and Parietal	Variable; improving to Broca's or Transcortical Aphasia

Figure 3–6. Lesion type and outcome in global aphasia.

evant information (Wallace & Stapleton, 1991). In the acute phase, the individual who performs better on auditory comprehension measures has a more favorable prognosis.

It is important to understand that persons with global aphasia are not mute. They have the ability to verbalize despite the extensive lesion, but utterances tend to be stereotypic, and they are unable to repeat. One utterance may be the extent of this person's speech output, for example, "Oh boy." This type of patient may also only produce neologistic speech, for example, "pifa, pifa." Although prosody may be within normal limits in this patient population, the verbal output has no syntactic or semantic value, and, therefore, the utterance is meaningless (de Bleser & Poeck, 1985). People with global aphasia rely most heavily on nonverbal communication

for understanding the message, for example, tone of voice, facial expression, and gestures (Herrmann, Koch, Johannsen-Horbach, & Wallesch, 1989).

Cognitively, the individual with global aphasia may demonstrate problems with abstract reasoning. Research has shown that there is a correlation between language ability and abstract reasoning in the globally aphasic patient. For example, nonverbal performance on the Raven's Colored Progressive Matrices (Raven, 1965) is impaired in this patient population (Collins, 1986). This test requires that the patient complete a sequence of geometric shapes and colors. People with Wernicke's aphasia and globally aphasic patients both scored equally low compared with other types of aphasic patients on pattern completion. It appears that the more posterior the lesion, the more this type of cognition is affected.

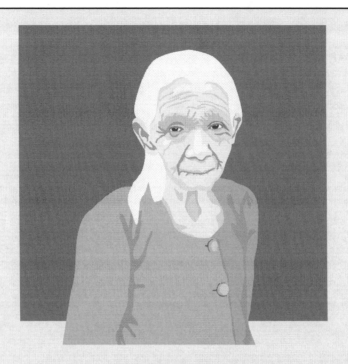

Case Scenario: Elizabeth

History and Physical (H & P): 85-year-old female, right-handed, admitted via ED with change in mental status. A CT scan revealed a massive left-sided CVA with right-sided hemiparesis and oral pharyngeal dysphagia.

Past Medical History (PMH): Gastrointestinal bleed, atrial fibrillation (A-fib), anemia, hypertension (HTN), irritable bowel syndrome (IBS), mitral valve regurgitation (MVR), history of gastric ulcers, and severe macular degeneration.

Social History: Widowed, four children, worked as a librarian; lives alone in first floor apartment in a senior citizens complex.

Surgical History: Left total knee replacement (left TKR)

A Functional Case Analysis for Elizabeth

Elizabeth has severe deficits in expressive language output (see Figure 3–7 for Elizabeth's Diagnostic Profile and Figure 3–8 for her ALD Target Model). Her utterances are meaningless and lack grammatical form. Furthermore, her ability to use the verbal modality is compromised by her apraxia of speech. Elizabeth relies on reading facial expressions and gestures in order to comprehend a message, so her therapist can use this as a foundation for rehabilitation. In addition, Elizabeth may be a candidate for an augmentative communication system (Steele, 2006) because she can match words and pictures with fairly consistent accuracy.

Language Expression	**Automatic Speech:** None.	**Repetition Ability:** None.	**Lexical Retrieval-Naming:** None.	**Conversational Ability:** No connected discourse and occasional meaningless utterances.	**Pragmatic Skills:** Cannot validly assess.	**Paraphasias:** Undetermined due to lack of intelligible output.
Speech	**Rate:** Nonverbal.	**Intelligibility:** Cannot assess secondary to nonverbal status.	**Prosody:** Cannot assess secondary to nonverbal status.	**Articulation:** Cannot assess secondary to nonverbal status.	**Fluency:** Absent.	
Auditory Comprehension	**Answering Yes/No Questions:** Mildly impaired for concrete/personal yes/no questions.	**Executing Commands:** Mildly impaired accuracy for simple commands.	**Understanding Stories & Paragraphs:** Poor.	**Understanding Conversational Speech:** Poor.	**Identifying Objects & Their Functions:** Mildly impaired but better with real objects.	
Reading	**Word-level Comprehension:** Moderate-severely impaired for sentences; better at CVC word level.	**Sentence-level Comprehension:** Poor.	**Oral Reading:** Unable to assess decoding skills due to unintelligible speech output.	**Oral Spelling:** Unable to assess oral spelling skills due to unintelligible speech output.		
Written Expression	**Copying:** Able to copy simple forms with the left hand.	**Writing to Dictation:** Could not form letters or numbers.	**Self-generated:** Attempts made, but unable to complete a word.	**Written Spelling:** Could not form letters or numbers.	**Drawing:** Can generate gross shapes but detailed features are missing.	
Cognition	**Attention/Concentration:** Limited and requires tactile cues.	**Visuospatial Skills:** Impaired for detailed drawing and personal navigation within a building.	**Memory:** Functional for procedural memory.	**Executive Functions:** Unable to determine due to receptive and expressive language impairments.		
Behavioral Symptoms	**Alertness:** Variable; optimal in the morning hours.	**Deficit Awareness:** Demonstrates variable levels of awareness.	**Frustration:** Frustrated when stimuli becomes too complex.	**Emotional Lability:** Patient's crying is likely due to frustration and not lability.	**Current Personality Characteristics:** Depressed and anxious.	

Figure 3–7. Diagnostic profile for Elizabeth.

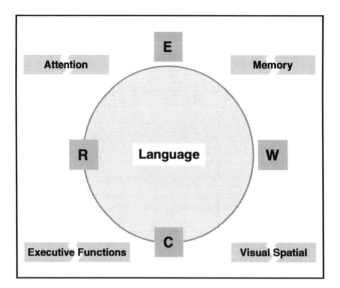

Figure 3–8. The Acquired Language Disorders Target Model for Elizabeth.

Elizabeth's auditory comprehension requires intervention, so that she can answer yes/no questions and follow basic directions with more reliability. This is crucial for the completion of her ADLs. Even with a home health aide present, Elizabeth still needs to be able to respond to concrete questions relating to her health and basic wants and needs. Cognitively, she appears to be able to attend during certain times of the day, more often in the morning hours. Her memory for family members, her biographical past, and rituals of self-care appear intact. Due to her limited executive functioning and severe language disorder, Elizabeth requires maximum supervision in the home environment. As a consequence, home care services for speech and language and other areas of need should be considered, as her social communication, communication of basic needs, and daily planning need to be addressed.

Critical Thinking/Learning Activity

- What information indicates that this patient has global aphasia?
- This patient would most likely be seen in outpatient therapy. Knowing that the insurance carrier will give you a limited number of sessions, how would you prioritize this patient's therapy goals to achieve long-term functional outcomes?
- What are the family counseling and education issues in this case, and how would you address them?
- How would you include the family/caregivers in this patient's treatment plan?

- Write a SOAP note on this patient. Assume that you are seeing the patient for the first time after the evaluation session. Include short-term therapeutic objectives in your note.
- What aspect of this patient's medical history made this patient susceptible to stroke?

Treatment Considerations

Elizabeth demonstrates severe receptive and expressive language impairment. She has severe buccofacial apraxia and apraxia of speech, further complicating her functional communication abilities. Therefore, speech production is not considered a viable mode of communication at this time. Answering yes/no questions is easier for Elizabeth when they pertain to emotionally charged information, family members, recent events, and her illness. Elizabeth can recognize objects and has some residual reading comprehension for basic words when printed in large letters with accompanying realistic pictures. She can also identify one of three pictured items, and she can copy simple line drawings.

- To improve ability to make her needs known, a computer-based program (Steele, 2006) may be beneficial. This speech-generating device provides large icons for vocabulary that speak in a human voice. This may be used to obtain basic core vocabulary.
- Attempt to convey messages and make needs known by generating simple line drawings.
- Attempt to build upon her ability to make simple line drawings as a form of communication.
- Use a trace and copy word recall strategy.
- Elizabeth attempts to understand speech by watching facial expressions and gestures. Therefore, optimize auditory comprehension by using facial expressions, voice, gesture, and pictures to follow basic, one-step directions.

Some Therapeutic Options

- AAC (for augmentative alternative communication) systems should be considered, for example, from simple communication boards to more complex word-picture systems
- VAT (Helm-Estabrooks, Fitzpatrick, & Barresi, 1982)
- PACE (Davis & Wilcox, 1985)
- Communicative Drawing Program (CDP; Helm-Estabrooks & Albert, 2004)
- Voluntary Control of Involuntary Utterances (VCIU; Helm & Barresi, 1980)
- NMAI (Richards, Singletary, Gonzalez-Rothi, & Koehler, 2002)

References

Albright, E., & Purves, B. (2008). Exploring Sentence-Shaper™: Treatment and augmentative possibilities. *Aphasiology, 22*(7–8), 741–752.

Alexander, M. P., & Schmitt, M. A. (1980). The aphasia syndrome of stroke in the left anterior cerebral artery territory. *Archives of Neurology, 37*, 97–100.

Barwood, C. H. S., Murdoch, B. E., Whelan, B-M., Lloyd, D., Riek, S., O'Sullivan, J. D., Coulthard, A., & Wong, A. (2012). Improved receptive and expressive language abilities in nonfluent aphasic stroke patients after application of rTMS: An open protocol case series. *Brain Stimulation, 5*(3), 274–286.

Basso, A. (2003). *Aphasia and its therapy.* New York, NY: Oxford University Press.

Basso, A., & Farabola, M. (1997). Comparison of improvement of aphasia in three patients withlesions in anterior, posterior, and antero-posterior language areas. *Neuropsychological Rehabilitation, 7*, 215–230.

Benson, D. F. (1979). Aphasia rehabilitation (editorial). *Archives of Neurology, 36*, 187–189.

Chapey, R., Duchan, J. F., Elman, R. J., Garcia, L. J., Kagan, A., Lyon, J., & Simmons-Mackie, N. (2008). Life-participation approach to aphasia: A statement of values for the future. In R. Chapey (Ed.), *Language intervention strategies in aphasia and related neurogenic communication disorders* (5th ed., pp. 403–449). Philadelphia, PA: Lippincott Williams & Wilkins.

Cherney, L. R. (2010). Oral reading for language in aphasia: Impact of aphasia severity on cross-modal outcomes in chronic nonfluent aphasia. *Seminars in Speech and Language, 31*(1), 42–51.

Choe, Y., Azuma, T., Mathy, P., Liss, J. M., & Edgar, J. (2007). The effect of home computer practice on naming in individuals with non-fluent aphasia and verbal apraxia. *Journal of Medical Speech-Language Pathology, 15*(4), 407–421.

Cimino-Knight, A. M., Hollingsworth, A. L., & Gonzales-Rothi, L. J. (2005). The transcortical aphasias. In L. L. LaPointe (Ed.), *Aphasia and related neurogenic language disorders* (3rd ed., pp.169–185). New York, NY: Thieme.

Collins, M. (1986). *Diagnosis and treatment of global aphasia.* San Diego, CA: College-Hill Press.

Collins, M. (2004). Global aphasia. In L. LaPointe (Ed.), *Aphasia and related neurogenic language disorders* (3rd ed., pp. 186–198). New York, NY: Thieme.

Damasio, H. (2008). Neural basis of language disorders. In R. Chapey (Ed.), *Language intervention strategies in aphasia and related neurogenic communication*

disorders (5th ed., pp. 20–41). Philadelphia, PA: Lippincott Williams & Wilkins.

Davis, G. A. (2007). *Aphasiology: Disorders and clinical practice* (2nd ed.). Boston, MA: Pearson.

Davis, G. A., & Wilcox, M. J. (1981). Incorporating parameters of natural conversation in aphasia treatment. In R. Chapey (Ed.), *Language intervention strategies in adult aphasia.* Baltimore, MD: Williams & Wilkins.

Davis, G. A., & Wilcox, M. (1985). *Adult aphasia rehabilitation: Applied pragmatics.* San Diego, CA: College-Hill Press.

de Bleser, R., & Poeck, K. (1985). Analysis of prosody in the spontaneous speech of patients with CV recurring utterances. *Cortex, 21*, 405–416.

Fink, R., Brecher, A., Montgomery, M., & Schwartz, M. (2003). *MossTalk.* Philadelphia, PA: Albert Einstein Healthcare Network.

Fridriksson, J. (2011). Measuring and inducing brain plasticity in chronic aphasia. *Journal of Communication Disorders, 44*, 557–563.

Goodglass, H., & Kaplan, E. (1982). *The assessment of aphasia and related disorders.* Philadelphia, PA: Lea & Febiger.

Hamilton, R. H., Chrysikou, E. G., & Coslett, B. (2011). Mechanisms of aphasia recovery after stroke and the role of noninvasive brain stimulation. *Brain and Language, 118*, 40–50.

Helm, N. A., & Barresi, B. (1980). Voluntary control of involuntary utterances: A treatment approach for severe aphasia. *Clinical Aphasiology, 10*, 308–315.

Helm-Estabrooks, N., & Albert, M. L. (2004). *Manual of aphasia and aphasia therapy* (2nd ed.). Austin, TX: Pro-Ed.

Helm-Estabrooks, N., Fitzpatrick, P. M., & Barresi, B. (1982). Visual action therapy for global aphasia. *Journal of Speech and Hearing Disorders, 47*, 385–389.

Helm-Estabrooks, N., & Nicholas, M. (2000). *Sentence production program for aphasia* (2nd ed.). Austin, TX: Pro-Ed.

Herrmann, M., Koch, U., Johannsen-Horbach, H., & Wallesch, C. W. (1989). Communicative skills in chronic and severe nonfluent aphasia. *Brain and Language, 37*, 339–352.

Johnson, A. F., & Jacobson, B. H. (2007). *Medical speech language pathology: A practioner's guide.* New York, NY: Thieme.

Kearns, K. (1985). Response elaboration training for patient-initiated utterances. In R. Brookshire (Ed.), *Clinical aphasiology conference proceedings* (pp. 196–204). Minneapolis, MN: BRK.

LaPointe, L. (2005). *Aphasia and related neurogenic language disorders* (3rd ed.). New York, NY: Thieme.

Lichtheim, L. (1895). On aphasia. *Brain, 7,* 433–484.

Marcotte, K., & Ansaldo, A. I. (2010). The neural correlates of semantic feature analysis in chronic aphasia: Discordant patterns according to the etiology. *Seminars in Speech and Language, 31*(1), 52–63.

Martin, P. I., Naeser, M. A., Ho, M., Doron, K. W., & Kurland, J. (2009). Overt naming fMRI pre- and post-TMS: Two nonfluent aphasia patients, with and without improved naming post-TMS. *Brain and Language, 111*(1), 20–35.

McKenna, P., & Warrington, E. K. (1978). Category specific naming preservation: A single-case study. *Journal of Neurology, Neurosurgery, and Psychiatry, 41,* 571–574.

Peach, A. R. (2008). Global aphasia: Identification and management. In R. Chapey (Ed.), *Language intervention strategies in aphasia and related neurogenic communication disorders* (5th ed., pp. 565–594). Philadelphia, PA: Lippincott Williams & Wilkins.

Raven, J. C. (1965). *Guide to using the colored progressive matrices.* London, UK: H. K. Lewis.

Richards, K., Singletary, F., Gonzalez-Rothi, L. J., & Koehler, S. (2002). Activation of intentional mechanism through utilization of non-symbolic movements in aphasia rehabilitation. *Journal of Rehabilitation Research and Development, 39,* 445–454.

Rosenbek, J. C., Kent, D. R., & LaPointe, L. L. (1989). Apraxia of speech: An overview and some perspectives. In J. C. Rosenbek, M. R. McNeil, & A. E. Aronson (Eds.), *Apraxia of speech* (pp. 1–28). San Diego, CA: College-Hill Press.

Schuell, H., Jenkins, J. H., & Jiménez-Pabón, E. (1964). *Aphasia in adults: Diagnosis, prognosis and treatment.* New York, NY: Harper & Row.

Sparks, R., Helm, N., & Albert, M. (1974). Aphasia rehabilitation resulting from melodic intonation therapy. *Cortex, 10,* 303–316.

Sparks, R., & Holland, A. (1976). Method: Melodic intonation therapy. *Journal of Speech and Hearing Disorders, 41,* 287–297.

Spinnler, H., & Vignolo, L. (1996). Impaired recognition of meaningful sounds in aphasia. *Cortex, 2,* 337–348.

Steele, R. D. (2006). AAC use and communicative improvements in chronic aphasia: Evidence comparing global with severe Broca's aphasia. *AAC Perspectives (ASHA SID-12), 15*(4), 18–22.

Thompson, C. K. (2008). Treatment of syntactic and morphologic deficits in agrammatic aphasia: Treatment of the underlying forms. In R. Chapey (Ed.), *Language intervention strategies in aphasia and related neurogenic communication disorders* (5th ed., pp. 735–755). Philadelphia, PA: Lippincott Williams & Wilkins.

Van Lancker, D., & Klein, K. (1990). Preserved recognition of familiar personal names in global aphasia. *Brain and Language, 39,* 511–529.

Wallace, G. L., & Stapleton, J. H. (1991). Analysis of auditory comprehension performance in individuals with severe aphasia. *Archives of Physical Medicine and Rehabilitation, 72,* 674–678.

Webb, W. G., & Adler, R. K. (2008). *Neurology for the speech-language pathologist.* St. Louis, MO: Mosby Elsevier.

Winhuisen, L., Thiel, A., Schumacher, B., Kessler, J., Rudoff, J., Haupt, W. F.(2005). Role of the contralateral inferior frontal gyrus in recovery of language function in post-stroke aphasia: A combined repetitive transcranial magnetic stimulation and positron emission tomography study. *Stroke, 36,* 1759–1763.

Chapter 4

THE FLUENT APHASIAS

Introduction

The fluent aphasias include the following subtypes: Wernicke's aphasia, transcortical sensory aphasia, conduction aphasia, and anomic aphasia. Although it is important to determine if a patient is presenting with a nonfluent or fluent type of aphasia, identifying a specific subtype is not always a simple matter. In fact, it is not uncommon for a clinician to evaluate a patient and to discover that the patient is presenting with characteristics of both fluent and nonfluent aspects of aphasia, which is typically a function of the site and extension of the lesion.

Fluent aphasias are characterized by a lesion posterior to the central sulcus (Rolandic fissure), which results in well-articulated speech with little or no content. One commonly encounters neologistic output, that is, jargon, which further complicates the patient's ability to convey a thought. Since self-monitoring skills are also poor in these patients, , their ability to self-correct their verbal output is not optimal, if it exists at all. Auditory comprehension may be compromised as the content of the incoming message becomes lengthy, more complex, and abstract. Finally, these patients also present with word-finding difficulties and repetition problems. All of these factors combine to create a very challenging therapeutic scenario for the speech-language pathologist (SLP). However, as patients begin to spontaneously recover and receive appropriate treatment, they tend to gain greater self-awareness,

thereby making therapy a more successful experience. There is evidence that the type of aphasia diagnosed at the time of onset, often evolves into another type within the same subgroup during the acute phase of recovery. This change often begins between 2 to 4 weeks post-onset. Cherney and Robey (2008, p. 187) reported that this occurred in 60% of cases based on descriptive criteria. These fluent patients were reclassified within the fluent aphasia domain and anomic aphasia was often the endpoint attained.

Because anomia is a pervasive symptom of fluent aphasia, the current work of Ferguson, Evans, and Raymer (2012) is pertinent. They report that lexical retrieval impairment is usually present in people with a fluent aphasia, as noted above. The problem can arise in the *semantic feature network,* the *lexical network,* and/or the *phonological network.* Planning treatment based on the results of the evaluation must be based not only on the patient's deficits, but on his or her strengths, that is, what is the *rehabilitation platform* upon which one can build a treatment plan.

In a case study by Davis, Harrington, and Baynes (2006), the authors investigated two main concerns. They questioned if intensive therapy to decrease production errors (paraphasias) by eliminating oral responses would improve naming with trained items; and additionally, if changes in naming could be correlated to changes in fMRI activation. After 4 weeks of intensive treatment focusing on semantic therapy (to discourage speech production errors such as paraphasias and empty speech), the study participant with Wernicke's aphasia improved in his use of nouns during narrative speech. Rather than working directly on naming and reducing paraphasic errors, therapy included more receptive tasks such as *sorting* (categorizing pictures by size, color, and functional use); *semantic judgment tasks* (giving a yes or no response to questions related to characteristics of the targets); and *definition to picture match* (pointing to one picture in a field of five that matched the verbal definition provided). The goal was not to name the target words but to have the patient choose characteristics of the target. By inhibiting competing targets (foil words that were similar to the actual target word such as *microscope* and *binoculars*), it was speculated that the patient would learn to inhibit semantic paraphasias. The patient in this case study did improve on targeted items that generalized to untrained items within the same categories. Lexical retrieval and structure also improved, and the patient used more nouns in narrative speech. Following treatment, fMRI results showed an increase in activation of the left inferior frontal cortex and increased activation in the inferior posterior temporal of the right hemisphere.

Intensive therapy in people with fluent aphasias has also shown promise. In a meta-analysis of 10 studies with 864 patients (Bhogal, Teasell, & Speechley, 2003), intense aphasia therapy (2 to 3 hours per day, 7 days a week for many months with both face-to-face direct therapy for 1 hour daily supplemented by homework with the family and volunteers) showed improvement for patients who suffered a stroke, even in cases with short-term treatment.

Patients with spoken word production deficits have benefited from the use of pantomime, iconic gestures, intention gestures, and pointing (Raymer, Singletary, Rodriguez, Ciampitti, Heilman & Rothi, 2006; Raymer & Thompson, 1991; Rose, 2006). found that individuals with more severe aphasia benefited from gesture training. Crosson et al. (2007) discovered that by using a nonsymbolic, circular, left-handed gesture (referred to as an intention gesture to prime initiation in the right hemisphere) improved word-finding with moderate to severe nonfluent aphasics. Patients with fluent aphasia are unable to monitor their verbal output effectively enough so that conversation becomes riddled with obstacles to mutual understanding and discourse. However, both communication partners will benefit from using gestures and pantomime to optimize the transmission of the intended message.

There have been concerns with both intention gestures and pantomimed gestures. Intention gestures require a meaningless motion without content, and pantomime gestures have been found to lack generalizability in conversation. In an attempt to determine carryover effects using these procedures for untrained words, Ferguson et al. (2012) investigated four individuals with chronic aphasia. Training consisted of intention gesture plus verbal production and pantomime gesture training plus verbal production using a crossover design. Training consisted of 10 sessions (2 to 3 per week) followed by a 1-week intermission and then a second training. Treatment continued until participants reached 90% accuracy for three sessions or until 10 sessions were completed. This was followed by a 1-month maintenance session for which three sets of 20 noun pictures were to be named. According to Ferguson et al. (2012), results indicated that intention gesture training increased verbal naming in two of the four participants (one with mild transcortical motor aphasia and the other with conduction aphasia). Pantomime gesture training helped three patients with naming (the participant with conduction aphasia and two with severe Broca's aphasia). Improvements were maintained at the 1-month follow-up visit. For example, pantomimes for words such as *hammer, Band-Aid, hat, apple,* and *zipper,* were among many words used as stimuli to train the patient in using pantomime. Pantomime training assisted the more severely impaired participants whereas intention gestures facilitated those with milder word production impairments. Overall, the left-handed pantomime gestures had the greatest effect on remediating word retrieval deficits in addition, those who made large verbal gains no longer needed the gestural support. The authors concluded that intention and pantomime gestures helped all participants improve their word retrieval, especially when the gestures were embedded into the flow of conversation. The clinical implications from these findings suggest that using pantomime and intention gestures are valid and valuable approaches for facilitating functional communication.

Wernicke's Type Aphasia

Characteristics

Carl Wernicke described the language disorder now bearing his name in 1908. Wernicke's aphasia is also referred to as *receptive aphasia, sensory aphasia,* and *posterior aphasia.* The lesion producing Wernicke's aphasia is at the anatomic intersection for all incoming auditory and visual information (Figure 4–1). Blood supply to this area is via the inferior division of the MCA (for middle cerebral artery). Wernicke's aphasia results from a lesion in the posterior third of the superior temporal gyrus; therefore, reading, writing, repetition, and other language functions are often impaired (Marshall, 2001, p. 435). The first variant of this type of aphasia is primarily due to temporal lesions, producing word deafness, and less impaired reading skills. Auditory comprehension for words in context is better than words in isolation. The second variant of this type of aphasia results from a more posterior lesion of the temporal gyrus, which affects the visual connections. As a consequence, reading comprehension is more impaired. Oral reading tends to be intact, but reading comprehension is affected. These patients will have difficulty recognizing letters by name and difficultly associating written words with their spoken counterparts. Writing is characterized by paragraphic jargon, similar to speech and spelling is severely impaired.

A hallmark of Wernicke's aphasia is a significant auditory comprehension problem with poor self-monitoring. Paraphasic speech is common and typically goes unnoticed by the speaker. The speech is effortless and melodic; however, there are verbal (semantic) and literal (phonemic) paraphasias, and in more severe cases neologisms are used, all of which go unnoticed due to poor self-monitoring skills. As a result, the person with Wernicke's aphasia has speech output with very low informational content. Articulation is unimpaired; however, they have poorly chosen words and poorly formed sentences, which tend to be paragrammatic, that is, they omit grammatical morphemes. Their self-initiated output tends to be more contextually appropriate than communication in dyadic discourse. This is due to their problems in the comprehension of the communicative partner's speech. The patient may also demonstrate a press for speech, or logorrhea. Hemiparesis is not common in this patient population as the lesion is posterior to motor functions mediated in the frontal lobes. In comparison with the other fluent aphasias, Wernicke's is the most severe and has the poorest prognosis. LaPointe (1997) reports that one marker of their prognosis for recovery is based on their auditory comprehension for single words. These patients can also demonstrate paranoid tendencies in addition to a general lack of awareness of their language difficulties. They can be resistant to therapy because they do not understand its value. Therefore, two primary goals with these patients are to improve auditory comprehension and self-monitoring of errors (Brookshire, 1997).

According to the Aphasia Center (http://www.theaphasiacenter.com), individuals with Wernicke's aphasia can be unsuccessful when direct treatment is initially provided. This is partially due to their phonological difficulties, paraphasias and neologisms. These patients typically do not attempt to repair their communication breakdowns and show little response to listener cues. They often need help with understanding what others say. Using written words, gestures, and intonation can initially assist with communication. An indirect type of treatment,

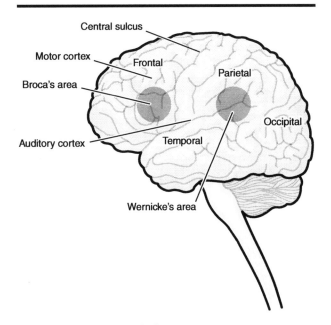

Figure 4–1. Wernicke's area.

contextual therapy, can also be helpful as it is less concerned with naming pictures and responding to questions than it is with helping the patient to be understood in the context of the interaction. The patient may be asked if he or she is talking about something (in particular), and once identified, no attempt would be made to have the patient repeat it. The patient is encouraged to write letters and words, having a notebook and pen readily available. In order to facilitate communication, some general suggested strategies for working with patients with a more severe fluent aphasia are included below:

■ Determine if the patient can read at any level. If so, pair auditory comprehension activities with written text to follow simple directions, answer yes or no questions, and identify objects and pictures.

■ Engage the patient in item or picture identification activities and follow verbal commands of increasing length and complexity. Use prepositions for placement of objects (under, on, before, after, etc.) and increase understanding of object functions (which one do we use to . . .) to add to the repertoire for auditory comprehension and direction following.

■ Use communication boards with pictures and try out the various Apps on iPad devices (or the like) to improve comprehension and communication in a variety of settings.

■ In addition, the SLP may decide to use a readily visible gestural "STOP" signal to help the person with fluent aphasia know that it is time to stop talking and to listen.

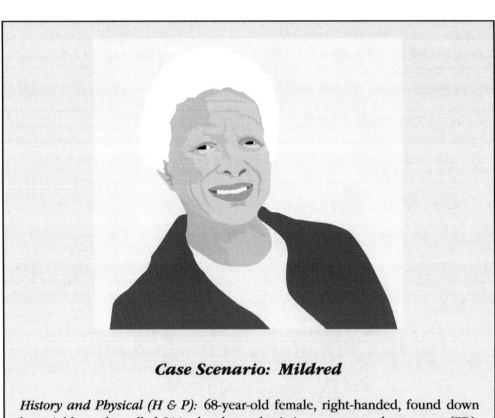

Case Scenario: Mildred

History and Physical (H & P): 68-year-old female, right-handed, found down by neighbor who called 911; alert but aphasic in emergency department (ED); preliminary CT scan revealed a CVA in the MCA distribution territory posterior to the central sulcus and superior to the sylvian fissure. There was no observable hemiparesis.

Past Medical History (PMH): Insulin Dependent Diabetes Mellitus (IDDM); hypertension; hyperlipidemia; A-fib; COPD; depression.

Social History: Widowed, lives alone; sedentary lifestyle; no family in area.

Surgical History: Cholesystectomy, appendectomy; hysterectomy.

A Functional Analysis of Mildred's Wernicke's Aphasia

Mildred's receptive language skills are significantly impaired (see Figure 4–2 for Mildred's Diagnostic Profile and Figure 4–3 for her ALD Target Model). As a consequence, she is unable to participate as a conversational partner for two primary reasons: (1) her logorrhea is unchecked due to her inability to self-monitor; and (2) her output is devoid of content. Therefore, her functional expressive abilities are limited. Mildred is unable to spell, so writing to communicate her needs is not possible. However, she has adequate graphomotor skills and visual perceptual skills for gross drawings, usable for communication purposes.

Cognitively, Mildred is able to attend to a task if it interests her and does not frustrate her. However, she may require tactile, verbal, and/or visual prompts for sustained attention. She wants to successfully convey messages and resorts to drawing, if prompted, when her communication partner conveys a lack of comprehension. Mildred's auditory-verbal memory span is reduced; however, visual memory is strength. Mildred is able to solve problems through action, not verbally (i.e., she can demonstrate a solution but is unable to convey it verbally due to her severely paraphasic output). For example, Mildred is able to recognize that a spilled liquid on the floor is to be avoided, so she walks around it. However, when she is asked to explain the solution, she points to the spill and says, "No, no, no watch out!" Her visuospatial skills for her gross drawings are functional, again, making this her strongest communication modality. An example of this is observed when Mildred wants something to drink and draws a crude representation of a cup while simultaneously saying, "It's a, I want it, it's a time, I want it a picka micka."

Critical Thinking/Learning Activity

- What information indicates that this is a person with Wernicke's aphasia?
- How would this patient's *press for speech* impact the patient's communicative effectiveness?
- What are the family counseling and education issues in this case, and how would you address them?
- What are the pros and cons of encouraging the use of an AAC device in this case?
- Write a SOAP note on this patient. Assume that you are seeing the patient for the first time after the evaluation session. Include three short-term therapeutic objectives in your note.

Language Expression

- **Automatic Speech:** Poor. Paraphasias noted in a counting sequence from 1-20; perseveration noted after the number 5.
- **Repetition Ability:** Poor for words and sentences.
- **Lexical Retrieval-Naming:** Circumlocutions and semantic paraphasias and neologisms noted on confrontation naming tasks.
- **Conversational Ability:** Devoid of content; press of speech with numerous paraphasias and neologisms; paragrammatic with omissions of tense markers, prefixes, etc.
- **Pragmatic Skills:** Poor awareness of turn-taking rules; inappropriate social language.
- **Paraphasias:** Frequent semantic, phonemic paraphasias and neologisms.

Speech

- **Rate:** WFL
- **Intelligibility:** WFL in all contexts.
- **Prosody:** Normal intonation patterns noted.
- **Articulation:** WFL
- **Fluency:** Logorrheic but devoid of content; "press of speech" noted; numerous paraphasias.

Auditory Comprehension

- **Answering Yes/No Questions:** Moderate ability to answer concrete questions and significant difficulty with abstract yes/no questions. Echolalia is present.
- **Executing Commands:** Moderate impairment at the simple one-step level.
- **Understanding Stories & Paragraphs:** Severely impaired.
- **Understanding Conversational Speech:** Severely impaired with an inability to self-monitor for errors.
- **Identifying Objects & Their Functions:** Moderately impaired when asked to point an object from a field of three.

Reading

- **Word-level Comprehension:** Severe alexia; sound-symbol disassociation; unable to read at the word level.
- **Sentence-level Comprehension:** Poor.
- **Oral Reading:** Difficulty associating written words with spoken counterparts and their meanings.
- **Oral Spelling:** Severely impaired.

Written Expression

- **Copying:** WFL given interest.
- **Writing to Dictation:** Breaks in the words are noted during writing to dictation.
- **Self-generated:** Writes with ease but letterforms are inconsistently correct; fluent paragraphic jargon similar to speech with no awareness of errors.
- **Written Spelling:** Severely impaired.
- **Drawing:** Functional for communicating ADL needs.

Cognition

- **Attention/Concentration:** Requires, tactile, verbal and/or visual prompts for sustained attention.
- **Visuospatial Skills:** WFL for ADL needs.
- **Memory:** Procedural memory appears intact for ADL needs; visual memory is a strength; semantic and episodic memory difficult to assess due to comprehension deficits.
- **Executive Functions:** Problem solving/judgment for safety purposes intact.

Behavioral Symptoms

- **Alertness:** More alert in the AM hours and when frustration is low.
- **Deficit Awareness:** No awareness of deficits (anosagnosia); poor self-monitoring of output.
- **Frustration:** More frustrated with others causing anger and lashing out verbally.
- **Emotional Lability:** None.
- **Current Personality Characteristics:** Depressed, anxious, angry, and tense which is dissimilar to her premorbid state.

Figure 4–2. Diagnostic profile for Mildred.

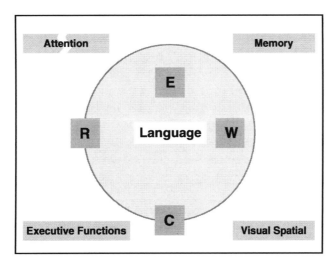

Figure 4–3. ALD Target Model for Mildred.

- Discuss the impact of this patient's depression on the patient's outcome for functional communication.

Treatment Considerations

The most important aspects of Mildred's treatment plan will include those that:

- Optimize her auditory comprehension so that she can participate, at the most basic level, in the social context around her.
- Give her a functional and efficacious means to communicate her wants and needs.
- Develop the strengths that she does have to facilitate both the receptive and expressive goals mentioned above.

Some general therapeutic objectives and techniques applicable to Mildred's profile include:

- Establish her ability to execute simple one-step commands by pairing speech with gestures and picture cues to augment understanding. This may help her caregivers in better meeting her ADL needs.
- Improve her ability to respond to simple, concrete, and personal yes or no questions to help her caregivers provide for her basic needs.
- Train Mildred to recognize the "STOP" hand gesture in order to facilitate a decrease in her press of speech. As a consequence, she may be able to process more effectively.

■ Optimize and facilitate Mildred's drawing skills so that she can supplement her verbal output with pictorial representations of her message. This can reduce her frustration and anxiety around the issue of not being understood by her communication partner.

Some Therapeutic Options

■ PACE (for Promoting Aphasics' Communicative Effectiveness; Edelman, 1987)
■ Schuell's Stimulation Facilitation Approach (Coelho, Sinotte, & Duffy, 2008)
■ LPAA (for Life Participation Approach to Aphasia; Chapey et al., 2008)
■ ACRT (for Anagram, Copy, and Recall Treatment; Helm-Estabrooks & Albert, 2004)

Transcortical Sensory Aphasia

Characteristics

Transcortical sensory aphasia (TSA) is a rare form of fluent aphasia. There is limited research about this form of aphasia in the rehabilitation literature. It is believed to result from vascular insufficiency in the MCA watershed area, that is, at the ends of the cerebral arteries. Wernicke's and Broca's areas remain intact and the arcuate fasciculus also remains undamaged, but the tissue surrounding them is infarcted.

TSA is characterized by fluent, well-articulated speech, with frequent neologisms and paraphasias, and discourse tends to be incoherent with numerous circumlocutions. These patients typically have a poor sense of the extent of their impairment. People with TSA have a more favorable communication prognosis than those with Wernicke's aphasia, which has a similar language profile. Individuals with TSA can repeat what is said to them by relying on the phonological system. For example, in these patients, performance improves on verbal repetition tasks because the arcuate fasiculus remains intact. Auditory comprehension deficits vary in magnitude, although most patients have severely limited language comprehension. Echolalia is often noted

and may deceive the listener into believing that the patient is responding somewhat appropriately. Word finding difficulties are common, and these patients tend to use many ready-made expressions, such as, "OK," "Ya know," "Oh, boy!," and so forth. Confrontation naming is often impaired with the patient giving meaningless responses (Goodglass & Kaplan, 2001). In summary, the most salient characteristics of TSA are intact repetition with limited comprehension and reduced propositional speech.

The neuroanatomical substrate for TSA is variable. For example, patients with early Alzheimer's dementia may present with symptoms similar to TSA as well as patients with vascular lesions of the left thalamic nuclei also present with TSA (Crosson, 1992). Left posterior temporal-parietal-occipital and thalamic areas are important for vocabulary knowledge in the semantic system, and these areas may be damaged in individuals with TSA. Thus, semantic dysfunction is often a concomitant feature of TSA. This is manifested as the inability to activate the semantic system for word output and the comprehension of meaning. As a consequence, coherent discourse and effective propositional speech are compromised.

In the TSA patient, repetition for words is usually easier than it is for sentences. Although they may be able to repeat the name of a common object, they are unable to name objects when they are seen or felt. They also have difficulty pointing to objects that are named for them. A patient with can translate a spoken sound to a written letter and this is very helpful because it permits them to communicate via writing despite spelling errors. These errors are characterized by the regularization of irregularly spelled words, that is, the patient may write the word ignoring spelling rules. For example, "face" may be written as "fas." Finally, any therapeutic approach to improve verbal output should utilize common words rather than abstract words and concepts.

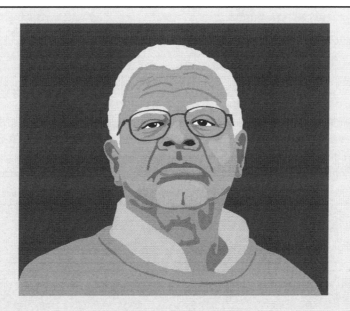

Case Scenario: John

History and Physical (H & P): 75-year-old, right-handed, African-American male, admitted to local psychiatric hospital. Hemiparesis was evident and the family noted that he had some sensory changes on the right side. On examination, he ambulated with maximum assistance. Family brought him to the hospital with echolalia and speaking in nonsense syllables that "sounded like foreign words." Blood pressure and heart rate were within normal limits for his age. He was unaware of his speech difficulty.

Past Medical History (PMH): The family reported the possibility of vascular dementia, and this was confirmed by the primary care physician via a telephone call from the ED.

Social History: Widowed, one adult daughter who lives nearby. John lives alone in an apartment complex that has an elevator. He has a few close friends in the complex.

Surgical History: Hernia surgery 5 years ago for inguinal tears. Cataract surgery was recently completed successfully in his left eye. The right eye is in need of cataract surgery.

A Functional Analysis of John's TSA

John's receptive language skills are the most impaired (see Figure 4–4 for John's Diagnostic Profile and Figure 4–5 for his ALD Target Model) Notice the similarities between John's TSA and Mildred's Wernicke's aphasias in this domain. Like Mildred, John was unable to effectively participate in any conversational exchanges because he was unable to self-monitor his speech errors and produced empty speech. Unlike Mildred, John was echolalic, which further complicated conversational success.

Expressively, John demonstrated normal syntax, but because of his word retrieval problems and paraphasias, his speech was empty of meaning. However, his automatic speech and repetition remained largely intact and would be important to consider in treatment planning. He was unable to use writing as a communication modality. He could recognize pictures. Therefore, creating an alternative means of communication for John using a portable picture book would be an efficacious method for augmenting his communication needs. Initially, John could benefit from starting with rote, automatic information, for example, days of the week, months of the year, numbers, and so forth.

According to John's primary care physician (PCP), his vascular disease has resulted in dementia. Therefore, further cognitive testing is indicated in this case. John's cognitive status is a critical factor in his functional success post-discharge and in outpatient therapy. If the cognitive testing demonstrates that John does have memory and executive function problems (i.e., problem-solving, reasoning, and judgment), then his ability to learn a new communication system may be compromised, especially as vascular dementia progresses. As a consequence, the clinician would need to develop other treatment options in order to facilitate functional communication. Cognitive assessment, as possible, is important for the therapeutic planning and progress monitoring in the person with aphasia.

Critical Thinking/Learning Activity

- How do you intend to establish a core vocabulary with John?
- What will you use to support his acquisition and comprehension of words?
- Which of John's strengths can you use to promote use of a core vocabulary?
- How will you advance John from the word level to the sentence level, receptively and expressively?
- John produces long paraphasic utterances that compromise his intended meaning. How will you facilitate the production of short, meaningful utterances so that John can become a functional communicator of his wants and needs?
- Do you view John's echolalia as a receptive or expressive deficit? Explain.

Language Expression

- **Automatic Speech:** WFL for counting, days of the week, alphabet. Able to repeat lengthy prayers and lyrics.
- **Repetition Ability:** WFL at word and phrase levels; however difficulty with longer sentences and abstract concepts.
- **Lexical Retrieval-Naming:** Confrontation naming is poor. Uses stereotypical phrases (i.e., "that a boy") and nonspecific words (i.e., "uh, um") as fillers and substitutions.
- **Conversational Ability:** Mild echolalia present in attempt to answer questions; running speech can be empty of meaning in long monologues.
- **Pragmatic Skills:** Turn-taking skills are functional; topic maintenance is impaired; proxemics is WFL; eye contact is WFL; initiating WFL.
- **Paraphasias:** Occasional neologisms, circumlocutions and paraphasias (especially semantic paraphasias) are present.

Speech

- **Rate:** WFL
- **Intelligibility:** WFL
- **Prosody:** Rate, rhythm, and intonation were WFL.
- **Articulation:** WFL
- **Fluency:** WFL

Auditory Comprehension

- **Answering Yes/No Questions:** WFL for concrete and personal yes/no questions; poor performance noted for abstract questions.
- **Executing Commands:** Poor performance; however, accuracy increases with visual cues.
- **Understanding Stories & Paragraphs:** Poor.
- **Understanding Conversational Speech:** Poor comprehension skills at the discourse level.
- **Identifying Objects & Their Functions:** Poor in a field of four or more objects.

Reading

- **Word-level Comprehension:** Able to match simple, regularly-spelled CVC words with pictures.
- **Sentence-level Comprehension:** Comprehension of written language severely impaired.
- **Oral Reading:** Spells aloud to facilitate oral reading at the CVC word level, with minimal success.
- **Oral Spelling:** Able to spell simple, CVC words aloud.

Written Expression

- **Copying:** WFL
- **Writing to Dictation:** Writing words and sentences to dictation is mildly impaired.
- **Self-generated:** Can write words only with occasional paraphasic errors.
- **Written Spelling:** Spelling is functional at the CVC level for regularly spelled words.
- **Drawing:** Can execute simple line drawings.

Cognition

- **Attention/Concentration:** Varies with time of day and medical status.
- **Visuospatial Skills:** Adequate for reading and writing with limited text.
- **Memory:** To be assessed.
- **Executive Functions:** To be assessed.

Behavioral Symptoms

- **Alertness:** Variable with more confusion noted in the evening.
- **Deficit Awareness:** No awareness of deficits (anosagnosia).
- **Frustration:** Demonstrates intermittent anger and frustration, especially when others do not seem to understand him.
- **Emotional Lability:** None noted.
- **Current Personality Characteristics:** Angry, frustrated, confused about his condition.

Figure 4–4. Diagnostic profile for John.

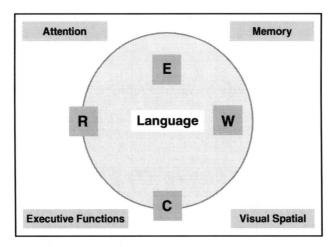

Figure 4–5. ALD Target Model for John.

Treatment Considerations

Persons with TSA tend to improve with repetition tasks. The list below will assist in determining how to use John's intact repetition therapeutically. Based on your findings, a treatment plan using repetition combined with another modality, at an appropriate level, may be developed.

- Compare repetition for single words versus sentences.
- Compare repetition for real versus nonwords.
- Compare repetition of common versus abstract words.
- Some general therapeutic techniques applicable to John's deficit profile include:
  - Pairing auditory input with another modality, typically visual support using pictures and words.
  - Reading aloud at the word level with pictured and written support (copying may support communication as another modality).
  - Providing visual support via pictures and matching that to written and verbally presented sentences for reducing paraphasic errors.
  - Using a verbal sequencing task (picture sequence cards) to facilitate cohesive discourse.
  - Based on John's ADL needs, build a core vocabulary for improving auditory comprehension and facilitating appropriate word use in functional contexts.

Some Therapeutic Options

- PACE (Edelman, 1987)
- Schuell's Stimulation Approach (Coelho, Sinotte, & Duffy, 2008)
- Supported Conversation
- LPAA (Chapey et al., 2008)
- ACRT (Helm-Estabrooks & Albert, 2004)

Conduction Aphasia

Characteristics

Conduction aphasia is a fluent aphasia and can result from a lesion to the cortical region connecting Broca's and Wernicke's area. This region incorporates the supramarginal gyrus and the white matter pathways of the arcuate fasiculus as well as the superior longitudinal fasiculus, sparing both Broca's and Wernicke's areas. Lesion localization has been controversial regarding conduction aphasia (Geschwind, 1965). Historically, the general assumption was that a lesion to the arcuate fasiculus would result in conduction aphasia (Anderson et al., 1999). However, Damasio (2001) indicated that the arcuate fasiculus does not need to be damaged for aphasia to be present. If the lesion is more posterior, the patient has more fluent speech. If the lesion is more anterior and inferior, speech is less fluent and contains phonemic paraphasias.

The most salient feature of conduction aphasia is a marked difficulty with repetition, especially for function words rather than nouns, in the presence of good auditory comprehension (Chapey & Hallowell, 2001). The conduction aphasic is able to produce complex syntactic structures in spontaneous speech. However, literal (phonemic) paraphasias will interfere with effective verbal communication, despite the appropriate syntactic structures. Speech production is characterized by good intonation and fluency, but because of word-finding difficulties, the clinician may observe hesitations in speech output as well as circumlocutions. Reading comprehension is intact, but oral reading is characterized by literal paraphasias, omission of words, and/or word substitutions. The person with conduction aphasia is able to recognize their errors, and they will try to self-correct. Typically, conduction aphasia will resolve to an anomic aphasia.

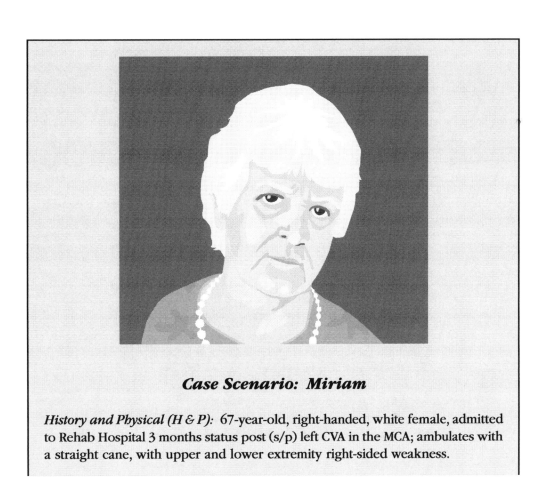

Case Scenario: Miriam

History and Physical (H & P): 67-year-old, right-handed, white female, admitted to Rehab Hospital 3 months status post (s/p) left CVA in the MCA; ambulates with a straight cane, with upper and lower extremity right-sided weakness.

Past Medical History (PMH): Hypertension (HTN), osteoporosis, s/p myocardial infarction (MI), history of (h/o) transient ischemic attacks (TIAs).

Social History: Married; two adult sons; husband retired policeman not supportive of patient's illness and needs; two-story home, eight steps to enter; attends an adult center during the day when at home. Patient stated that she was "depressed" over her CVA and the impact it had on her ADLs (activities of daily living).

Surgical History: Unremarkable.

A Functional Analysis of Miriam's Aphasia

In general, Miriam's ability to understand conversation is good with some diminished capacity in group settings (see Figure 4–6 for Miriam's Diagnostic Profile and Figure 4–7 for her ALD Target Model) She is able to interact appropriately with a conversational partner although she is often frustrated by her word finding difficulties. She tries repeatedly to find the correct word, but this is often a struggle and she becomes angry with herself. As a consequence, Miriam's verbal communication has many interruptions. Word finding and paraphasias are prevalent, making conversation challenging for both Miriam and her communication partner.

Cognitively, Miriam attends well and appears to have intact memory for information and events. She is usually correct with her answers to questions about facts and stories from the immediate and more remote past. Visuospatial skills are adequate as Miriam is able to copy and draw, and she can recall print for letters and common words. Executive functioning appears within normal limits. She functions appropriately in most social settings and is able to make her needs known. She takes care of family demands for basic cooking, light cleaning, and is planning to return to her card-game group in the community where she lives.

Critical Thinking/Learning Activity

- What characteristics of this patient's language disorder indicate that she has features of conduction aphasia?
- What are some psychosocial factors that could impact this patient's ability to effectively participate in therapy?
- What are the family counseling and educational issues in this case, and what objectives would you target?
- How would you implement an interdisciplinary plan with this patient, and which other services would you include?
- Discuss an activity and materials that you believe would target several of the short-term objectives listed in the above section.

Language Expression						
Automatic Speech: WFL for counting, reciting the alphabet, stating days and months of the year.	**Repetition Ability:** Repeating phrases moderately impaired; difficulties with multisyllabic words and with more abstract words; Spontaneous speech better than repetition. Repetition of numbers is easier than for words.	**Lexical Retrieval-Naming:** Frequent anomia, especially on confrontation naming, with attempts to self-correct.	**Conversational Ability:** Syntax is WFL. Ability to converse with paraphasias noted; at the conversational level, speech was circumlocutory and paraphasic. Miriam hesitates after brief runs of fluent speech.	**Fluency:** Fluent; average phrase length is 7+ words. Demonstrates episodes logorrhea; tries to produce repeated approximations to self-correct speech errors. [May be mistaken for apraxia of speech]	**Pragmatic Skills:** WFL	**Paraphasias:** Verbal output characterized by literal (phonemic) paraphasias.

Speech			
Rate: WFL	**Intelligibility:** WFL	**Prosody:** WFL for inflection, rhythm, and stress of speech.	**Articulation:** WFL

Auditory Comprehension				
Answering Yes/No Questions: WFL for concrete and abstract questions.	**Executing Commands:** WFL	**Understanding Stories & Paragraphs:** Comprehension for sentences is intact. Difficulty with grammatical morphemes (tense, plurals).	**Understanding Conversational Speech:** WFL; group settings pose some difficulty.	**Identifying Objects & Their Functions:** WFL

Reading			
Word-level Comprehension: WFL	**Sentence-level Comprehension:** WFL	**Oral Reading:** Minimal difficulty reading aloud at the sentence level.	**Oral Spelling:** Paraphasic errors noted on words > 4 letters in length.

Written Expression				
Copying: WFL	**Writing to Dictation:** Able to write common words to dictation.	**Self-generated:** Writing contains spelling errors; however, words are mostly accurate in context.	**Written Spelling:** Syllables in words are inconsistently transposed.	**Drawing:** WFL

Cognition			
Attention/Concentration: WFL	**Visuospatial Skills:** WFL	**Memory:** Long-term memory and working memory intact for procedural, semantic, and episodic systems.	**Executive Functions:** Planning and reasoning WFL for ADL needs.

Behavioral Symptoms				
Alertness: Depressed mood, however alert and cooperative for therapy.	**Deficit Awareness:** Keenly aware of speech production difficulty.	**Frustration:** Significant frustration noted.	**Emotional Lability:** None.	**Current Personality Characteristics:** Depressed with feelings of hopelessness; not consistent with her premorbid personality.

Figure 4–6. Diagnostic profile for Miriam.

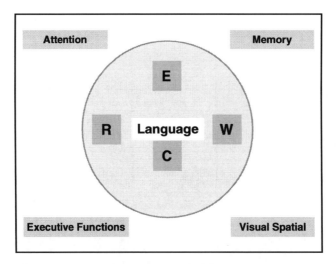

Figure 4–7. ALD Target Model for Miriam.

Treatment Considerations

Miriam's speech is characterized by many phonemic paraphasias; however, her prognosis for becoming a functional communicator is good. Good self-monitoring skills are an asset to her treatment although she is often frustrated by her awareness of her paraphasic speech and word finding difficulties. Repetition also presents a challenge once the words become multisyllabic, that is, greater than three to four syllables. Her good auditory comprehension and ability to write are assets to be used in program planning. Therapeutic intervention will begin where Miriam feels successful and increase in small steps, extending from concrete to more abstract stimuli. Here are some suggestions:

- Increase ability to retrieve words through: word associations, pictures, gestural cues, and sentence stem fill-ins. Avoid phonemic cues, as they are often paraphasic.
- Decrease paraphasic errors by self-monitoring and using a readily available picture-based dictionary.
- Improve repetition ability starting with easy, one-syllable words and progressing to less common multisyllabic words with written word cues, unison production, and syllable taps. However, if success is limited, consider whether repetition is a functional goal worth continuing.
- Improve sequencing of phonemes to reduce metathesis (transposing sounds and syllables within a word).
- Improve writing ability by using printed syllables on separate cards to be organized in the correct sequence and then copied.

Some Therapeutic Options

- LPAA (Chapey et al., 2008)
- RET (for Response Elaboration Training) to improve content words used to describe a picture (Kearns & Scher, 1988)
- Narrative story cards to facilitate accurate recall of information and optimize discourse skills for daily needs (Helm-Estabrooks & Nicholas, 2003)
- Divergent word retrieval to stimulate word retrieval by asking the patient to visualize and name as many of a specific category (animals, food, transportation, etc.) as can be recalled (Chapey & Hallowell, 2001)

Anomic Aphasia

Characteristics

Word finding difficulties, also referred to as anomia or lexical retrieval difficulty, accompany most types of aphasia. However, when the individual has a disproportionately greater difficulty naming than other language difficulties, it is referred to as anomic aphasia. This deficit becomes most noticeable when the individual attempts confrontation naming, that is, naming an entity when a visual image is presented. These individuals often use circumlocutions and are frustrated by their inability to name things. However, the inability to retrieve words and names for objects can be severe enough to completely halt the flow of speech and severely restrict discourse. Other salient features of anomic aphasia include fluent speech with the exception of intermittent hesitations. This halt in the flow of fluent speech is a direct result of the word-finding problem. For most people with anomic aphasia, morphology, syntax, and auditory comprehension are normal.

Anomia is generally caused by damage to the left inferior temporal cortex. If the damage occurs in the posterior portion of the inferior temporal cortex, pure anomia is more likely to be observed. Pure anomia results when access to phonological word forms is impaired. If the damage occurs in the more anterior portion of the temporal lobe, then semantic anomia is noted. This type of anomia is a result of a degradation of semantic knowledge. It also has been reported that the more anterior the lesion, the more severe the anomia. There is some suggestion

that if the lesion extends into more anterior regions, the anomia will worsen. This is due to a disconnection between the areas critical for access of phonological word forms and areas of preserved semantic knowledge (Antonucci, Beeson, & Rapcsak, 2004).

Although patients with lesions in the left temporal pole can experience deficits in retrieving proper names for people, they maintain the ability to recognize them. Larger lesions may further affect the ability to name and often include difficulty naming animals and tools (Tranel, Logan, Frank, & Damasio, 1997).

Research by Lorenz and Nickels (2007), investigated two primary cueing strategies (orthographic/letters and phonological/sounds) to determine if one type was superior in helping those with word-finding difficulty following stroke. Three people with chronic aphasia and anomia participated in the study to determine if using the initial letter of a word or the initial sound of the target word best facilitated naming. In one participant, both orthographic and phonological cues had similar results. In the other two, orthographic cues were most beneficial. Initial letter cues were equally effective in supporting irregularly spelled words such as *knife*, as they were for regularly spelled word such as *king*. The authors concluded that initial letter cues appear effective in treating anomia as they provide strong and enduring effects, regardless of the patient's ability to benefit from initial phoneme cues. Although there were only three participants in the study, it is worthwhile to note that naming skills may be improved by showing the first letter as a cue for target words when working with individuals who have lexical-retrieval difficulties.

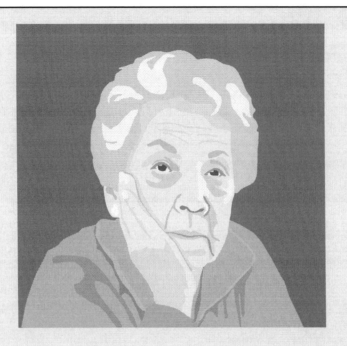

Case Scenario: Sophie

History and Physical (H & P): Sophie is a 63-year-old white female admitted to the ED via EMS; found on first floor of her home, sitting in a chair; lethargic, slurred speech; disoriented.

Past Medical History (PMH): Hypertension, hyperlipidemia, IDDM, osteoarthritis.

Social History: Lives alone in two-story home, two blocks away from daughter and her family. Retired school teacher.

Surgical History: s/p right total hip replacement (THR); s/p angioplasty with stent in left anterior descending artery (LAD).

A Functional Analysis of Sophie's Aphasia

Sophie's ability to comprehend language in both verbal and written forms is within functional limits (see Figure 4–8 for Sophie's Diagnostic Profile and Figure 4–9 for her ALD Target Model). Reading ability is normal at sentence and paragraph levels. Her confrontational naming ability and word finding during discourse remain a challenge. However, Sophie can express herself to make her needs and wants known, even though she has a tendency to use circumlocutions to convey ideas. Speech rate and prosody are normal and intelligibility is good, but fluency is impacted by her word-finding difficulties. As a consequence, Sophie has many pauses and self-correcting attempts during telephone conversations in public encounters, for example, shopping, banking, and managing public transportation exchanges.

Language Expression

Automatic Speech:	Repetition Ability:	Lexical Retrieval-Naming:	Conversational Ability:	Pragmatic Skills:	Paraphasias:
WFL for counting, days of the week, alphabet.	Normal repetition for words, phrases and sentences.	Impaired for confrontation naming and lexical retrieval during discourse; circumlocutions noted.	WFL; however, word finding difficulties impact speech fluency in conversation.	WFL	None.

Speech

Rate:	Intelligibility:	Prosody:	Articulation:	Fluency:
WFL	WFL	WFL	WFL	Impacted by word-finding difficulty.

Auditory Comprehension

Answering Yes/No Questions:	Executing Commands:	Understanding Stories & Paragraphs:	Understanding Conversational Speech:	Identifying Objects & Their Functions:
WFL	WFL	WNL	Comprehension for sentences and discourse is WFL.	WNL

Reading

Word-level Comprehension:	Sentence-level Comprehension:	Oral Reading:	Oral Spelling:
WFL	WFL	WFL	Letter substitutions noted in minimal pairs, e.g., mat for hat.

Written Expression

Copying:	Writing to Dictation:	Self-generated:	Written Spelling:	Drawing:
WFL	WFL	Affected by word-finding difficulty.	WFL for basic words.	WFL

Cognition

Attention/Concentration:	Visuospatial Skills:	Memory:	Executive Functions:
WFL	WFL	Long-term memory and working memory intact for procedural, semantic, and episodic systems.	WFL

Behavioral Symptoms

Alertness:	Deficit awareness:	Frustration:	Emotional Lability:	Current Personality Characteristics:
WFL	Keen awareness of deficits.	Demonstrates extreme frustration with inability to retrieve desired words.	None.	Pleasant and apologetic for her word-finding problems.

Figure 4–8. Diagnostic profile for Sophie.

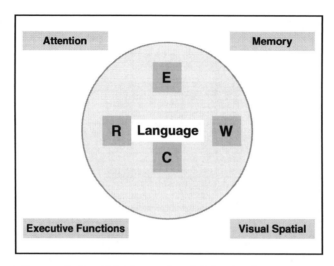

Figure 4–9. ALD Target Model for Sophie.

Sophie's writing skills are good. She can write sentences but has some lexical retrieval difficulty in this domain as well. When she cannot think of a needed word, she may ask the listener for help as she struggles. Although this can be an effective compensatory strategy, it is not always practical in public venues. Therefore, this causes more frustration for Sophie in that she knows she can find the means to express her ideas, but cannot readily use them in certain public scenarios.

Cognitively, Sophie displays good attention to tasks and can concentrate, especially if the task is of interest to her. Her memory skills for her ADL appear to be functioning within normal limits, and she is able to recall basic information from events in the recent and distant past. She recalls how to cook her favorite meals and is able to manage her money and pay bills. Planning and judgment appear to be intact for common household tasks and chores, making appointments, and organizing her day. Sophie maintains a vibrant social network with her family and friends who are supportive of her rehabilitation goals. Although she is keenly aware of her deficits, she maintains a pleasant demeanor and continues to improve her functional communication skills by being actively engaged in her therapy program.

Critical Thinking/Learning Activity

■ People with anomic aphasia can be classified into treatment categories that are semantically based, phonologically based, and self-cued (Boyle, 2004).
■ How would you attempt to determine the most beneficial treatment for your patient?

- What will you use to support semantic and phonemic cuing?
- Which of Sophie's strengths can you use to promote word finding (lexical retrieval)?
- How will you advance Sophie's conversational skills with a variety of communication partners?
- Do you view Sophie's word finding difficulties as a receptive or expressive deficit? Explain.

Treatment Considerations

Some general therapeutic objectives and techniques applicable to Sophie's deficit profile include:

- Improve lexical retrieval to request information and assistance using semantic feature analysis (SFA). For each word she cannot access, the category to which the item belongs, its action, physical properties, location, and associated features, will be sought.
- Increase engagement in conversation with designated people using comprehension tasks that facilitate oral naming. For word finding difficulties, supportive pictures and a written list of functional words to view will be provided.
- Make needs and wants known with semantic and phonemic self-cuing to increase word finding. Provide words following circumlocutions.
- Based on Sophie's needed activities of daily living (ADL), make her needs and wants known for use during conversation and begin facilitating their use in functional contexts.

Some Therapeutic Options

- Response-Contingent Small Step Treatment (RCSST; Bollinger & Stout, 1976)
- PACE (Li et al., 1988)
- SFA (Coelho, McHugh, & Boyle, 2000)
- Semantic Cueing Treatment (SCT; Wambaugh et al., 2001)
- Phonological Cueing Treatment (PCT; Wambaugh et al., 2001)
- Cognitive Neuropsychological Models of Lexical Processing (Raymer & Rothi, 2001)
- Semantic Judgment Questions, Written Word to Picture Matching, and Naming to Definitions (Drew & Thompson, 1999)

References

Anderson, J., Gilmore, R., Roper, S., Crosson, B., Bauer, R. M., Nadeau, S., . . . Heilman, K. (1999). Conduction aphasia and the arcuate fasciculus: A reexamination of the Wernicke-Geschwind model. *Brain and Language, 70*, 1–12.

Antonucci, S. M., Beeson, P. M., & Rapcsak, S. Z. (2004). Anomia in patients with left inferior temporal lobe lesions. *Aphasiology, 18*, 543–554.

Bhogal, S. K., Teasell, R., & Speechley, M. (2003). Intensity of aphasia therapy, impact on recovery. *Stroke, 34*, 987–993.

Bollinger, R. L., & Stout, C. E. (1976). Response-contingent small-step treatment: Performance-based communication intervention. *Journal of Speech and Hearing Disorders, 41*, 40–51.

Boyle, M. (2004). Semantic feature analysis: The evidence for treating lexical impairments in aphasia. In *Aphasia: Treatment for lexical and sentence production skills*. Rockville, MD: American Speech-Language-Hearing Association.

Brookshire, R. H. (1997). *Introduction to neurogenic communication disorders*. New York, NY: Mosby.

Chapey, R., Duchan, J. F., Elman, R. J., Garcia, L. J., Kagan, A., Lyon, J. G., & Simmons-Mackie, N. (2008). Life-participation approach to aphasia: A statement of values for the future. In R. Chapey (Ed.), *Language intervention strategies in aphasia and related neurogenic communication disorders* (5th ed., pp. 279–289). Philadelphia, PA: Lippincott Williams & Wilkins.

Chapey, R., & Hallowell, B. (2001). Introduction to language intervention strategies in adult aphasia. In R. Chapey (Ed.), *Language intervention strategies in aphasia and related neurogenic communication disorders* (4th ed., pp. 3–19). Philadelphia, PA: Lippincott, Williams & Wilkins.

Cherney, L. R., & Robey, R. R. (2008). Aphasia treatment: Recovery, progrnosis, and clinical effectiveness. In In R. Chapey (Ed.), *Language intervention strategies in aphasia and related neurogenic communication disorders* (5th ed., pp. 186–243). Philadelphia, PA: Lippincott Williams & Wilkins.

Coelho, C. S., McHugh, R., & Boyle, M. (2000). Semantic feature analysis as a treatment for aphasic dysnomia: A replication. *Aphasiology, 14*, 133–142.

Coelho, C. A., Sinotte, M. P., & Duffy, J. R. (2008). Schuell's stimulation approach to rehabilitation. In R. Chapey (Ed.), *Language intervention strategies in aphasia and related neurogenic communication disorders* (5th ed., pp. 403–449). Philadelphia, PA: Lippincott Williams & Wilkins.

Crosson, B. (1992). *Subcortical function in language and memory*. New York, NY: Oxford University Press.

Crosson, B., Fabrizio, K. S., Singletary, F., Cato, M. A., Wierenga, C. E., Parkinson, R. B., & Rothi, L. J. G. (2007). Treatment of naming in non-fluent aphasia through manipulation of intention and attention: A phase 1 comparison of two novel treatments. *Journal of International Neuropsychological Society, 13*, 582–594.

Damasio, H. (2001). Neural basis of language disorders. In R. Chapey (Ed.), *Language intervention strategies in adult aphasia and related neurogenic communication disorders* (4th ed., pp. 18–36). Philadelphia, PA: Lippincott Williams & Wilkins.

Davis, C. H., Harrington, G., & Baynes, K. (2006). Intensive semantic intervention in fluent aphasia: A pilot study with fMRI. *Aphasiology, 20*, 59–83.

Drew, R. L., & Thompson, C. K. (1999). Model-based semantic treatment for naming in aphasia. *Journal of Speech, Language, and Hearing Research, 4*, 972–990.

Edelman, G. (1987). *P.A.C.E.: Promoting aphasics' communicative effectiveness*. Bicester, UK: Winslow Press.

Ferguson, N. F., Evans, K., & Raymer, A. M. (2012). A comparison of intention and pantomime gesture treatment for noun retrieval in people with aphasia. *American Journal of Speech-Language Pathology, 21*, 126–139.

Geschwind, N. (1965). Disconnection syndromes in animals and man. *Brain, 88*, 237–294.

Goodglass, H., & Kaplan, E. (2001). *The assessment of aphasia and related disorders*. Philadelphia, PA: Lea & Febiger.

Helm-Estabrooks, N., & Albert, M. L. (2004). *Anagram, copy, and recall therapy. Manual of aphasia and aphasia therapy* (2nd ed). Austin, TX: Pro-Ed.

Helm-Estabrooks, N., & Nicholas, M. (2003). *Narrative story cards*. Austin, TX: Pro-Ed.

Kearnes, K., & Scher, G. (1988). The generalization of response elaboration training. In T. Prescott (Ed.), *Clinical aphasiology conference proceedings* (Vol. 18, pp. 223–245). Boston, MA: College-Hill.

LaPointe, L. L. (1997). *Aphasia and related neurogenic language disorders* (2nd ed.). New York, NY: Thieme.

Li, E. C., Kitselman, K., Dusatko, D., & Spinelli, C. (1988). The efficacy of PACE in the remediation of naming deficits. *Journal of Communication Disorders, 21*, 491–503.

Lorenz, A., & Nickels, L. (2007). Orthographic cueing in anomic aphasia: How does it work? *Aphasiology, 21,* 670–686.

Marshall, R. C. (2001). Early management of Wernicke's aphasia: A context-based approach. In R. Chapey (Ed.), *Language intervention strategies in aphasia and related neurogenic communication disorders* (4th ed., pp. 507–530). Philadelphia, PA: Lippincott Williams & Wilkins.

Raymer, A. M., & Rothi, L. J. G. (2001). Cognitive approaches to impairments of word comprehension and production. In R. Chapey (Ed.), *Language intervention strategies in aphasia and related neurogenic communication disorders* (4th ed., pp. 524–550). Baltimore, MD: Lippincott Williams & Wilkins.

Raymer, A. M., Singletary, F., Rodriguez, A., Ciampitti, M., Heilman, K. M., & Rothi, L.J.G. (2006). Effects of gesture + verb treatment for noun and verb retrieval in aphasia. *Journal of the International Neuropsychological Society, 12,* 867–882.

Raymer, A. M., & Thompson, C. K. (1991). Effects of verbal plus gestural treatment in a patient with aphasia and severe apraxia of speech. In T. E. Prescott (Ed.), *Clinical Aphasiology, 12,* 285–297. Austin, TX: Pro-Ed.

Rose, M. L. (2006). The utility of arm and hand gestures in the treatment of aphasia. *Advances in Speech-Language Pathology, 8,* 92–109.

Tranel, D., Logan, C. G., Frank, R. J., & Damasio, A. R. (1997). Explaining category-related effects in the retrieval of conceptual and lexical knowledge for concrete entities: Operationalization and analysis of factors. *Neuropsychologia, 35,* 1329–1339.

Wambaugh, J. L., Linebaugh, C. W., Doyle, P. J., Martinez, A. L., Kalinyak-Flisar, M., & Spencer, K. A. (2001). Effects of two cueing treatments on lexical retrieval treatments in aphasic speakers with different levels of deficit. *Aphasiology, 15,* 933–950.

Chapter 5

OTHER APHASIC SYNDROMES

Subcortical Aphasia

Introduction

Understanding subcortical aphasias can be challenging even for the most seasoned clinicians due to individual differences in cortical and subcortical architecture as well as interpretation of research findings. Nadeau and Crosson (1997) wrote a seminal, comprehensive review of the thinking at the time regarding subcortical aphasias, specifically striatocapsular infarcts, that is, nonthalamic. Out of 33 reported cases, there were 17 with no aphasia. A primary conclusion of their review was that aphasia due to nonthalamic subcortical lesions results from a combination of thalamic disconnection and cortical dysfunction related to persistent ischemia or infarct. These lesions could not be visualized by conventional MRI or CT scans of the time.

However, as a result of more refined imaging techniques, a better understanding of *subcortical aphasia* emerged (Webb, Adler, & Love, 2008). For example, magnetic resonance diffusion-weighted imaging (DWI) was able to visualize small cortical infarcts not visible on conventional MRI or CT scans (Han et al., 2003). These authors proposed that subcortical aphasias are due to smaller, previously unidentifiable cortical infarcts. Although this may not explain all subcortical aphasias, the interest lies in the fact that DWI and magnetic resonance perfusion-weighted imaging (PWI) have clarified the role of cortical lesions in subcortical aphasias (Hillis et al., 2004).

More recently, Hillis et al. (2004) studied 24 patients with acute left caudate nucleus infarcts (nonthalamic) on diffusion-weighted imaging (DWI). They found that the stroke in these patients was caused by *cortical hypoperfusion* due to stenosis of the large vessels. That is, the subcortical stroke was due to the cortical hypoperfusion preventing blood flow to the subcortical region. They found that in 14 patients with aphasia, 13 had hypoperfusion of at least one cortical region. The other patient had hypoperfusion of the left occipital lobe only, and no aphasia. In the 10 patients that did *not* have aphasia, none of them had hypoperfusion of a cortical region. The severity and type of the resulting aphasia was statistically associated with hypoperfusion of a specific region of infarct. This investigation only included patients with nonthalamic infarcts, but patients who sustain a thalamic infarct may present differently. These patients, according to Hillis et al. (2004), present with fluent, anomic speech, possible paraphasias, good comprehension, and repetition. The site of lesion associated with these language characteristics tends to be in the left pulvinar or ventrolateral thalamus.

The subcortical aphasias are often divided into two general groups, thalamic and nonthalamic types (Davis, 2007; Nadeau & Rothi, 2001). Kuljic-Obradovic (2003) further divides the classification into three groups: thalamic aphasia, striatocapsular aphasia, and aphasia with white matter paraventricular lesions. First, the subcortical structures are many, and they comprise a complex functional network supporting communication. Second, the range of communicative impairment noted in people with subcortical aphasias is variable based on the anatomical location and size of the lesion.

According to Vigneau et al. (2006), the left hemispheric language functions are *not* modular in nature, but rather form large-scale architectural networks with subcortical structures. For example, Vukovic et al. (2012) analyzed the acoustic and perceptual aspects of phonation in 60 men with aphasia—20 with subcortical aphasia, 20 with Broca's aphasia, and 20 with Wernicke's aphasia, and an additional 20 age-matched controls with no neurological history, using the Multidimensional Voice Program. They found that all the groups were impaired on the acoustic and perceptual measures. However, those with subcortical aphasia were more impaired than the other aphasic groups on the entire neurocognitive system of articulation-phonological language processing. The authors feel that this may be due to lesions in the globus pallidus, suggesting a link with the striatal vocal area (Wise, Greene, Buchel, & Scott, 1999). In discussing their findings, the authors state that thalamic lesions can even lead to temporary muteness, then followed by aphasia. Thus, the message for the clinician is that in some subcortical thalamic aphasias, the patient may not have speech especially in the acute phase of the stroke. Furthermore, it may be that the person presenting with a subcortical aphasia may not perceive sound production in the same way as a normal listener.

The information above demonstrates that there is a lack of conclusive evidence regarding the nature and etiology of subcortical aphasias as well as variability in the research findings. Both of these factors foster clinical ambiguity in diagnosing the type of aphasia.

Characteristics of the Subcortical Aphasias

These two types of subcortical aphasia—nonthalamic and thalamic—have critical differences with the exception of spared repetition, which is preserved in both types. Individuals that have *striatocapsular* involvement and *white matter periventricular* lesions generally experience a lack of speech flu-

ency, literal (phonemic) paraphasias, but generally preserved comprehension and naming. Individuals with thalamic aphasia generally experience fluent speech output but have impaired comprehension, naming and verbal (semantic) paraphasias (Kuljic-Obradovic, 2003)

A brief review of the neuroanatomical substrates to these aphasias is in order (Figure 5–1). The primary subcortical areas include the *internal capsule* (white matter pathways), the *basal ganglia*, and the thalamus. The internal capsule is a passageway for motor and sensory fiber tracts leaving the cortex and is located between the thalamus and the lenticular nuclei. The lenticular nuclei comprise a part of the basal ganglia. The *caudate nucleus* and the *putamen* make up the lenticular nuclei, and together the *caudate* and the *putamen* are called the *striatum*. It is in the region of the *capsulostriatum*—the internal capsule, the caudate nucleus, and the putamen—that most subcortical infarcts generally occur.

The role of the *nonthalamic structures* below the perisylvian region in normal and impaired language processes is controversial. The actual controversy lies not in the fact that it is possible to sustain language impairment due to lesions in this region; it is the variability in nature and degree of those impairments that raises some questions (Kennedy & Murdoch, 1993; Nadeau & Crosson, 1997). Some authors have reported differences in the language impairment of those patients with *anterior* striatocapsular lesions versus those with *posterior* striatocapsular lesions (Cappa, Cavallotti, Guidotti, Papagno, & Vignolo, 1983; Murdoch, Thompson, Fraser, & Harrison, 1986; Naeser et al., 1982). However, Kennedy and Murdoch (1993) described cases in which the differences in language difficulties could not be attributed to an anterior-posterior distinction, leaving this controversy unresolved.

The basal ganglia and thalamus are connected to the cerebral cortex by a series of white matter circuits called the *cortico-striato-pallido-thalamocortical loops*. The thalamus is a nucleus located deep in the cerebrum. It is connected to motor, sensory, and association areas of the cortex. It is a primary relay station for information entering and leaving the cerebral cortex. For example, a hallmark of thalamic

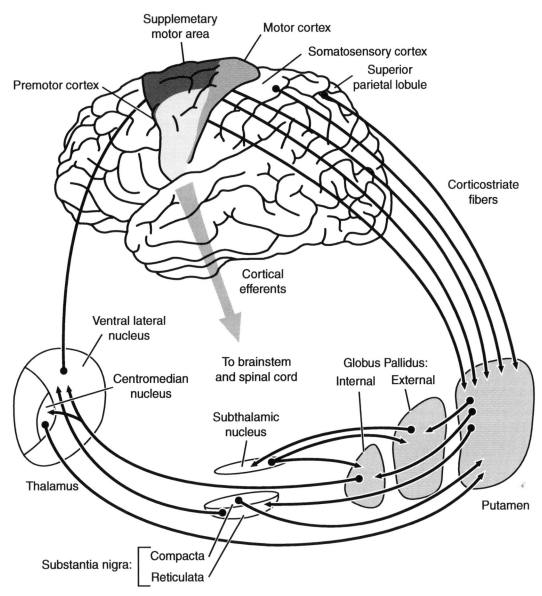

Figure 5–1. A schematic of subcortical pathways. (Adapted from Bhatnagar, 2002, p. 256.)

aphasia is poor attention. This is thought to be due to a lesion in the white fibers connecting the thalamus to the prefrontal cortex (Davis, 2007, p. 48). Aphasias due to thalamic lesions are better understood and better documented compared with aphasias that are due to nonthalamic subcortical lesions. As noted above, a reason for this discrepancy is that the nonthalamic lesions had not been visible on imaging studies (Chapey, 2001, p. 460). The clinical profile for thalamic aphasia is more unitary, and as a consequence, a clinician would be able to determine the existence of a thalamic aphasia more easily. For a thorough and succinct review of the subcortical aphasias, see Kent (2004). We have also provided a summary table (Table 5–1), for further clarification.

Table 5–1. Comparative Thoughts on the Subcortical Aphasias

Citation	Conceptualization of the Subcortical Aphasias

Bhatnagar, C. (2013). *Neuroscience for the study of communicative disorders* (4th ed., pp. 447–448). Baltimore, MD: Lippincott Williams & Wilkins.	1. Subcortical aphasias are defined by the site of lesion and not by aphasic characteristics.
	
	 2. Subcortical lesions disrupt the connections to the cortical language regions.
	
	 3. The most common type is *anterior subcortical aphasia syndrome.*
	    a. Seen in patients with lesions in the caudate, anterior limb of the internal capsule, and anterior putamen.
	    b. Characteristics: Speech is dysarthric and nonfluent, and mild comprehension and repetition impairments exist.
	
	 4. Lesions of the *dominant thalamus* produce a thalamic aphasia characterized by:
	    a. Fluent aphasia with paraphasic errors.
	    b. "Relatively spared" auditory comprehension.
	    c. A dichotomy may be observed in speech fluency in that when the patient is awake, speech is intact, but paraphasic when drowsy.
	
	 5. The thalamus may play a role in activating the language cortex, so lesions to the thalamus may actually cause the language area to sleep.
	
	 6. Subcortical lesions may also involve the temporal isthmus with connections to Wernicke's area, possibly interfering with auditory comprehension.

Papathanasiou, I., Coppens, P., & Portagas, C. (2013). *Aphasia and related communication disorders.* Burlington, MA: Jones & Bartlett Publishing.	1. Subcortical aphasia is not a unitary entity, and variability exists among patients.
	
	 2. Lesions in the head of the left caudate and anterior limb of the internal capsule produce an aphasia with the following characteristics:
	    a. Auditory comprehension deficits
	    b. Dysarthria
	    c. Motor impairments
	
	 3. Thalamic aphasia is characterized by:
	    a. Nonfluent speech.
	    b. Spared auditory comprehension.
	    c. Sometimes complete suppression of speech at onset.
	    d. Low vocal volume (later in recovery).
	    e. Severe reduction of spontaneous speech, restricted mainly to direct questions only.
	    f. Semantic paraphasias.
	
	 Note: Compare this description of thalamic aphasia with Bhatnagar's above.

Table 5–1. *continued*

Citation	Conceptualization of the Subcortical Aphasias

Nadeau, S. E., & Gonzalez Rothi, L. (2008). Rehabilitation of subcortical aphasia. In Roberta Chapey (Ed.), *Language intervention strategies in aphasia and related neurogenic communication disorders* (5th ed.). Baltimore, MD: Lippincott Williams & Wilkins.	1. Aphasia is an indirect consequence of subcortical lesions.
	2. Aphasia is usually caused by ischemic strokes.
	3. Cortical projections to the thalamus are as extensive as those from the thalamus to the cortex (Nadeau, 2001).
	4. Thalamus is a regulated, or gate-relay device.
	5. Thalamic aphasia:
	  a. Spares repetition.
	  b. Spares procedural knowledge underlying phonological processing.
	  c. Anomia is noted in spontaneous speech.
	  d. Normal grammar.
	  e. Normal articulation.
	  f. In the worst cases, moderate auditory comprehension deficits may be noted.
	6. Nonthalamic aphasia:
	  a. The *striatocapsular* complex, that is, the head of the caudate, the putamen, and anterior limb of the internal capsule.
	  b. Because of cortical connections, reductions in cortical blood flow associated with a lesion to this subcortical region will produce an aphasia consistent with the cortical reduction. Subcortical lesion affecting blood flow to Wernicke's area will produce an aphasia resembling a fluent, Wernicke's type aphasia.
	  c. Commonly include impairment in:
	    i. Grammatical function
	    ii. Phonologic function
	    iii. Lexical-semantic function

Murdoch, B. E. (2004). Language disorders in adults: Subcortical involvement. In Raymond E. Kent (Ed.), *The MIT encyclopedia of communication disorders.* Cambridge, MA: The MIT Press	1. Nonthalamic lesions: Controversy and uncertainty surround the role of the striatocapsular complex in producing aphasias.
	  a. Difference between *anterior* striatocapsular and *posterior* striatocapsular lesions.
	  b. Anterior lesions: Good comprehension, slow, but grammatical speech.
	  c. Poste*rior* lesions: Poor comprehension, fluent, Wernicke's type output.
	2. Some common impairments of subcortical aphasias, in general, noted by researchers:
	  a. Confrontation naming
	  b. Repetition
	  c. Auditory comprehension
	  d. Reading comprehension

continues

Table 5–1. *continued*

Citation	Conceptualization of the Subcortical Aphasias
Murdoch, B. E. (2004) *continued*	3. Thalamic lesions produce aphasia of a *mixed transcortical* type. a. Preserved repetition b. Variable but often good comprehension c. Reduction in spontaneous speech output d. Anomia e. Semantic paraphasias. 4. "Contemporary theories suggest that the role of subcortical structures in language is essentially neuroregulatory, relying on quantitative neuronal activity"(Murdoch, p. 317).

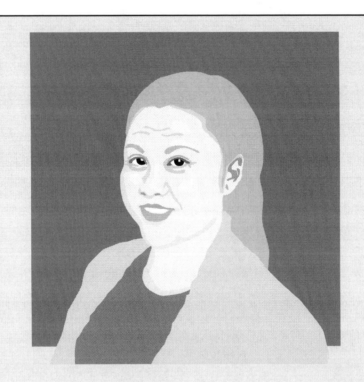

Case Scenario: Winnie

History and Physical (H & P): 63-year-old, right-handed, Vietnamese female, admitted to local hospital. Numbness in the right arm and shoulder; lethargy. On examination, her level of alertness was significantly reduced. Family brought her to the hospital describing her as "babbling and sleepy." Blood pressure in the emergency department (ED) was 130/85 and heart rate was 92. She did not seem to understand the questions asked of her.

Past Medical History (PMH): Winnie has no prior history of stroke. Her PMH includes hyperlipidemia and hypertension (HTN). She is compliant with all medications.

Social History: Lives with her husband and her son and his family in a two-story row home in Philadelphia. Winnie speaks proficient English as a second language. She has been in the United States since 1977. Completed required schooling in South Vietnam.

Surgical History: Unremarkable.

A Functional Analysis of Winnie's Subcortical Aphasia

In the acute phase of the stroke, Winnie presented with extreme lethargy, often dozing off during the middle of a communicative interaction (see Figure 5–2 for Winnie's Diagnostic Profile and Figure 5–3 for her ALD Target Model)Her lethargy complicates her already compromised ability to process auditory information, especially at the conversational level. It is important for the clinician to understand the impact that Winnie's level of alertness has on her auditory processing skills and to adjust the therapy accordingly. Although Winnie speaks fluently, her speech is characterized by numerous semantic paraphasias. From a functional perspective, Winnie's paraphasic output can be circumvented if the listener uses the context of the exchange to facilitate appropriate word selection. She is very aware of her receptive and expressive deficits, but appears almost indifferent to them. Reading is impaired at the paragraph level, but is functional at the word and phrase levels. The clinician may want to consider using Winnie's reading skills at the word/phrase level to promote growth in other deficit areas. Because the written word is static, and not fleeting like the speech signal, Winnie processes and attends better to this type of stimuli. This can help her process information for communication purposes. Therapeutically, the clinician can pair the written word with the speech signal to optimize Winnie's comprehension of more difficult material, if necessary. Winnie's difficulty maintaining attention affects all areas of cognition. To complicate matters, Winnie demonstrates memory deficits for declarative functioning. In other words, her procedural motor memory for activities such as dressing, cooking, and grooming are less impaired than her ability to talk about them. This is an instance where the written word and/or pictures can facilitate procedural functioning. Visuospatial skills are functional but are optimized with large print and pictures. Using simple drawings and bold print as well as pictures with emotional valence are suggested. Winnie's ability to solve problems associated with her activities of daily living (ADLs) will vary based on her procedural memory and the number of steps involved completing the task. Therefore, Winnie may not be able to manage some of her ADLs such as cooking independently. However, every patient is different, so this admonishment is merely cautionary. Her functional profile will change in a positive direction as her level of alertness increases.

Language Expression

- **Automatic Speech:** WFL for counting, days of the week, alphabet with a verbal prompt to facilitate initiation.
- **Repetition Ability:** WFL for words and sentences, however some paraphasias noted.
- **Lexical Retrieval-Naming:** Confrontation naming is moderate-severely impaired.
- **Conversational Ability:** Syntax WFL at sentence level. However, her lethargy and paraphasias complicate her functional discourse.
- **Pragmatic Skills:** Affected by lethargy and difficulty maintaining the communication dyad.
- **Paraphasias:** Semantic paraphasias present.

Speech

- **Rate:** Slowed rate, hesitant speech.
- **Intelligibility:** WFL
- **Prosody:** Reduced intonation contours; may be secondary to lethargy.
- **Articulation:** WFL
- **Fluency:** Speech output is borderline fluent (6-8 words per utterance), with semantic paraphasias.

Auditory Comprehension

- **Answering Yes/No Questions:** Response accuracy affected by level of alertness.
- **Executing Commands:** Able to execute one-step commands when alert.
- **Understanding Stories & Paragraphs:** Impaired due to inability to maintain attention and concentration.
- **Understanding Conversational Speech:** Severely impaired at the conversational level due to lethargy and inattentiveness
- **Identifying Objects & Their Functions:** Able to name and identify common objects when alert and attentive.

Reading

- **Word-level Comprehension:** WFL for common words in large print.
- **Sentence-level Comprehension:** Moderately impaired at the paragraph level due to lack of attention at the time of assessment.
- **Oral Reading:** Reading aloud is slow and labored.
- **Oral Spelling:** Some difficulty spelling commonly used words; may be secondary to problems with declarative memory.

Written Expression

- **Copying:** WFL
- **Writing to Dictation:** Paragraphic errors noted.
- **Self-generated:** Functional for ADL needs: signature, address, names of family.
- **Written Spelling:** Paragraphic errors.
- **Drawing:** Able to execute simple line drawings when alert.

Cognition

- **Attention/Concentration:** Poor.
- **Visuospatial Skills:** Functional but optimized with large print and pictures.
- **Memory:** Declarative functioning is impaired; procedural motor memory for ADLs is less impaired.
- **Executive Functions:** Cannot assess secondary to lethargy and inattention.

Behavioral Symptoms

- **Alertness:** Lethargic, but not oppositional. Cooperative, as able.
- **Deficit Awareness:** She is aware of her communication deficits as indicated by yes/no responses to questions.
- **Frustration:** None noted at the time of assessment.
- **Emotional Lability:** None noted.
- **Current Personality Characteristics:** Cannot determine at the time of assessment due to lethargy.

Figure 5–2. Diagnostic profile for Winnie.

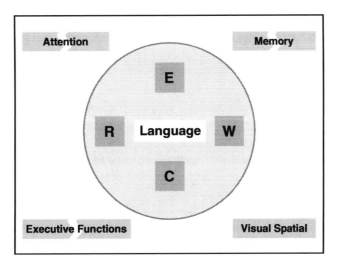

Figure 5–3. Acquired Language Disorders Target Model for Winnie.

Critical Thinking/Learning Activity

1. What would you do to determine if Winnie's processing deficit is an aphasic symptom or simply a complication of her lethargy?
2. Why will Winnie benefit from multimodality cueing?
3. Which of Winnie's strengths can you use to facilitate improvement in her weaker areas?
4. Given her symptoms, what type of subcortical aphasia does Winnie exhibit?
5. Why would you want to facilitate Winnie's self-monitoring of her speech output?

Treatment Considerations

Winnie's lethargy will affect her ability to participate in the therapy, especially in the acute phase. Therefore, the clinician's first task is to arouse the patient to a level of alertness (LOA) that supports her ability to participate in therapy. Daily monitoring of her LOA is essential for determining when to initiate direct intervention. Noting the changes in her gaze, eye contact, facial expression, and so forth, are practical ways to monitor her LOA prior to each session. The three primary areas that need to be addressed in this case in order to optimize Winnie's functional communication are:

- Word retrieval
- Auditory comprehension
- Semantic paraphasias

Once her LOA supports direct treatment, consider the following:

- It is important to demonstrate patience. Winnie may need more time to process a simple command and respond.
- Supplement information presented auditorily with pictures and words in large print format. This will optimize her response by engaging her visual attention system.
- Train Winnie in the use of self-cuing strategies to compensate for her word retrieval deficit. For example, you can teach her how to use phonemic self-cues to facilitate word retrieval. You can also instruct her in self-cuing with descriptive cues, that is, describe the object's characteristics, but this may be more difficult for her due to her semantic paraphasias.
- Contextual cues methods can be effective, that is, avoid confrontation naming approaches but use and talk about objects in a functional context related to a purpose. For example, talk about getting dressed for the day and facilitate discussion about the necessary items needed to accomplish this activity of daily living. Consider cotreating with occupational therapy during morning ADL treatment.
- To develop the ability to self-monitor, speech output is essential in a patient presenting with semantic paraphasias. This can be very challenging for the clinician depending on the severity of the auditory comprehension impairment. However, there are a few things that you can do to optimize this function. First, always use an auditory alerting signal to increase Winnie's attention to the incoming signal. This can be a tap on the desk or even a statement such as "Winnie, listen." If you ask Winnie an open-ended question such as, "What do you put on your feet?," and she answers "hat" instead of "shoe" try the following method. First, ask her if "hat" was correct. If she says, "No," you can facilitate the target word with a phonemic cue. On the other hand, if she said, "Yes," indicating her inability to self-monitor, then provides the correct word accompanied by a picture or real object of the target. The clinician can heighten her awareness of her errors by feeding back the incorrect word choices with a questioning intonation. Be sure to instruct Winnie to "listen to herself very carefully" so that she can pick out her incorrect word choices. She would then use her self-cuing techniques for naming that you trained. Notice how self-monitoring and naming are entwined in this case and in many others that you will encounter.

Some Therapeutic Options

- Schuell's Stimulation Approach to Rehabilitation (Duffy & Coelho, 2001)
- Cognitive Stimulation: Stimulation of Recognition/Comprehension, Memory and Thinking (Chapey, 2001)
- Any program that works on the parallel distributed processing (PDP) model of language function (Chapey, 2001)

Primary Progressive Aphasia

Introduction

Primary Progressive Aphasia (PPA) can be classified as a clinical syndrome with three variants based on motor speech, linguistic, and cognitive features (Wilson et al., 2010). The three variants of PPA are *nonfluent*, *semantic*, and *logopenic*. Patients presenting with the nonfluent variant had speech characterized by slow rate, articulatory distortions, paragrammatism with limited linguistic complexity. For those presenting with the semantic type of PPA, their speech was characterized by a normal rate, but very few syntactic and articulatory errors. However, they exhibit increased lexical retrieval deficits. In patients with the logopenic variant, speech rate was more normalized. Articulatory distortions and syntactic errors were less evident, and lexical retrieval was less impaired. Cortical atrophy was linked to both anterior and posterior language areas in individuals with reduced speech rate. Deficits in the frontal area were linked to motor speech impairment and syntactic abnormalities, and lexical retrieval deficits were associated with anterior and inferior temporal regions. Lesions in the posterior temporal regions were linked to phonological errors and disruptions to speech fluency. These findings reveal the multidimensional aspects of PPA.

Characteristics

PPA is of unknown etiology and is progressive and currently untreatable. It is a form of dementia characterized by a degeneration of the language functions, reading, writing, speaking, and comprehension. Onset is insidious with a gradual and slow decline. PPA can be associated with other neurologic symptoms and these include: dysarthria, dysphagia, oral apraxia, right central facial droop or weakness, right extremity weakness, and limb apraxia (Kavrie & Duffy, 1994; McNeil, 1998). On autopsy, other pathologic diagnoses have been associated with PPA. These include progressive supranuclear palsy, corticobasal degeneration, corticonigral degeneration, amyotrophic lateral sclerosis (ALS), and Creutzfeldt-Jacob disease (Mandel, Alexander, & Carpenter, 1989). It is also known as a slowly progressive aphasia. Initially, memory and other cognitive abilities, as well as personality, remain intact. However, over time, other mental faculties begin to deteriorate. This is considered a precursor to dementia or Alzheimer's disease, and onset tends to be in younger people with symptoms often beginning in the fifth decade of life. The average age of onset tends to be around 60 years and the incidence is higher in males than females. The site of degeneration in PPA is usually in the left frontotemporal-parietal region (perisylvian). Patients with early signs of PPA initially present with word finding difficulties in both speaking and writing tasks. They also demonstrate semantic word substitutions (*car/bus*); phonemic word substitutions (*pin/bin*); and circumlocutions ("I went to the place that you buy the paper," referring to "I went to the newsstand"). In the early stages of this process, they can maintain normal activities of daily living because memory and other cognitive skills are still intact. These patients have difficulty following conversations and participating in groups. They have diminished use of expressive language, and their verbal output can be devoid of meaning. Later in the disease process, they demonstrate difficulty with numbers and performing simple mathematical calculations. PPA is often known as a cortical degeneration syndrome (Caselli, 1995). Research has found that that any type of aphasic symptom is possible and that individuals at earlier stages tend to sound fluent. However, as the disease progresses, individuals progress to a more nonfluent expressive profile (Weintraub, Rubin, & Mesulam, 1990).

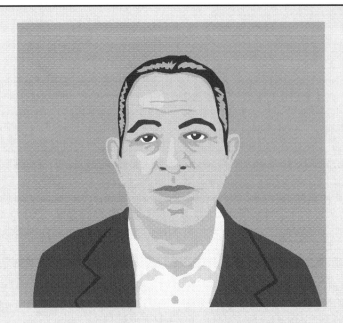

Case Scenario: Luis

History and Physical (H & P): 58-year-old, right-handed, Hispanic male, taken to physician's office by daughter who complained of his speech and language difficulties; right extremity clumsiness; no gross physical weakness; noted difficulty with word finding; articulation of speech unclear with sound substitutions. Luis is cognitively intact according to his daughter.

Past Medical History (PMH): Patient complains of language difficulty over 2 years; previous imaging studies have identified focal atrophy in language zone; slight HTN but otherwise in good health.

Social History: Widower with one adult daughter; lives with daughter in two-bedroom apartment; worked as a retail clerk at a local home improvement store (duties now limited to stock clerk due to difficulty communicating). Patient is cognitively intact and does not believe he is having any difficulty with his mental abilities; independent in most ADLs (activities of daily living) at home and at work.

Surgical History: Hernia repair 10 years prior.

A Functional Analysis of Luis's Primary Progressive Aphasia

Luis's ability to understand language is intact (see Figure 5–4 for Luis' Diagnostic Profile and Figure 5–5 for his ALD Target Model). He enjoys interacting with others in conversation although he is often frustrated by his word finding difficulties and reduced speech intelligibility. Despite his frustration and looming depression, Luis remains motivated to improve his functional communication.

Language Expression

- **Automatic Speech:** WFL for counting, reciting the alphabet, stating days and months of the year.
- **Repetition Ability:** Repetition of multisyllabic words is impaired.
- **Lexical Retrieval-Naming:** Difficulty with lexical retrieval. Often states he knows what he wants to say but can't find the words.
- **Conversational Ability:** Unable to carry on a fluent conversation.
- **Pragmatic Skills:** Understands the rules of conversation but his word-finding, and verbal nonfluency affect his pragmatic language.
- **Paraphasias:** Semantic paraphasias are present with similarly categorized words often substituted.

Speech

- **Rate:** Slow rate of speech.
- **Intelligibility:** WFL in known and unknown contexts.
- **Prosody:** Aprosodic speech with inappropriate inflection, rhythm, and stress.
- **Articulation:** Mild spastic dysarthria characterized by articulatory distortions and dysprosody.
- **Fluency:** Diminished use of expressive language. Average phrase length varies but is generally 4 words or less.

Auditory Comprehension

- **Answering Yes/No Questions:** WFL for concrete and personal questions.
- **Executing Commands:** WFL
- **Understanding Stories & Paragraphs:** Comprehension for words and sentences is relatively intact. Paragraph length material is good for concrete concepts.
- **Understanding Conversational Speech:** Relatively intact; however comprehension is impaired at the conversational level with multiple conversational partners.
- **Identifying Objects & Their Functions:** WFL

Reading

- **Word-level Comprehension:** WFL
- **Sentence-level Comprehension:** WFL
- **Oral Reading:** Oral reading is WFL but deteriorates as word length increases.

Written Expression

- **Copying:** WFL for common words.
- **Writing to Dictation:** WFL for basic words.
- **Self-generated:** Characterized by semantic and phonological paraphasias.
- **Written Spelling:** Paragraphic.
- **Oral Spelling:** Able to spell common words when given the word verbally.
- **Drawing:** WFL

Cognition

- **Attention/Concentration:** WFL
- **Visuospatial Skills:** Can read print and identify photos and pictures.
- **Memory:** Procedural, semantic and episodic WFL for ADLs.
- **Executive Functions:** Problem solving skills and reasoning intact for ADL needs.

Behavioral Symptoms

- **Alertness:** WFL
- **Deficit Awareness:** Aware of speech production and language difficulties and attempts to self-correct.
- **Frustration:** Very frustrated and becoming depressed. Motivated to improve.
- **Emotional Lability:** None noted.
- **Current Personality Characteristics:** Pleasant, sociable, and motivated to improve.

Figure 5–4. Diagnostic profile for Luis.

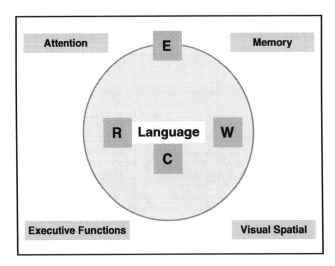

Figure 5–5. Acquired Language Disorders Target Model for Luis.

He is aware of his speech and language difficulties and tries to self-correct; however, his family is skeptical about his true understanding of the progressive nature of this disease process. Cognitively, Luis demonstrates good attentional skills and is very willing to work in therapy. His episodic, semantic, and procedural memory systems for ADLs are functioning within normal limits at this time, based on his activities in the home. Visuospatial skills appear intact, and he is able to read, print, and identify photos and pictures. Currently, Luis demonstrates normal problem-solving skills and can reason to make appropriate decisions during the day at home. For example, Luis can dress and groom himself and can prepare a simple meal independently. He still plays poker and rummy with his close friends regularly, with an adaptive tray for card organization and manipulation.

Critical Thinking/Learning Activity

- Given that this patient has articulation difficulties and oral apraxia, what information in his history helps to differentiate apraxia from dysarthria?
- In what ways does this patient resemble a nonfluent aphasic?
- What would be your rationale for providing treatment or not providing treatment to Luis? Select a position and defend it based on the information about PPA and Luis's profile.
- What kind of counseling and education would you provide to Luis's family? Please include content information as well as emotional support.

Treatment Considerations

Luis is strong in many communication areas. His auditory comprehension and reading comprehension are near normal. He is able to understand linguistic material at the paragraph level and is able to follow a conversation with one communication partner. Luis is able to count, name the days of the week and the months of the year, which are important for ADL needs. His sentence length is four words or fewer. Luis's primary weaknesses are his dysarthria and his word finding difficulties. These two deficits combine to reduce Luis's ability to be a functional communicator in all social contexts. However, a complication in Luis's case that is not found in the other aphasic syndromes is that PPA is progressive and degenerative. Because Luis has a strong social support network, is motivated to engage in treatment, and has other cognitive strengths (attention and memory), treatment should be considered. Because of the nature of Luis's profile, the clinician needs to have multiple foci of treatment, which are:

- Maintaining functional communication over the long term of the disease process, as possible, using any modality available to Luis.
- Building on Luis's stronger language skills to optimize his functional communication in the short term.
- Establishing an alternative communication method, for example, gesture or augmentative devices.
- Train Luis in the use of compensatory speech strategies to increase his speech intelligibility in known and unknown contexts.
- Facilitate word finding ability to reduce frustration and increase verbal fluency
- Provide ongoing family counseling and education regarding the goals and procedures of therapy across the course of the disease.

Some Therapeutic Options

- Lexical-Semantic Activation Inhibition Treatment (L-SAIT; McNeil, Small, Masterson, & Fossett, 1995)
- SFA (for Semantic Feature Analysis; Boyle & Coelho, 1995)
- AAC devices and software
- LPAA (for Life Participation Approach to Aphasia; Chapey et al., 2008)
- Speech conservation strategies to optimize intelligibility
- Back to the Drawing Board (Morgan & Helm-Estabrooks, 1987)
- Support group for patients and families dealing with PPA

Acquired Alexia and Agraphia

Characteristics

To explain the processes of alexia, it is necessary to provide the reader with some fundamental knowledge of normal reading. The goal in reading is for words to be comprehended via print, yet it is possible for a person to read without obtaining any meaning from the text. However, initially, in order to read with meaning, one must connect letters to sounds that blend together to form words or read a word as a whole unit. Words then activate semantic knowledge, and the written text can be understood. Once this process becomes automatic, an individual typically reads fluently via whole word recognition. The following sections introduce the three routes of normal reading. With this knowledge, the reader should better comprehend the processes of phonological alexia, surface alexia, and deep alexia.

Characteristics of Normal Reading

The visual information presented as words on the page is projected to the extrastriate cortex in the right occipital lobe. Early visual analysis (EVA) of words can be interpreted via three types of reading routes: *phonic*, *direct*, and *lexical*. For the phonic route, there is an EVA for letters. This requires learning abstract symbols as graphemes (written letters corresponding to sounds in a language). Here, visual information travels via the corpus callosum to the left temporal lobe for phonemic coding. After the letters are parsed or separated for individual coding, graphemes are connected with phonemes (sounds for the letters) to be blended into words. Auditory cues help decipher the word through the angular gyrus and the supramarginal gyrus. For example, children learning to read the word *cat* via the *phonic route* will learn the corresponding sound for each letter. After the letters are parsed for individual coding, they are blended together to sound out the word *cat* and connect it with its real-life object. If the *direct route* is used, the EVA works with whole words. Whole word recognition travels to Broca's area through the arcuate fasciculus. The word can then be read aloud. If the *lexical route* is used, the

EVA works with a *morphological decomposer*. In this context, for example, a young child learning to read the word *teacher* will decompose the *–er* morpheme as the lexical marker for "one who teaches." Another example of morphological decomposition is in the morph *–ology,* meaning "the study of," being separated from the morph attached to it—rheumatology, biology, morphology, and so forth. Therefore in the lexical route, these words produce semantic representations for comprehension of the written word. Ultimately, the insular cortex automatizes the process to permit rapid automatic word recognition with comprehension. Information is sent to the frontal lobes for output, that is, reading aloud (Duffy & Geschwind, 1985). It is important to understand that the phonic, direct, and lexical routes are operating simultaneously in a normal, fluent reader.

Alexia

An individual can have a breakdown in any of the three reading routes. A breakdown in the phonic route produces a phonological alexia; a breakdown in the direct route may lead to surface alexia; and a breakdown in the lexical route may lead to a deep alexia. *Graphemes*, or letters corresponding to the sounds of a language, are converted to sounds which can be read. The graphemes also activate the semantic system when read and understood. A foundational process necessary for reading and writing requires the ability to turn sounds into letters, that is, phonemes into graphemes, so that the meaning of a word can be activated, and thus understood by the reader.

According to Chapey (2001), the semantic system is at the central point in the reading and writing process (p. 573). She depicts both *lexical-semantic* and *sublexical* routes for both reading and writing. There are three primary routes that can activate the semantic system: the *visual representation* (object or picture), the *phonological input lexicon route* (sound-to-letter correspondence), and the *graphemic input lexicon route* (letter-to-sound correspondence). The visual representation route uses a visual object or picture to convey meaning. This direct path allows a person to see an image, for example, a flower, and know what it is. The phonological input lexicon route converts a phoneme into a letter that can be written and read. This does not guarantee meaning. The third route is the graphemic input lexicon. Letters in print correspond to sounds that can then be read. This activates the semantic system when the word is understood.

Neurologic disease or damage can impair processing of the reading-writing system, so that comprehension and production of written words are no longer possible. Word length, word frequency, and the concrete nature of the word itself all contribute to the problems individuals have with reading.

There are two broad classifications of alexia: central and peripheral. Central alexia is found in the presence of aphasia. Normal readers read by sound and by sight, that is, by sounding out words and by recognizing words. For example, recognizing the word *the,* yet sounding out the word *bibliography,* based on sound pattern and spelling rules in English. For a person with central alexia, there is impairment in using these two reading routes, producing the observable alexia. Table 5–2 provides a review of the types of central alexia, damage incurred, and salient features (Beeson & Hillis, 2001). Table 5–3 provides an overview of peripheral alexia profiles.

Peripheral alexia is defined as reading difficulties that occur without a concomitant aphasia. There are five types of peripheral alexia. A patient with global alexia reads very slowly and/or inaccurately, but can recognize letters, and numbers can be spared. A patient with pure alexia cannot read words and needs a letter-by-letter strategy to do so. When the patient spells the word aloud, reading comprehension is better. Hemianopic alexia is characterized by an inability to read prefixes and suffixes; and in a neglect alexia, prefixes are more in error than suffixes. The patient presenting with an attentional alexia will crowd letters together and merge words.

Leff et al. (2001) investigated single-word reading in patients with hemianopsia and pure alexia. Pure alexia has been defined as a severe disturbance in reading comprehension with linguistically accurate writing, normal oral spelling, and the absence of aphasia or dementia. Pure alexia results from an inability to map letters in a familiar sequence to mental representation of the word. For those with pure alexia, it is a right hemianopsia that may impede single-word reading due to an inability to

see letters at the end of a word. The work of Leff et al. (2001) demonstrated patients with hemianopic alexia activating the left occipitotemporal junction, although there was lack of input from the ipsilateral primary and prestriate visual cortex. Therefore, it was determined that destruction of the left occipitotemporal junction can result in a severe impairment of word recognition or pure alexia. It has been noted that alexia resulting from a middle cerebral artery (MCA) stroke accompanies a generalized language disorder. A person with a mild naming deficit may also have pure alexia if it is associated with a left posterior cerebral artery infarct. Although rare, there have been reported cases of pure alexia without hemianopsia, and for those individuals, there was often a generalized language disorder (Iragui & Kritchevsky, 1991; Sinn & Blanken, 1999).

Agraphia

Agraphia (or dysgraphia) is a term used to indicate a writing impairment. Agraphia reflects a lexical-semantic breakdown. Links between written words and their meanings are impaired. Letters and sound associations are often affected. Deep agraphia involves impairment with written semantics. High-frequency words, high-imagery words, and nouns are often written with greater ease. Patients presenting with deep agraphia make substitutions of one word for another word, although semantically related (i.e., table for chair). In that situation, there is a disturbance in sublexical and lexical processes required for spelling.

Lexical agraphia, also known as surface agraphia, is a written impairment in which the person relies heavily on sound-to-letter conversions. Words with irregular spellings are often written as they sound ("right" written as "rit"). Phonological agraphia is the term used to describe the impairment experienced by a person who cannot write non-words (for example, "prask") due to sublexical sound-to-letter conversion problems; however, patients with phonological agraphia can write familiar words.

Surface agraphia is another term used to describe an acquired writing impairment whereby the person reads by converting each letter to a sound so that irregularly spelled words are not pronounced correctly.

Table 5–2. Types of Central Alexia

Central Alexia	Damage	Salient Features
Phonological Alexia (reads by sight)	▪ Cannot sound out the phonemes associated with the graphemes, so the meaning of words cannot be obtained (impaired graphemic input lexicon)	▪ Cannot sound out words ▪ Sound-symbol disassociation ▪ Relies on word shape to facilitate reading ▪ Uses memory as a strategy to facilitate reading. ▪ May benefit from retraining letter-to-sound correspondence
Surface Alexia (reads by sound)	▪ Impaired representation of translating the way the word looks to its meaning (graphemic input lexicon) ▪ A variant of this is difficulty noted when the person regularizes irregularly spelled words (impaired phonological output lexicon)	▪ Visually perceived words that were once familiar are no longer identifiable or meaningful ▪ Relies heavily on sounding out words letter by letter to facilitate reading ▪ Irregular words such as "rhythm" are difficult ▪ Has difficulty making reading "automatic" ▪ May regularize a word that is spelled irregularly ("yacht" may be read as "yet") ▪ Typically seen in individuals with progressive language deterioration or other neurodegenerative processes ▪ May benefit from work on phoneme-grapheme pairs to sound out letters in words (establish a key word for each letter) ▪ High-frequency words are easier ▪ Written words may cue speech output (reading aloud)
Deep Alexia (both sound and sight routes damaged)	▪ Difficulty recognizing written words, understanding their meaning, and sounding out words using letter-to-sound conversions (semantics and letter-to-sound correspondence impairment)	▪ There may be semantic errors in oral reading, visual errors for words that look similar, and substitutions of words within a word class ▪ Nouns are more easily read compared with adjectives due to their conceptual saliency ▪ Adjectives are easier than verbs, and verbs are easier than function words ▪ Abstract, low-frequency words are most difficult ▪ Error words may be linked to the target word through association (e.g., reading *dinner* as *food*). ▪ May benefit from methods to associate sounds with letters

Table 5–3. Types of Peripheral Alexia

Peripheral Subtype	Damage	Salient Features
Global	- Left ventrolateral occipitotemporal cortex (VLOT) or splenium of corpus callosum	- Slow or inaccurate letter naming - Can recognize letters and often numbers
Pure Alexia (Alexia without Agraphia)	- Left VLOT or connections - Can see the letters but cannot identify the group of letters as a visual word with meaning (impaired access to graphemic input lexicon)	- Slow and inaccurate reading, short words are easier - Cannot recognize strings of letters as words, although knows the letters - Writing is intact - Spelling the word helps identify it - Usually benefits from letter-by-letter reading with shorter words easier or palm tracing (using tactile cues to imprint traced letters on the palm of the hand) - May benefit from brief exposure to single words with repeated reading aloud
Hemianopic	- Homonymous hemianopia, often macular-splitting, often postgeniculate	- Slow but accurate text reading - May miss prefix or suffix - Left-sided more disabling than when in right visual fields
Neglect	- Right parietal lobe	- Errors on prefixes more frequent than on suffixes
Attentional	- Left parietal lobe	- Words merged - Letter crowding - Reads better with isolated words

For example, the word "know" may be read with the /k/ audible. Patients presenting with surface agraphia can spell regular and nonsense words using phoneme-to-graphemes conversion, but they misspell irregular words and homophones, e.g. "sweet" and "suite." Barriere (2002) indicated in most people with aphasia, writing is the most impaired language function. Most often, patients with Broca's aphasia or a transcortical motor aphasia have nonfluent agraphia and difficulty spelling (Duffy & Ulrich, 1976). Patients who do not have aphasia but have agraphia and alexia usually have parietal lobe lesions (Roeltgen, 1997).

Various treatment approaches can be found in Barriere (2002). One example is that of Beeson, Rewega, Vail, and Rapcsak (2000), in which thegoal was to help the patients problem-solve their spelling errors. In their research with patients who had spelling difficulties with a mild anomia, they taught them to use plausible misspellings gathered from sound-to-letter conversions. After writing words as they sounded, the task was to teach to patients to carefully monitor and self-correct spelling errors by considering their knowledge of the lexicon. They used an electronic speller that was able to accept plausible misspellings. Another fruitful treatment approach for individuals with Wernicke's aphasia and deficits at the level of graphemic output is the Anagram, Copy, and Recall Treatment, ACRT (Beeson, 1999). See Appendix D for a full description of this program.

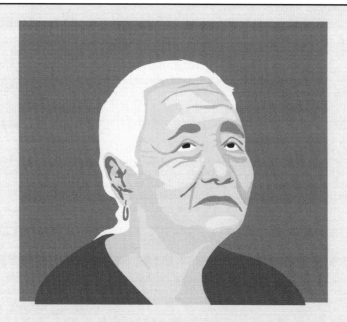

Case Scenario: Sue

History and Physical (H & P): 69-year-old, right-handed, Asian female, referred for outpatient cognitive-linguistic therapy 6 months status post (s/p), fell while shoveling snow; patient suffered a left hemispheric stoke in the distribution area of the posterior cerebral artery (PCA).

Past Medical History (PMH): HTN, Diabetes Mellitus Type II, hypercholesterolemia; family history of cardiac problems.

Social History: Divorced; no children; lives alone with two cats; worked part-time as a teacher's aid in a local elementary school. Patient upset about inability to work with children reading at school. ADLs (activities of daily living) are within normal limits (WNL).

Surgical History: Unremarkable.

A Functional Analysis of Sue's Alexia

Sue's reading skills are significantly impaired and should be the focus of her therapy (see Figure 5–6 for Sue's Diagnostic Profile and Figure 5–7 for her ADL Target Model.) The therapist will need to decide if her approach will be restitutive or substitutive based on the residual reading that Sue still possesses. She is unable to participate in her favorite avocation—reading. Combining therapy for her word retrieval problem with therapy for her alexia would be efficient. Furthermore, the natural relationship between writing/reading/naming will facilitate growth in each. The therapist will have to deal with Sue's frustration and anger over her impairment, especially as reading held such a prominent place in her life.

Language Expression

- **Automatic Speech:** WFL for counting, reciting the alphabet, stating days, and months of the year.
- **Repetition Ability:** Repeating phrases and sentences are WFL.
- **Lexical Retrieval-Naming:** Able to retrieve words with relative ease in discourse, however confrontation naming is a problem.
- **Conversational Ability:** Syntax is WNL.
- **Pragmatic Skills:** All social language skills WFL.
- **Paraphasias:** None.

Speech

- **Rate:** WFL when not reading.
- **Intelligibility:** WFL when not reading.
- **Prosody:** WFL for inflection, rhythm, and stress of speech during conversation.
- **Articulation:** WFL when not reading.
- **Fluency:** WFL; average phrase length is 8+ words. Fluent speech output with ability to self-correct.

Auditory Comprehension

- **Answering Yes/No Questions:** WFL
- **Executing Commands:** WFL
- **Understanding Stories & Paragraphs:** WFL
- **Understanding Conversational Speech:** Comprehension for words and sentences is intact. Can engage in conversational dialogue with minimal difficulty.
- **Identifying Objects & Their Functions:** WFL

Reading

- **Word-level Comprehension:** Compromised with difficulty processing word forms as a whole unit. Slow and inaccurate reading attempted with moderate-severe difficulty reading words. Short, common, and concrete words may be understood.
- **Sentence-level Comprehension:** Impaired due to the reliance on sounding out words letter by letter. To facilitate rereading.
- **Oral Reading:** Present difficulty reading aloud especially with irregularly spelled words, abstract words, and at the sentence level. Inaccurate pronunciation of those words attempted. Slow and labored. Some residual whole-word reading retained.
- **Oral Spelling:** WFL for spelling concrete regularly spelled words' often relies on spelling letters to read words.

Written Expression

- **Copying:** WFL
- **Writing to Dictation:** WFL
- **Self-generated:** Writing is unaffected. Performs at same level prior to illness. Can write letters and take notes as necessary.
- **Written Spelling:** WFL for regularly spelled words.
- **Drawing:** WFL

Cognition

- **Attention/Concentration:** WFL
- **Visuospatial Skills:** WFL
- **Memory:** WFL
- **Executive Functions:** WFL

Behavioral Symptoms

- **Alertness:** WFL
- **Deficit Awareness:** Aware of reading difficulty and attempts to improve daily using closed-caption television at home.
- **Frustration:** Frustrated with inability to return to work as a teacher's aid.
- **Emotional Lability:** None.
- **Current Personality Characteristics:** Frustrated, angry, and sad.

Figure 5–6. Diagnostic profile for Sue.

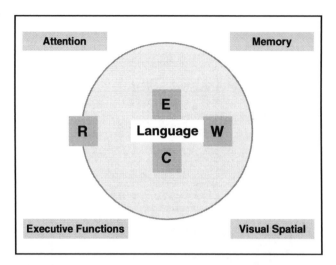

Figure 5–7. Acquired Language Disorders Target Model for Sue.

As a consequence, the therapist may want to point out the small successes that Sue makes, counseling her that these building blocks are crucial for any restitution of her reading ability. Sue's cognitive abilities are within functional limits that allow her to understand the implications of her deficits. This is advantageous from a treatment perspective.

Critical Thinking/Learning Activity

- What information indicates that this is a person with a pure alexia?
- How will Sue's reading problems affect her activities of daily living?
- What are the family counseling and education issues in this case, and how would you address them?
- Prepare a script reflecting a conversation between you and a caregiver who is trying to understand the complexity of Sue's reading problem.
- Write a SOAP note on this patient. Assume that you are seeing her for the first time after the evaluation session. Include three of the Short-Term Therapeutic Objectives in your note.

Treatment Considerations

Sue demonstrates functional receptive and expressive verbal language abilities. She is able to communicate effectively with her friends, watch TV with comprehension, and engage in normal phone conversations. Her speech is intelligible in all known and unknown contexts. However, her alexia has had a significant impact on her ability to return to work at the school and enjoy her favorite pastime: reading.

■ There are two general types of treatment for alexia—*restitutive* and *substitutive.*

■ Restitutive Treatment approaches are designed to restore the impaired ability to its premorbid level. This is done by facilitating the underlying processes of reading.

   1. Present written words on cards and present them rapidly to discourage letter-by-letter reading.

   2. Use any method and materials that force the patient into relying on the residual whole-word skills that they may have.

■ Substitutive Treatment approaches are designed to compensate for the absent reading skills.

   1. Allow the patient to write the letter as she reads it, that is, use a kinesthetic modality to support the oral reading.

   2. Use any multimodality approach—tactile, tactile-kinesthetic, and visual—that can support the patient's reading of a letter or word.

Some Therapeutic Options

■ Consider using the ACRT (Beeson, 1999)

■ Successful blending in a phonological reading treatment for deep alexia (Friedman & Lott, 2002)

■ Computer-provided reading treatments (Katz & Wertz, 1997)

■ Oral Reading for Language in Aphasia with Virtual Therapist (ORLA VT; Cherney et al., 2005)

   ■ Alexia Treatments in Perspectives on Neurophysiology and Neurogenic Speech and Language Disorders (Greenwald & George, 2002)

   ■ A Treatment Sequence for Phonological Alexia/Agraphia (Beeson, Rising, Kim, & Rapcsak, 2010) See review in Appendix E at the end of this text.

   ■ Concurrent Treatment for Reading and Spelling in Aphasia (CART and ORT; Beeson, Rising, & Volk, 2003; Orjada & Beeson, 2005)

References

Beeson, P. (1999). Treating acquired writing impairment: Strengthening graphemic representations. *Aphasiology, 13,* 767–785.

Beeson, P. M., & Hillis, A. E. (2001). Comprehension and production of written words. In R. Chapey (Ed.), *Language intervention strategies in aphasia and related neurogenic communication disorders* (4th ed., pp. 572–604). Philadelphia, PA: Lippincott Williams & Wilkins.

Beeson, P. M., Rewega, M., Vail, S., & Rapcsak, S. (2000). Problem-solving approach to agraphia treatment: Interactive uses of lexical and sublexical spelling routes. *Aphasiology, 14,* 551–565.

Beeson, P. M., Rising, K., Kim, E. S., & Rapcsak, S. Z. (2010). A treatment sequence for phonological alexia/agraphia. *Journal of Speech, Language, and Hearing Research, 53,* 450–468.

Beeson, P. M., Rising, K, & Volk, J. (2003). Writing treatment for severe aphasia: Who benefits. *Journal of Speech, Language and Hearing Research, 46,* 1038–1060.

Bhatnagar, C. (2013). *Neuroscience for the study of communicative disorders* (4th ed., pp. 447–448). Baltimore, MD: Lippincott Williams & Wilkins.

Boyle, M., & Coelho, C. A. (1995). Application of semantic feature analysis as a treatment for aphasic dysnomia. *American Journal of Speech-Language Pathology, 4*, 94–98.

Cappa, S. F., Cavallotti, G., Guidotti, M., Papagno, C., & Vignolo, L. A. (1983). Subcortical aphasia: Two clinical CT scan correlation studies. *Cortex, 19*, 227–241.

Caselli, R. J. (1995). Focal and asymmetric cortical degeneration syndromes. *Neurologist, 1*(1), 1–19.

Chapey, R. (Ed.). (2001). *Language intervention strategies in aphasia and related neurogenic communication disorders* (4th ed.). Philadelphia, PA: Lippincott Williams & Wilkins.

Chapey, R., Duchan, J. F., Elman, R. J., Garcia, L. J., Kagan, A., Lyon, J. G., & Simmons-Mackie, N. (2008). Life-participation approach to aphasia: A statement of values for the future. In R. Chapey (Ed.), *Language intervention strategies in aphasia and related neurogenic communication* (5th ed., pp. 279–289). Philadelphia, PA: Lippincott Williams & Wilkins.

Cherney, L. R., Babbitt, E. M., Cole, R., Van Vuuren, S., Hurwitz, R., Lee, J., & Ngampatipatpong, N. (2005). Oral reading for language in aphasia with virtual therapist. *The Center for Spoken Language Research (CSLR)*. Retrieved from http://clear.colorado.edu/start/orla/orla.html

Davis, G. A. (2007). Cognitive pragmatics of language disorders in adults. *Seminars in Speech and Language, 28*(2), 111–121.

Duffy, J. R., & Coelho, C. A. (2001). Schuell's stimulation approach to rehabilitation. In R. Chapey (Ed.), *Language intervention strategies in aphasia and related neurogenic communication disorders* (4th ed., pp. 403–449). Philadelphia, PA: Lippincott Williams & Wilkins.

Duffy, F. H., & Geschwind, N. (1985). *Dyslexia: A neuroscientific approach to clinical evaluation*. Boston, MA: Little, Brown & Company.

Duffy, R., & Ulrich, S. (1976). A comparison of impairments in verbal comprehension in speech, reading and writing in adult aphasics. *Journal of Speech and Hearing Disorders, 4*, 110–119.

Friedman, R., & Lott, N. (2002). Successful blending in a phonological reading treatment for deep aphasia. *Aphasiology, 16*(3), 355–372.

Greenwald, M., & George, P. (2002). Alexia. *Perspectives on Neurophysiology and Neurogenic Speech and Language Disorders, 12*(1), 4–13.

Han, M., Kang, D., Bae, H., Oh, G., & Jeong, S. (2003). Aphasia in striatocapsular infarction may be explained by concomitant small cortical infarctions of cortical language zones. *Stroke, 34*, 259.

Hillis, A. E., Work, M., Barker, P. B., Jacobs, M. A., Breese, E. L., & Maurer, K. (2004). Re-examining the brain regions crucial for orchestrating speech articulation. *Brain, 127*(Pt. 7), 1479–1487.

Iragui, V. J., & Kritchevsky, M. (1991). Alexia without agraphia or hemianopia in parietal infarction. *Journal of Neurology, Neurosurgery, and Psychiatry, 54*, 841–842.

Katz, R., & Wertz, R. (1997). The efficacy of computer-provided reading treatment for chronic aphasic adults. *Journal of Speech, Language, and Hearing Research, 40*, 493–507.

Kavrie, S. H., & Duffy, J. R. (1994). *Primary progressive apraxia of speech*. Paper presented at the annual convention of the American Speech-Language-Hearing Association, New Orleans, Louisiana.

Kennedy, M., & Murdoch, B. (1993). Chronic aphasia subsequent to striato-capsular and thalamic lesions in the left hemisphere. *Brain and Language, 44*(3), 284–295.

Kent, R. D. (Ed.). (2004). *The MIT encyclopedia of communication disorders*. Cambridge, MA: Massachusetts Institute of Technology.

Kuljic-Obradovic, D. C. (2003). Subcortical aphasia: Three different language disorder syndromes? *European Journal of Neurology, 10*(4), 445–448.

Leff, A. P., Crewes, H., Plant, G. T., Scott, S. K., Kennard, C., Wise, R. J. (2001). The functional anatomy of single-word reading in patients with hemianopic and pure alexia. *Brain, 124*(Pt. 3), 510–521.

Mandel, A., Alexander, M., & Carpenter, S. (1989). Creutzfeldt-Jakob disease presenting as isolated aphasia. *Neurology, 39*, 55.

McNeil, M. R. (1998). The case of the lawyer's lugubrious language: Dysarthria plus primary progressive aphasia or dysarthria plus dementia? *Seminars in Speech and Language, 19*(1), 49–57.

McNeil, M. R., Small, S. L., Masterson, R. J., & Fossett, T. R. D. (1995). Behavioral and pharmacological treatment of lexical-semantic deficits in a single patient with primary progressive aphasia. *American Journal of Speech-Language Pathology, 4*, 76–87.

Morgan, A. L., & Helm-Estabrooks, N. (1987). Back to the drawing board: A treatment program for nonverbal aphasic patients. *Clinical Aphasiology, 16*, 34–39.

Murdoch, B., Thompson, D., Fraser, S., & Harrison, L. (1986). Aphasia following non-haemorraghic lesions in the left striato-capsular region. *Australian Journal of Human Communication Disorders, 14*(2), 5–21.

Nadeau, S., & Crosson, B. (1997). Subcortical aphasia, *Brain and Language, 58*(3), 355–402.

Nadeau, S. E., & Rothi, L. J. G. (2001). Rehabilitation of subcortical aphasia. In R. Chapey (Ed.), *Language intervention strategies in aphasia and related neurogenic communication disorders* (4th ed.). Philadelphia, PA: Lippincott Williams & Wilkins.

Naeser, M., Alexander, M., Helm-Estabrooks, N., Levine, N., Laughlin S., & Geschwind, N. (1982). Aphasia with predominantly subcortical lesion sites: Description of three capsular/putaminal aphasia syndromes. *Neurology, 39*(1), 2–14.

Orjada, S. A., & Beeson, P. M. (2005). Concurrent treatment for reading and spelling in aphasia. *Aphasiology, 19*, 341–351.

Roeltgen, D. P. (1997). Agraphia. In T. E. Feinberg & M. J. Farah (Eds.), *Behavioral neurology and neuropsychology.* New York, NY: McGraw-Hill.

Sinn, H., & Blanken, G. (1999). Visual errors in acquired dyslexia: Evidence for cascaded lexical processing. *Cognitive Neuropsychology, 16*, 631–653.

Vigneau, M., Beaucousin, V., Hervé, P. Y., Duffau, H., Crivello, F., Houdé, O. Mazoyer, B., & Tzourio-Mazoyer, N. (2006). Meta-analyzing left hemisphere language areas: Phonology, semantics, and sentence processing. *NeuroImage, 30*, 1414–1432

Vukovic, M., Sujic, R., Petrovic-Lazic, M., Miller, N., Milutinovic, D., Babac, S., & Vukovic, I. (2012). Analysis of voice impairment in aphasia after stroke-underlying neuroanatomical substrates. *Brain and Language, 123*(1), 22–29.

Webb, W. G., Adler, R. K., & Love, R. J. (2008). *Neurology for the speech- language pathologist.* St. Louis, MO: Mosby Elsevier.

Wilson, S. M., Henry, M. L., Besbris, M., Ogar, J. M., Dronkers, N. F., Jarrold, W., . . . Gomo-Tempini, M. L. (2010). Connected speech production in three variants of primary progressive aphasia. *Brain, 133*(7), 2069–2088.

Weintraub, S., Rubin, N. P., & Mesulam, M. M. (1990). Primary progressive aphasia: Longitudinal course, neurological profile and language features. *Archives of Neurology, 47*(12), 1329–1335.

Wise, R. J., Greene, J., Büchel, C., Scott, S. K. (1999). Brain regions involved in articulation. *Lancet, 353*(9158), 1057–1061.

Chapter 6

RIGHT HEMISPHERE DISORDER

Introduction

Individuals with right hemisphere disorder (RHD) typically do not have language problems as seen in those with aphasia. However, it is now well-established that unilateral damage to the right hemisphere can cause extralinguistic and paralinguistic deficits, which then produce communication impairment. Nevertheless, a referral for a cognitive-linguistic evaluation is not assured. In a retrospective study, Blake, Duffy, Myers, & Tompkins (2002) reviewed the medical charts of 123 patients who were admitted to an inpatient rehabilitation unit for RHD and found that only 45% were referred for speech-language pathology services, despite the fact that they presented with treatable communication and cognitive deficits. This suggests that referrals for speech-language pathology services are inadequate and underused in this clinical population.

The etiology of RHD can be stroke, trauma, tumor, or degenerative disease and damage to the right cortical and subcortical structures is more diffuse than with left hemispheric damage. The consequence of this is more widespread dysfunction. As noted above, people with RHD do not demonstrate frank language impairment, but do demonstrate deficits in areas related to communication. *Extralinguistic impairments* include poor attentional skills, memory deficits, and visualspatial difficulties. *Paralinguistic impairments* include pragmatic abnormalities: incohesive discourse, and tangential and circumlocutionary verbal output. It can be seen that a patient with a clinical presentation that includes these types of deficits will have problems in social

discourse on a daily basis. Furthermore, these extralinguistic and paralinguistic impairments can affect the patient's ability to be adequately assessed and, as a consequence, produce an inconclusive or incorrect language picture. Thus, the clinician must be alert to the presence of these features during the assessment.

Characteristics

Not all patients will present with the same communicative characteristics (Tompkins & Fassbinder, 2004), and this causes problems for experimental design, data analysis, and combined with small sample sizes, affects the value of the results. Therefore, obtaining a valid representation of the communication disorder associated with right hemisphere brain damage has been challenging. Despite this, research has been able to provide the clinician with both verbal and nonverbal findings applicable to this population.

The patient with a RHD presents with perceptual, cognitive, and emotional deficits. Interpretation of linguistic and nonlinguistic information is problematic as they do not readily use context clues and have difficulty identifying what is important information in a communicative event from that which is unimportant. Following conversational rules is difficult, and their speech can sound robotic due to an inability to vary prosody to reflect their emotional state at the time. Judgment and problem-solving abilities are also challenged. Nonlinguistic deficits are a hallmark in RHD. These patients may be disoriented to time and place, and have visuospatial deficits such as a left-sided neglect. Further complicating matters, the majority of RHD patients fail to recognize their own deficits (anosagnosia). In many cases, the patient with RHD does not fully understand the extent of their disorder.

Communication Deficits

The following list comprises deficits commonly associated with RHD:

- Difficulty organizing information
- Impaired discourse
- Difficulty summarizing information in a meaningful way
- Impulsivity in their responses
- Tangential and circumlocutionary speech
- Using unnecessary detail in verbal communication
- Difficulty deciding what is relevant versus what is irrelevant to the context of the communicative event
- Difficulty using contextual cues
- Literal interpretation of idioms and indirect requests
- Pragmatic deficits, for example, speaker's intentions, understanding other's motivation, and following conventions of conversation
- Reduced sensitivity to facial expression, gestures, body language, and the emotional content within verbal language
- Difficulty understanding inferences based on context clues.

RHD and Pragmatic Impairment

Pragmatic impairment as a result of damage to the right hemisphere is challenging to both the researcher and the clinician. For the researcher, uncovering the relationship between the right hemisphere and its paralinguistic functions is still ongoing and still unclear, and for the clinician, efficacious treatment techniques addressing the pragmatics of the communication dyad in this population remain elusive due to the variability and oftentimes subtle manifestations that alter the individual's communi-

cation. Weed (2011) suggests that an *emergentist* approach to understanding pragmatics has value and explanatory power, especially in patients with RHD.

Perkins (2005a, 2005b) introduced the idea that pragmatics is not an individual ability, but must be treated as a mutually constructed or emergent phenomenon between two people in conversation. Their mutual goal is to communicate a message. This is not only true for normally functioning people, but also in clinical populations whose language functions are impaired. For example, if a clinician asks a client, "What did you do today?," and the client responds by saying, "Work," Perkins considers this the client's attempt to maintain the conversational flow, and as such is a complete answer despite the desire for more details and ongoing discourse. Grice (1975), considered the founder of the study of pragmatics, would disagree in the sense that the client's response violates the principal of "quantity" in that not enough information is provided to encourage continued discourse. The important difference between using a *Gricean Model* to explain the clinical findings and *Perkin's Emergentist Model* is that for Perkins, conversation is viewed from the bottom-up and not from the top-down as it is for Grice (Weed, 2011). Grice prefers a logical framework in order to understand pragmatics, but Perkins prefers to start with the cognitive and biological elements that are readily available to the speakers. Furthermore, Perkins wants to account for both healthy pragmatics and pragmatics of the impaired individual, whereas Grice is not so inclined.

Perkins introduces the idea of *equilibrium* to the conversational dyad. *Equilibrium* can happen within an individual or between the two members of the communication dyad. *Disequilibrium* occurs when a speaker is unable to adequately express the desired idea due to linguistic impairment. In cases like this, the speaker may resort to gestures or facial expressions, and the therapist may decide to use a yes/no format versus an open-ended format in order to achieve a successful conversational outcome. Here one can see the mutually constructed feature that Perkins proposes in the emergentist model.

Finally, Perkins believes that pragmatics is based on three *interacting components*: *higher-level cognition* (e.g., theory of mind (ToM), *perception* (auditory and visual), and *motor function*, yet another example of Perkins' departure from the Gricean model of pragmatics. Of these elements, the role of ToM is not yet firmly decided in patients with RHD (Weed, 2011).

Weed (2011) proposed that conversational analysis (CA) can be applied to study pragmatics of people affected by RHD, primarily because CA takes the conversation between two or more speakers as its point of departure. This type of analysis could generate a clearer understanding of the conversational elements between an impaired individual (e.g., a RHD patient and a nonimpaired speaker). This in turn can lead to more refined and focused interventions for discourse and pragmatic difficulties in those patients.

The Role of Auditory Perception, Visual Perception, and Motor Perception in Pragmatics

Myers (1999) reported that people with RHD have problems understanding prosody and producing contextually-appropriate prosodic patterns. To use the prosodic information of any given speaker, the listener must be able to infer meaning from it as well as distinguish one pattern from any other. The right hemisphere seems to play a role in these functions (Weed, 2011).

As far as the role of visual perception in pragmatics, Weed (2011) reports on studies that firmly support the role of the right hemisphere for gleaning information from faces and facial expressions of the conversational partner. The *fusiform face area* (FFA) and the *occipital face area* are implicated, and both seem to be right-lateralized. In addition, Weed, McGregor, Feidbaek Nielsen, Roepstorff, and Frith (2010) reported on RHD patients who had difficulty on a mental-state attribution task that was based on motor cues. Their findings complemented previous findings of other researchers who indicated that the perception of complex motion, biological motion, and intentional motion were impaired in RHD patients (see Weed, 2011).

In summary, the research on pragmatics in RHD patients does point to an important role for the right hemisphere in processing faces, perceiving auditory information, and interpreting complex motion. The Target Model introduced in this text recommends that the clinician include visuospatial skills, higher level cognitive functions, as well as auditory processing into the assessment process. We also recommend, based on the current research, that the clinician probe the RHD patient's ability to process complex motion, by examining whether they can interpret motion cues (gesture and facial cues) in a conversational dyad.

Visual-Perceptual Deficits

The person with a right hemisphere syndrome can present with an array of visual-perceptual impairments. *Visual agnosias* can manifest as an inability to recognize objects or colors. The patient will see and even handle an object, for example, a blue cup, yet not be able to tell what it is. This can have a very significant impact on the patient's activities of daily living(ADLs). *Prosopagnosia* is defined as the inability to recognize faces, regardless of how familiar those faces are. Here again, one can see the devastating effects that this type of problem can have on a patient and his or her caregivers. Furthermore, this type of patient may also be unable to read facial expressions, for example, happy, sad, surprised, or angry. Difficulty with visual imagery can also have serious social consequences. *Simultagnosia* is a disorder in which the patient cannot process the entire visual scene before him or her, but only attends to one part of the whole. Thus, the person misses the meaning of the image before him or her. *Visual integration deficits* are also observed with this population. Patients with this disorder are unable to form a cohesive visual percept from the stimuli before them. The visual image is not processed as integrated whole, but rather as separate pieces. This problem along with *spatial disorientation* can affect the patient's ability to move around in space safely and efficiently.

Visuomotor Deficits

Associated with visual-perceptual problems are *visuomotor deficits*. The RHD patient may have difficulty dressing himself or herself as the patient is unable to orient his or her body to the placement of the clothing during dressing. From a diagnostic perspective, the patient will not be able to produce an accurate and correct clock drawing, and will be unable to construct objects in space, for example, build a tower of blocks or draw to express his or her needs. Both the drawings and the constructions will be inaccurate, indicating to the clinician that there is a visuomotor deficit present.

Auditory Perceptual Deficits

Although auditory perceptual deficits are more often observed with bilateral lesions, it is possible that the RHD patient will present with some type of auditory perceptual difficulty. *Sound localization* difficulty may be observed as well as *auditory agnosia,* that is, an inability to home in on the source of the auditory signal in space and the inability to recognize the sound as something familiar and/or meaningful. These patients also demonstrate problems with *discriminating prosodic patterns,* similar to the way that they are unable to discriminate facial expressions to convey meaning. The inability to perceive music appropriately is also a feature associated with RHD patients, and this may be a factor in the functional life of a patient, which should always be considered when planning treatment.

Cognitive Deficits

Attentional problems are very prevalent in this population. To sustain a dyadic communication, both partners must be attentive to the speech signal of the other. If the attention of one partner falters, then the probability that a successful communicative event will occur drops significantly. Furthermore, many patients with RHD present with left-sided neglect, or just an inattention to the left side. This can complicate the existing attentional problem because the patient is not able to make eye contact with the communication partner, unless he or she is on the patient's right side. A thorough chart review and diagnostic evaluation will highlight either of these issues for the speech-language pathologist.

The RHD patient may present with both *working memory* and *long-term memory* problems.

Working memory is critical to functional language processing, and long-term memory is necessary in order to access past knowledge and events. Deficits in both of these areas, although not directly related to speech and language, will affect the patient's ability to participate in social communication.

Clinicians working with RHD patients find that executive functioning is noticeably impaired. The neurophysiologic correlates to the relationship between the right hemisphere, and executive functioning is most commonly seen in these patients who are experiencing *planning difficulties,* impaired *problem-solving skills,* and difficulty *integrating* information. The role of attention in all of these functions is a critical element to performing them successfully, and as noted above, these patients have significant attentional problems (Patterson & Chapey, 2008).

As noted above, there are several non-linguistic deficits that often are encountered in persons with RHD. These primarily include left neglect, arousal deficits, and attention deficits including selective attention, more pronounced in the acute phase of the stroke. Myers (1998) reports that there tends to be less orientation to the environment in general. These patients also tend to have slower reaction times to both visual and auditory input, and in general, more intense stimulation is needed to facilitate attention than in a normally functioning individual. Because RHD patients tend to have reduced performance accuracy over time, attention for tasks is best when it is shorter in duration (Bub, Audet, & Lecours, 1990). Research indicates that if distracters are present, the person with RDH exhibits slower performance and less accuracy in their responses. Neglect also increases when greater attention is required to complete a task (Kaplan et al., 1991).

Another performance deficit of RHD is the patient's difficulty integrating components into a whole. For example, the individual may draw a tire above the car instead of under the car indicating that they understand the components but have difficulty organizing them together into a coherent unit. Difficulty integrating and organizing information may also impact the patient's ability to express himself or herself clearly in narrative form. These patients also tend to be tangential in their expressions, likely due to their difficulty staying on topic and getting to the point (Chapey, 2008).

Finally, it is worth mentioning that these paralinguistic and extralinguistic deficits are also associated with emotional factors. The clinician will note very soon after meeting an RHD patient that there is a flat facial affect, mirrored by a flat emotional affect. They have difficulty conveying emotions, and consequently, appear distant and remote. These patients also have an impaired ability to process and produce appropriate prosodic patterns as well as facial expressions that further complicate their social interactions post-stroke.

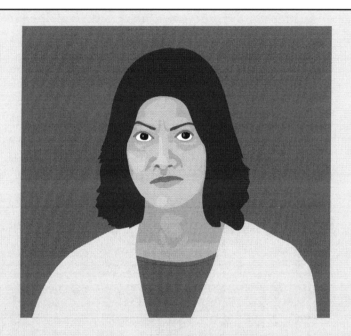

Case Scenario: Debra

History and Physical (H & P): 37-year old female, right-handed, admitted via Emergency Department with twitching of the left hand and left upper extremity weakness. A CT scan revealed an infarct in the right frontal area, highly suggestive of a cerebrovascular accident. Family reported seizure-like movements × 1 at bedtime. Left-sided hemiparesis was also noted; left neglect noted.

Past Medical History (PMH): Right partial thyroidectomy, insomnia, chronic bronchitis; difficulty with gait, urinary incontinence.

Social History: Married; one child (21 months old); PhD professor at a local university

Surgical History: status post (s/p) Thyroidectomy for a benign neoplasm.

A Functional Analysis of Debra

Debra's primary deficit areas are extralinguistic, prosodic, and cognitive (see Figure 6–1 for Debra's Diagnostic Profile and Figure 6–2 for her ADL Target Model).

Figure 6–1. Diagnostic profile for Debra.

Language Expression	**Automatic Speech:** WFL, able to count to 20, recite the alphabet, and name days and months of the year. **Repetition Ability:** WFL; difficulty noted with lengthy sentences (may be related to attentional deficit). **Lexical Retrieval-Naming:** WFL for confrontation naming and in conversation. **Conversational Ability:** Verbose, disorganized conversation with tangential and circumlocutionary output. Syntax WFL. **Pragmatic Skills:** Inappropriate turn-taking noted; her tangential output affects listener's attention. **Paraphasias:** None.
Speech	**Rate:** Slow. **Intelligibility:** Good at conversational level in both known and unknown contexts. **Prosody:** Poor; flattened intonation with reduced stress patterns. **Articulation:** Mild consonantal distortions noted. **Fluency:** WFL
Auditory Comprehension	**Answering Yes/No Questions:** WFL for simple and abstract questions. **Executing Commands:** WFL **Understanding Stories & Paragraphs:** WFL at word, phrase, and sentence levels. **Understanding Conversational Speech:** Affected by inattentiveness. **Identifying Objects & Their Functions:** WFL
Reading	**Word-level Comprehension:** WFL **Sentence-level Comprehension:** Functional at the sentence and paragraph levels. However, unable to state the central theme of a complex paragraph. **Oral Reading:** WFL for monosyllabic and multisyllabic words; however, errors noted at sentence level due to neglect and inattentiveness.
Written Expression	**Copying:** WFL **Writing to Dictation:** WFL for words and sentences. **Self-generated:** Writing functional sentences and notes WFL. **Written Spelling:** WFL for words and sentences. **Oral Spelling:** WFL for monosyllabic words. **Drawing:** WFL for simple line drawings.
Cognition	**Attention/Concentration:** Poor; attention deteriorates with fatigue. **Visuospatial Skills:** Left neglect noted. **Memory:** Episodic memory, procedural memory, and semantic memory all WFL. **Executive Functions:** Difficulty with verbal problem-solving due to tangential output.
Behavioral Symptoms	**Alertness:** WFL when well-rested. **Deficit Awareness:** No awareness of deficits (anosagnosia). **Frustration:** Impatient and impulsive with noticeable frustration if listener offers corrections. **Emotional Lability:** None. **Current Personality Characteristics:** Depressed; lacks motivation; impulsive with her responses.

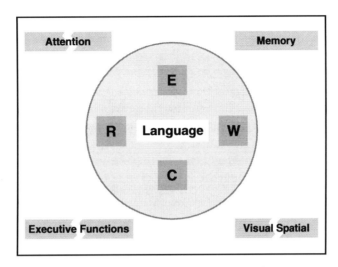

Figure 6–2. Acquired Language Disorders Target Model for Debra.

She is unable to process facial expressions, gestures, and body language. This interferes with her functional communication as nuanced meanings are missed, making her interpretations of the message very concrete and literal. Furthermore, she cannot accurately determine the speaker's intentions, which can easily produce misinterpretations. As Debra also has a left-sided neglect, she will not attend to people and/or objects located on her left side. Communication partners who are not aware that Debra has a left-sided neglect may feel as though Debra is ignoring them. Debra is also very dysprosodic making her sound robotic. Therefore, one aspect of her therapy must focus on developing proper pitch variations. This lack of appropriate intonation contours combined with Debra's flat affect make her a very challenging communication partner.

Her therapy also should focus directly on attention and neglect as well as the affective and prosodic components of communication. The goals for Debra would be to increase appropriate content in her communication; to improve her inferential abilities so she can make meaning of more than just the facts; and to facilitate her ability to generate meaning given ADL scenarios. For example, if a visitor walks into Debra's room and does not immediately greet her, she may not be able to correctly interpret that person's intentions, that is, she may believe that the visitor is angry with her. Therefore, helping Debra to develop alternate possibilities for people's behavior may assist her return to the social fabric of life. As noted above, Debra's inferential skills are weak, and she has difficulty connecting an outcome to previous sequential events. For example, if you tell her that you went outside and then you came back in and were wet, one would infer that it was raining outside. However, Debra may not be able to make that inference and would need some facilitation in order to understand the inferential process. Also, reviewing the steps involved in completing a task verbally and in writing and then discussing the sequence prior to attempting the task may help facilitate functional problem-solving for ADL needs. For example, rehearsing and writing out the sequence of steps involved in a common household task, for example, making coffee or preparing a meal will be helpful. Similar scenarios, increasing in complexity and length, would be appropriate.

Cognitively, Debra has difficulty attending to stimuli and maintaining her focus. She is distractible and impulsive in her responses, and this is further complicated by fatigue. Visuospatial skills are compromised due to left visual neglect. Finally, Debra also presents with impairment in problem-solving, and this is partially due to tangential thinking. Her episodic procedural and semantic memory systems are within functional limits (WFL) for activities of daily living (ADL) needs.

Critical Thinking/Learning Activity

- What information indicates that this patient has RHD?
- This patient would most likely be seen in acute rehabilitation and then for outpatient therapy. Knowing that the insurance carrier will give you a limited number of sessions, how would you prioritize this patient's functional outcomes?
- What are the family counseling and education issues in this case, and how would you address them?
- How would you include the family/caregivers in this patient's treatment plan?
- Write a SOAP note on this patient. Assume that you are seeing the patient for the first time after the evaluation session. Include three short-term therapeutic objectives in your note.

Treatment Considerations

Debra is a functional communicator. She can carry on a conversation; however, her flat affect and reduced intonation contours interfere with the social interaction during the communication event. As a consequence, Debra appears disinterested and distracted during conversation. Although she is 100% intelligible in known and unknown contexts, Debra's speech is still characterized by articulatory distortions and a slow rate. Her voice is breathy and, therefore, she can be difficult to hear. Therefore, treatment must focus on the paralinguistic and extralinguistic aspects of her communication disorder, as well as her speech production.

- Use contrastive stress drills with visual support to represent rising and/or falling intonation patterns. For example, in the sentence "I want to eat," Debra must accent the appropriate word to respond to a "wh–" question such as, "*Who* wants to eat?" or "*What* do you want to do?" These provide Debra with a graphic representation of the intonation contour to facilitate her accurate production. Model as necessary.

- Increase loudness by providing visual feedback in the form of a sound level meter placed within Debra's view.
- Increase focus and attention using trail-making tasks and/or mazes. These tasks involve connecting letters or numbers in sequence across a page using a pencil.
- Improve Debra's ability to locate the left margin of a newspaper or magazine article by having her find the highlighted left margin, for example, a thick yellow line drawn down the left side of the page.

Some Therapeutic Options

- Motoric-imitative treatment and cognitive-linguistic treatment (Rosenbek et al., 2004; Leon et al., 2005). The treatments have been based on theories that aprosodia is caused by motor programming deficits and a reduction in the ability to access emotionally charged words with prosody.
- Psychoeducationally Based Program (Klonoff, Sheperd, O'Brien, Chiapello, & Hodak, 1990) investigated the appropriate use of context in pragmatics and discourse. Problems understanding discourse are often due to the abstract, nonliteral aspects of information. The program attempts to enhance independence through individual and group treatment focusing on emotional issues and pragmatics. Cognitive flexibility and visuospatial problem solving are also reinforced.
- Group Sessions focusing on Debra's attentional and affectual deficits.
- Dysarthria therapy focusing on increasing loudness, articulatory distortions, and rate of speech.
- Task-oriented treatments: These treatment approaches provide the patient with compensatory techniques useful for achieving a functional goal.
- Process-oriented treatments: These treatment approaches optimize functional skills by working on the building blocks of those skills, that is, working on the parts of a skill and build the patient's skill set toward the whole.

References

Blake, M. L., Duffy, J. R., Myers, P. S., & Tompkins, C. A. (2002). Prevalence and patterns of right hemisphere cognitive communicative deficits: Retrospective data from an inpatient rehabilitation unit. *Aphasiology, 16*, 537–548.

Bub, D., Audet, T., & Lecours, A. R. (1990). Re-evaluating the effect of unilateral brain damage on simple reaction time to auditory stimulation. *Cortex, 26*, 227–237.

Chapey, R. (2008). *Language intervention strategies in aphasia and related neurogenic communication disorders* (5th ed.). Philadelphia, PA: Lippincott Williams & Wilkins.

Grice, H. (1975). Logic and conversation in P. Cole and J. Morgan. *Syntax and Semantics, 3*, 41–58.

Kaplan, R. F., Verfaillie, M., Meadows, M. E., Caplan, L. R., Peasin, M. S., & deWitt, L. D. (1991). Changing attentional demands in left hemispatial neglect. *Archives of Neurology, 48,* 1263–1266.

Klonoff, P. S., Sheperd, J. C., O'Brien, K. P., Chiapello, D. A., & Hodak, J. A. (1990). Rehabilitation and outcome of right-hemisphere stroke patients: Challenges to traditional diagnostic and treatment methods. *Neuropsychology, 4,* 147–163.

Leon, S. A., Rosenbek, J. C., Crucian, G. P., Hieber, B., Holiway, B., & Rodriguez, A. D. (2005). Active treatments for aprosodia secondary to right hemisphere stroke. *Journal of Rehabilitation Research and Development, 42,* 93–102.

Myers, P. S. (1998). *Right hemisphere damage: Disorders of communication and cognition.* San Diego, CA: Singular.

Myers, P. S. (1999). *Right hemisphere damage: Disorders of communication and cognition.* San Diego, CA: Singular.

Patterson, J. P., & Chapey, R. (2008). Assessment of language disorders in adults. In R. Chapey (Ed.), *Language intervention strategies in aphasia and related neurogenic communication disorders* (5th ed., pp. 64–160). Philadelphia, PA: Lippincott Williams & Wilkins.

Perkins, M. (2005a). Clinical pragmatics: An emergentist perspective. *Clinical Linguistics and Phonetics, 19,* 363–366.

Perkins, M. (2005b). Pragmatic ability and disability as emergent phenomena. *Clinical Linguistics and Phonetics, 19,* 367–377.

Rosenbek, J. C., Crucian, G. P., Leon, S. A., Hieber, B., Rodriguez, A. D., & Holiway, B. (2004). Novel treatments for expressive aprosodia: A phase I investigation of cognitive linguistic and imitative interventions. *Journal of the International Neuropsychological Society, 10,* 786–793.

Tompkins, C. A., & Fassbinder, W. (2004). Right hemisphere language disorders. In R. D. Kent (Ed.), *The MIT encyclopedia of communication disorders* (pp. 388–392). Cambridge, MA: MIT Press.

Weed, E. (2011). What's left to learn about right hemisphere damage and pragmatic impairment? *Aphasiology, 25,* 872–889.

Weed, E., McGregor, W., Feidbaek Nielsen, J., Roepstorff, A., & Frith, U. (2010). Theory of mind in adults with right hemisphere damage: What's the story? *Brain and Language, 113,* 65–72.

Chapter 7

TRAUMATIC BRAIN INJURY

Introduction

Traumatic brain injury (TBI) is caused by a closed head injury, a penetrating head injury, or a deceleration injury that disrupt normal functioning of the brain. The severity of TBI is variable, ranging from mild, with a brief loss of consciousness and mental ability, to severe with coma and/or amnesia. In some cases, long-term disability results, and the person is not able to return to his or her premorbid lifestyle. The most common causes of brain injury are motor vehicle accidents, recreational accidents that typically occur during sports, and through acts of violence. The risk of TBI is greater for males between the ages of 15 and 19 and for children of either gender between 0 to 4 years of age (Webb & Adler, 2008). Neimeier (2010) reports that the incidence of TBI is higher in people under 5 years of age and above 85 years of age. Of 1.4 million people who experience a TBI annually in the United States, approximately 50,000 die, 235,000 are hospitalized, and 1.1 million are seen in an emergency room and then released. The World Health Organization (WHO) estimates that 70% to 90% are treated for mild TBI (mTBI; Polito, Thompson, & DeFina, 2010). Vos et al. (2012) report that 10% of mTBIs produce intracranial complications, and only 1% require neurosurgical intervention. Intracranial abnormalities may include life-threatening hematomas. The recommended time for observation is minimally 12 to 24 hours. Medical personnel also attempt to determine if any one of six clinical signs are present. These include headache, vomiting, short-term memory loss, physical signs of trauma above the clavicles, seizure, and intoxication. Any one of these findings is often associated with an abnormal CT scan.

There is an urgent need to treat members of U.S. troops diagnosed with mTBI and post traumatic stress disorder (PTSD). The increase in incidence of TBI in the United States is primarily due to brain injuries sustained in the war zones, for example, due to improvised explosive device (IED) explosions, gunshot wounds, and other blast related injuries. Recent data in the Rand Report indicate that 320,000 of the 1.64 million U.S. troops engaged in "Operation Enduring Freedom" and "Operation Iraqi Freedom" sustained a mild to moderate brain injury. The Department of Defense (DoD) reports that 70% of TBIs are caused by the blast wave transmitted from the source (Neimeier, 2010).

Characteristics

Individuals with TBI often present with a wide range of symptoms and disabilities. There is a physiologic disruption of brain functioning immediately following a TBI. Most patients will experience an altered state of consciousness at the time of the injury. Some patients will lapse into a coma immediately, whereas others may gradually evolve into that state of consciousness. The majority of patients experience loss of memory for the events directly before the injury (retrograde amnesia) or after it (anterograde amnesia). Depending on the level of severity of the brain injury, the patient also may sustain focal or diffuse neurologic deficits and/or cognitive-linguistic impairment. Agitation is very common in the head injured patient. It can begin at the scene of the accident as combativeness and continue throughout the stages of recovery. The primary mechanisms of injury leading to TBI are illustrated in Figure 7–1. For soldiers returning from war, there can be symptoms that are missed due to their subclinical nature, for example, headaches, memory problems, and irritability, and as a consequence, the individual may not seek help for these symptoms. PTSD may also be a consequence of TBI in this population. In 2011, the Veterans Administration treated over 100,000 veterans from the Iraq and Afghanistan wars for PTSD. Common symptoms of PTSD include nightmares, flashbacks, emotional numbness, difficulty sleeping, depression, and other physical and mental health problems. Rage surfaces in soldiers who avoid dealing with emotions (Guy, 2012). The speech-language pathologist (SLP) will need to be aware of the ramifications of PTSD during evaluation and treatment, being especially careful to be sensitive about the patient's history. PTSD can affect a patient's performance, and the clinician must be observant and attentive during the session to insure accuracy of performance, that is, that the patient's performance is due to their current skill level ver-

sus their PTSD. Appropriate referrals to other health care professionals must be considered as well.

Types of Brain Injury

Although any change in brain neurophysiology and/or structure can be considered traumatic, the term *TBI* is much more specific in reference. The three most common types of TBI are due to: open head injury, closed head injury, and deceleration injuries. Stroke, hypoxia, tumors, infections, and toxic/metabolic processes are not considered TBI in this context, despite the changes in brain functioning that ensue. Table 7–1 describes the three types of head injury most typically associated with TBI.

The term *coup injury* refers to the injury at the point of contact. For example, if one sustains a blow to the left side of the head, and only the left hemisphere is affected, then the patient has experienced a coup injury. If, however, the patient sustains damage in the right hemisphere after a blow to the left side of the head, then that is termed a *contrecoup injury*. Thus, these two lesion sites arise from the original blow to the brain (coup injury), and the other contusion is a result of the brain rebounding off the skull at the site opposite of impact (con-

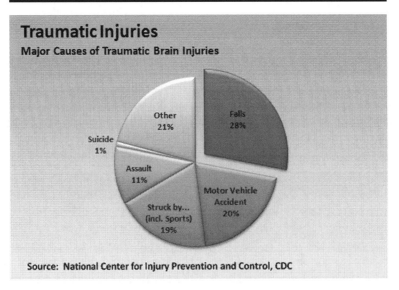

Figure 7–1. Primary mechanisms of injury causing TBI (Langlois, Rutland-Brown, & Thomas, 2006).

Table 7–1. Causes and Characteristics of TBI

Common Causes of TBI	Characteristics
Open Head Injury Example: Gunshot wound (GSW) to the head	Penetration of the skull (missile wound) with a direct injury to the brain. There is large focal damage, and effects can be life-threatening. About 30% to 40% of patients experience seizures.
Closed Head Injury Examples: Assault with a blunt object; motor vehicle accident (MVA); falls	There is no penetration of the skull. Indirect force to the head is caused by rotation and/or deceleration. There is focal damage with the possibility of diffuse axonal injury. About 5% experience seizures. Coup and contrecoup injuries.
Deceleration Injuries Example: Head-on motor vehicle accident	Because of a sudden deceleration, the brain continues to move inside the skull as it moves at a different rate than the skull because it is soft. There tends to be diffuse axonal shearing, contusions, and brain swelling due to repeated back and forth motion inside the skull. If axons tear, the neurons die.

trecoup injury). Shearing forces occur if there is a rapid and forceful motion of the head, which is often the case in auto accidents. For example, in an auto accident, the patient's brain still may be moving in an anterior-posterior direction after the car has stopped. Such movement can cause *diffuse axonal injury* due to tearing of axons and the myelin sheath covering them.

There is also a loss of consciousness accompanied by swelling (edema) of the brain and vascular damage deep within the brain. If pressure in the skull is not stopped through surgery, cooling, medication, or by other medical intervention, the brain will swell to the point that it is pushed down through the opening at the skull's base (the foramen magnum). This is referred to as *brain herniation*. As a consequence, the brainstem nuclei controlling breathing and heart functions will be compressed, and the person will die. Abnormal posturing may result from brain herniation, and there are two types that can be observed in people with TBI: *decorticate posturing*, due to unilateral or bilateral corticospinal tract damage; or *decerebrate posturing*, which indicates that there is swelling of the upper brainstem. The severity and duration of these abnormal postures contribute to the favorability of the patient's long-term outcome, that is, the longer the duration and the more severe the posturing, then the poorer the long-term prognosis (Springhouse, 2007). Figure 7–2 illustrates the two types of abnormal posturing.

Symptoms Related to Localization of the TBI

TBI often results in diffuse damage to cortical and subcortical regions depending on the mechanism of injury. However, certain areas are more affected due to direct insult. Those who have sustained a right hemispheric injury may experience sensory impairment on the left side of the body, left inattention, poor awareness of limitations, impaired math skills, and impaired memory for nonverbal information. Left hemispheric injury affects language and right-sided motor skills, with impaired memory for nonverbal information. For patients with bilateral frontal involvement, executive functions are generally impaired, for example, disinhibition, social appropriateness, difficulty controlling emotions, poor at initiating tasks, and poor self-regulation. Diffuse axonal injury (DAI) leads to poorer performance when tasks become more complex.

Prognostic Considerations in Head Injury

The clinician working with a patient who has TBI status post (s/p) head injury will need to consider five general variables in relation to functional outcome: premorbid intelligence, age at the time of

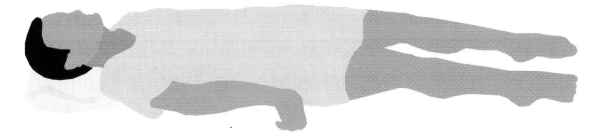

A. Extension posturing (decerebrate rigidity)

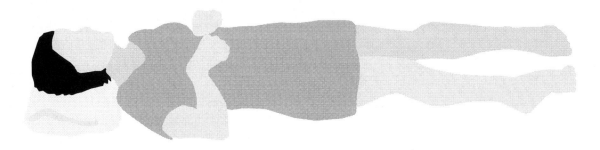

B. Abnormal flexion (decorticate rigidity)

Figure 7–2. Decerebrate and decorticate postures. **A.** Extension posturing (decerebrate rigidity). **B.** Abnormal flexion (decorticate rigidity).

injury, duration of coma, posttraumatic amnesia, and medical complications during the hospital stay. There are other variables that also can impact functional outcome, such as gender and initial Glasgow Coma Scale (GCS) score (Brown et al., 2005), so if the clinician is attentive to all of these factors, a very reasonable prognostic picture for the patient can be formulated.

Premorbid Intelligence

Kesler, Adams, Blasey, and Bigler (2003) tested the concept of cognitive reserve in 24 patients with brain injury. Cognitive reserve has been postulated as the factor to explain the individual difference in functional outcomes. Using MRI imaging, the authors measured total intracranial volume and ventricle-to-brain ratio. They also looked at educational level and premorbid standardized testing and compared it with the subject's cognitive outcome postinjury. Their results found that larger premorbid brain volume and higher education level may decrease vulnerability to cognitive deficits following TBI, consistent with the notion of a cognitive reserve.

Age at the Time of Injury

Age at the time of injury appears to be a strong indicator of morbidity and functional outcome (Wetzel & Squire, 1982). If the patient is 40 years of age or under, a good outcome is predicted in most cases. However, if the patient is over 50, the outcome is poorer—and poorer still if the patient is over 60 years of age (Brain Trauma Foundation, 2000a).

Duration of Coma

There are two factors to consider in relation to coma: duration of coma and depth of coma. Duration is measured in weeks, and there appears to be a direct and linear relationship between recovery and the duration of the coma. Depth of coma is based on the GCS score. Patients whose coma lasts less than 2 weeks have better prognosis for full recovery than those whose coma lasts longer than 2 weeks (Brain Trauma Foundation, 2000b). When the patient is first encountered by medical professionals, and the GCS is administered within 24 hours of the injury, those with a score less than 8 are at a higher risk than those with a score greater than 8. If the GCS is administered 24 hours after the injury, a score of 5 or less indicates a poor outcome, and greater than 5 is predictive of a good outcome (Brain Trauma Foundation, 2000b).

Posttraumatic Amnesia

Another prognosticator for recovery after head injury is the duration of amnesia. Typically, people who sustain head injury have no memory of the actual event. However, as they recover, they may be able to go back in time and begin to remember events closer and closer to the actual incident. If the posttraumatic amnesia is less than 2 weeks prior to patient's admission to the hospital, then the prognosis for a fuller recovery is better. This is dependent on the severity of the injury, the type of injury, and the communication skills of the patient. The clinician can monitor this amnesia, which will help in prognostication and even therapy planning. Table 7–2 provides expectations for full recovery given the amount of time with posttraumatic amnesia.

Medical Complications

To obtain a rapid clinical picture of the patient, the first assessment tool used by medical professionals on their first encounter with the head injured patient is the GCS (Jennett & Bond, 1975). This typically occurs in the field, that is, at the scene of the accident or injury, as the patient is being stabilized

Table 7–2. Relationship Between Duration of Posttraumatic Amnesia and Recovery Time

Time of Posttraumatic Amnesia Experienced	Time Expected for Full Recovery
Less than 5 minutes	1 month
5 to 60 minutes	3 months
1 to 24 hours	1 year
1 to 7 days	1 to 2 years
8 to 28 days	Residual deficits remain

for transport. However, the GCS also can be administered by EMTs in the helicopter transporting the patient to the hospital, or in the emergency department upon arrival to the hospital. The patient is rated according to his eye opening response, verbal response, and motor response. These scores are then tallied, and a score is obtained. The highest score obtainable on the GCS is 15. The lowest score obtainable is 3. Teasdale and Jennett (1974) describe a GCS score of 3 to 8 as severe TBI, 9 to 12 as moderate TBI, and 13 to 15 as mTBI. It is important to remember that a patient may improve despite a low GCS score; however, it is generally held that a score between 8 and 15 represents a more favorable diagnosis. Table 7–3 shows the rating scale of the GCS.

Dawodu (2007) further refines the criteria for severity of brain injury as follows:

A diagnosis of mild brain injury is made when:

- The GCS score is greater than 12.
- There are no abnormalities noted on the CT scan.
- There are no operative lesions.
- The length of stay in the hospital is less than 48 hours.

A diagnosis of moderate brain injury is made when:

- The GCS score is from 9 to 12.
- There are abnormal CT scan findings.
- There exists anoperative intracranial lesion.
- The length of stay in the hospital is at least 48 hours.

Table 7–3. The Glasgow Coma Scale

Eye Opening Response	Spontaneous—open with blinking at baseline	4 points
	Opens to verbal command, speech, or shout	3 points
	Opens to pain, not applied to face	2 points
	None	1 point
Verbal Response	Oriented	5 points
	Confused conversation, but able to answer questions	4 points
	Inappropriate responses, words discernible	3points
	Incomprehensible speech	2 points
	None	1point
Motor Response	Obeys commands for movement	6points
	Purposeful movement to painful stimulus	5 points
	Withdraws from pain	4 points
	Abnormal (spastic) flexion, decorticate posture	3 points
	Extensor (rigid) response, decerebrate posture	2 points
	None	1 point

A diagnosis of severe brain injury is made when:

■ The GCS score is below 9 within 48 hours of the injury.

Medical complications after TBI are common and myriad. Of course, the level of severity of the initial head injury plays a role in the extent and nature of these problems, that is, the more severe, the more likely those complications will arise post injury. We briefly summarize below the medical complications that the speech-language pathologist will most likely encounter in the acute care and rehab phases of the patient's hospitalization: post-traumatic seizures, hydrocephalus, and spasticity.

Posttraumatic Seizures

Posttraumatic seizures (PTS) are a common complication of TBI and most commonly occur after moderate and severe head injury. Seizures are classified based on how soon after the initial injury they occur: immediate seizures occur within 24 hours of the injury, early seizures occur in 2 to 7 days post-injury, and late seizures occur any time after day 7 post-injury (Pangilinan, 2008). Late onset posttraumatic seizures occur in 5% to 19% of those with brain injury, and approximately one-third to one-half of all brain-injured patients develop them (Bushnik, Englander, & Duong, 2004).

Hydrocephalus

The four ventricles of the brain compose the ventricular system, whose function is to keep the brain and spinal cord bathed in cerebral spinal fluid (CSF). The CSF circulates continuously and is reabsorbed back into the bloodstream. Hydrocephalus occurs when the CSF cannot exit the ventricles, builds up there, and causes significant pressure on the adjacent cortical areas. In TBI, the two most common types of hydrocephalus are *communicating* and *noncommunicating*. If there is an obstruction in the subarachnoid space, preventing the free flow of CSF, communicating hydrocephalus results, and this is the most common type found in TBI. An obstruction in the ventricular system that prevents the CSF from exiting the fourth ventricle results noncommunicating hydrocephalus (Parcell, Ponsford, Rajaratnam, & Redman, 2006).

Spasticity

Elovic and Zafonte (2001) found that in one inpatient rehabilitation unit, 25% of the patients demonstrated spasticity. Spasticity is a sign of upper motor neuron damage, whereas rigidity is a sign of basal ganglia involvement. The important fact that the speech-language clinician must keep in mind is that some medications used to reduce spasticity and rigidity may cause cognitive deficits, especially the use of baclofen, tizanidine, clonidine, and benzodiazepines (Pangilinan, 2008).

Cognitive-Linguistic Impairment Due to TBI

There are three major deficit areas that result from TBI. These are neurologic/physical impairments, cognitive/intellectual impairments, and emotional/behavioral impairments. Neurologically, there may be coordination problems, epilepsy, paresis (unilateral or bilateral), sensory, and/or perceptual impairments, to name a few. Cognitive impairment also may arise and includes deficits of memory, intellectual quotient, processing speed, attention, executive functioning, and/or communication problems. Emotional and behavioral complications are very common in this population. The person may display personality changes, difficulty self-monitoring, a lack of motivation, impulsivity, aggression, disinhibition, anxiety, and/or depression, with limited awareness. Language deficits occur in one-third of severe TBI survivors, but rarely evident in cases of mTBI. Table 7–4 summarizes the deficit areas and offers some treatment considerations.

In children, outcomes are impacted by the severity of the TBI, and the site and size of the lesion and age. Children with mTBI generally make the most improvements within 6 months post injury, whereas those with severe TBI and more diffuse damage tend to make gradual improvements over an 18-month postinjury time frame. Children with brain injury often recover more readily because the language areas have greater brain plasticity. As individuals age, the areas become more specialized and less resilient (Szaflarski, 2006).

Establishing Goals for the Therapeutic Course

During the acute phase of the hospitalization, a primary goal is to assess the severity of the patient's injury. A professional team composed of a speech-language pathologist, occupational and physical therapists, social work, and medicine are initially necessary to evaluate and chart the course of functional treatment. The typical evaluation approach for these patients at this stage is to administer a formal assessment, if they are able to participate, in order to delineate deficit areas. Although this may be a controversial practice, in our clinical experience it is important to establish a baseline in order to measure the patient's cognitive-linguistic recovery over time. Furthermore, because patients do not remain in the acute care setting as long as they once did, supplying information to the clinicians and rehab team at the next level of care is important for this patient's rehabilitation program. Assessment must also include the Rancho Los Amigos Level of Cognitive Functioning Scale (RLA) level, again, to facilitate a common ground of communication between the members of the patient's team. The evaluator must also consider the duration of the patient's coma and be certain to review the physician and nursing notes for the latest GCS assessment. Hearing, balance, vision, motor skills, sensory status, cognitive skills, and other social effects of the TBI must be noted. Neimeier (2010) suggests using a "What Am I Forgetting" Questionnaire as part of the evaluation process. This is a simple five-question form to evaluate if the patient has the ability to recall names of familiar people; identify where they have placed personal objects; what they ate during the day; temporal and spatial orientation (today's date); and a brief overview of their daily schedule. It is important to monitor changes in behavior and cognitive-linguistic skills during this stage and report on the patient's progress in the chart.

Table 7–4. Primary Deficits in TBI and Areas for Treatment

Primary Type of Deficits	Treatment Considerations
Cognitive-Communication	Word finding is a major deficit in severe TBI and can be seen in mild cases, although to a lesser degree of impairment. There is difficulty organizing and sequencing information. Speech is often tangential, and the patient is unable to differentiate relevant from irrelevant information when formulating a discourse. Expressing and comprehending humor can be impaired. Understanding of abstract language and expression is often limited. Synthesizing written information can also be impaired.
	Pragmatic language is often impaired, for example, eye contact, affect, use of gestures, and understanding of body language and facial expressions are deficient. Pragmatic deficits also include topic selection and maintenance, expression of complex ideas, and making inappropriate comments. Narrative discourse is incohesive. Automatic and overlearned language is often unaffected.
Academic	There is difficulty organizing, integrating, and generalizing information to another context. Self-awareness of problems is limited, and there is poor planning ability. Self-monitoring of errors and behaviors are weak.
	An individual is often ready for school when they can attend to a task for 15 to 20 minutes, and they can tolerate 20 to 30 minutes of stimulation. They should also be able to function in a group of two or more and engage in meaningful communication with the ability to follow basic directions. There should be an interest in learning.
Executive Functioning	Three areas must be considered: executing cognitive plans, managing time, and self-regulating. A fully functioning individual needs to possess the ability to organize and sequence plans and initiate activities to work toward goals. They also should work toward estimating time and creating schedules to carry out activities and change plans if needed. In order to self-regulate, the individual must judge their own behavior to complete tasks, control impulses, work without perseveration, and act independently.
Memory	During the sensory store stage, stimuli enter the system (visual, auditory, tactile, emotional, etc.) and disappear. Short-term working memory is limited and tends to last 20 seconds or less. It is assisted by rehearsal, visuospatial sketchpad, and decision-making. Long-term memory lasts from minutes to years. Consolidation must occur for this to work for later recall. Three memory systems, semantic knowledge, episodic or event-based, and procedural are important to communication.

Postconcussive Syndrome

Postconcussive syndrome (PCS) has been identified as a sequela to mild brain injury in some cases (Legome & Wu, 2006). Mild injury is characterized by a brief loss of consciousness and/or posttraumatic amnesia and the patient may also demonstrate disorientation. Interestingly, more men sustain mild brain injury, but the incidence of PCS is higher in women. Fifty percent of mild brain injury patients are between the ages of 15 and 34. The PCS patient may also present with a GCS of 13 to 15 (Legome & Wu, 2006). Legome and Wu (2006) also report that between 29% to 90% of patients will experience PCS symptoms after mild brain injury, and these patients tend not to report to the emergency department (ED) immediately after the injury. Approximately 15% of PCS patients will continue to report problems 12 months after the injury, which may be refractory to treatment, leaving the patient with a lifelong disability (Legome & Wu, 2006).

Ponsford et al. (2012) set out to determine the influence of preinjury factors, injury-related factors, and postinjury factors on outcomes of mTBI. Findings indicated that an individual's anxiety response to postinjury symptoms was an important factor in the acute phase. Female individuals' anxiety levels 1-week post injury combined with any preinjury psychiatric problems were most often associated with PCS following mTBI. When PCS was diagnosed, it was most often related to PTSD symptoms, life stressors, anxiety, pain, and memory and concentration difficulties.

For this population, treatment recommendations include cognitive rehabilitation with an emphasis on attentional and communication skills. Cognitive-behavioral therapy (CBT), and desensitization to reduce hypersensitivity have also been used as have neurosensory retraining for visual-vestibular dysfunction and drug therapy for headaches and sleep disturbance . It is also important that these patients receive compensatory training for functional skills related to personal and vocational responsibilities, that is, the clinician should provide strategies to optimize the patient's success with daily living activities and job-related duties, focusing on organizational skills, time management, problem solving, and other executive functions that would positively impact daily life. An important factor to keep in mind is that all treatment must be individualized. Furthermore, incorporating direct instruction, that is, reading, writing, and social skills, and strategy-based instruction, for, self-monitoring the integration of learned strategies, planning, and sequencing, must include reinforcement and modeling (Sohlberg, Ehlhardt, & Kennedy, 2005).

The diagnosis of PCS remains controversial. However, Legome and Wu (2006) feel that if headache, dizziness, fatigue, irritability, impaired memory and concentration, insomnia, and lowered tolerance for noise and light continues after the injury, than the diagnosis can be made. Legome and Wu (2006) believe that PCS can at least be loosely defined as a persistence of these symptoms within several weeks after the initial insult. Kalinian (2008) states that PCS is a "cluster of cognitive, behavioral, and emotional symptoms that occur after a blow, a fall, or hit to the head" (p. 1). The most common symptoms of PCS are:

- Persistent low-grade headaches that linger
- Attentional difficulties or problems concentrating
- Difficulty remembering things
- Problems with planning and organization
- A new and noticeable slowness in thinking
- Disorientation resulting in getting lost more easily
- Reduced energy level
- Changes in the senses of smell and/or taste
- Tinnitus
- Changes in behavior and personality such as anxiety, depression, irritability, sleep abnormalities, changes in appetite, and changes in libido.

Diagnostic testing of patients with PCS may identify weaknesses in the following areas:

- Vocabulary
- Short-term and immediate memory
- Attention
- Cognitive flexibility
- Information processing
- Object recall
- Drawing
- Mathematics

The clinician must present detailed prophylactic counseling and education to the caregivers regarding PCS. In the case of children, the clinician should consider giving a copy of the evaluation report to the child's teachers (with parental permission) so that any special programming can be arranged. Follow-up cognitive-linguistic testing should also be considered approximately 6 weeks s/p discharge to monitor the trends in the recovery process and to rule out the emergence of any new impairments.

Mild TBI (mTBI)

Mild brain injury is characterized by a brief change in consciousness (less than 20 to 30 minutes) or mental status resulting from an acute injury from some mechanical energy applied to the head. Hospitalization is generally less than 72 hours, with a GCS greater than 12. Numminen (2011) supports the use of more sophisticated methods to determine mTBI. Symptom-based criteria are currently used as guidelines for determining the incidence of mTBI. Often loss of consciousness (LOC) and posttraumatic amnesia (PTA) are required for diagnosing mTBI. When these criteria are not required, the incidence rate tends to drop by one-third. Estimated incidence also reflects patients who receive treatment at a hospital. Often, patients who visit outpatient clinics are not counted. In the United States, approximately 25% of individuals do not seek medical treatment following a mTBI. Such information is either self-reported or provided by another who identified a loss of consciousness in someone they knew. On the other hand, according to the WHO (World Health Organization), confusion and disorientation are the only symptoms determined as relevant in the diagnosis of mTBI without other transient neurological abnormalities (Numminen, 2011).

Symptoms of mTBI generally include headaches, dizziness, poor concentration, mental slowness, difficulty engaging in divided attention, memory difficulties, visual disturbance, fatigue, irritability, depression, anxiety, and alcohol intolerance (Carroll et al., 2004). Poorer cognitive performance regarding reaction time, processing speed, and memory are more often associated with intracranial abnormalities. The presence of other health problems, life stressors, and psychiatric illness prior to a mTBI tends to predict poorer outcomes 3 months after the injury. Although the prevalence of mTBI is 100 to 300 out of 100,000 annually (Hirtz et al., 2007), most cases make a complete recovery within 3 months of the injury. Approximately 15% to 25% experience ongoing symptoms (Carroll et al., 2004). Coping strategies for reducing anxiety have been found helpful in minimizing the effects of mTBI over time.

The clinician must be alert to those patients who experience very mild cognitive-linguistic impairment upon initial testing. Presently, CT scans, MRIs, neuropsychological testing, and rating scales have not been sensitive enough to accurately assess mTBI. With mTBI, there is excessive hyperexcit-ability and cortical stimulation that leads to neuro-degeneration and cell death (Hovda, 2007). Hovda stated that surviving cells are in a state of dysfunction and suggested multimodal brain-mapping to appropriately assess brain integrity. Hovda further recommended identification of neuromarkers for electrical, magnetic, metabolic, and chemical functions. Spectroscopy with MRI, fMRI, and EEG testing can provide information about the individual's ability to focus attention, process information, and execute specific tasks—all important to the therapeutic process. Such testing is also helpful in differentiating PTSD from mTBI.

According to Ozen and Fernandes (2012), individuals with mTBI often experience working memory impairment and attention/concentration difficulties that go undetected on standard neuropsychological tests. In their study of 26 undergraduate college students who suffered an mTBI, at least 6 months prior to their investigation, they were found to have higher state anxiety levels and slowed information processing compared with 31 students in the control group. Although task accuracy rates were similar between the groups, results suggested that individuals with mTBI may delay their responses on cognitively demanding tasks to improve accuracy. Patients with posttraumatic amnesia lasting less than 7 days who received regular outpatient follow-up visits had significantly less social disability and fewer postconcussive symptoms 6 months after the injury, than those who did not receive the services (Wade, King, Wenden, Crawford, & Caldwell, 1998).

Slower information processing and increased frontal lobe activation has been found 1-month post mTBI on tasks involving working memory. Researchers speculate that additional frontal lobe resources for processing are activated in order to successfully complete such tasks after mTBI. Young adults with mTBI, often due to sports injuries, experienced slowing when attempting higher order cognitive tasks compared with control peers. The slower information processing is associated with microstructural axonal damage, detected using diffusion tensor imaging (Niogi et al., 2008).

New treatments for mTBI include individualized protocols established from the International Brain Research Foundation (IBRF) to reduce dysfunction by changing amplitude, frequency, and coherence of the brain's electrical activity. Transcranial magnetic stimulation (TMI) and transcranial direct current stimulation (tDCS) attempt to alleviate persistent symptoms of mTBI by changing neuronal firing with low-amplitude direct currents.

Rating Scales for Functional Outcomes

The GCS is designed to provide the first responders and the medical team with a clinical picture of the patient immediately after the injury and for the early stage of the hospitalization. It does not address the cognitive, linguistic, behavioral, and functional outcomes as well as two other scales: the RLA (for Rancho Los Amigos Level of Cognitive Functioning Scale; Northeast Center for Special Care, 2007and the Disability Rating Scale (DRS; Rappaport, Hall, Hopkins, Belleza, & Cope, 1982). We review the scales and their functions below.

Rancho Los Amigos (RLA)

Currently, there are 10 levels of function that are defined by the patient's behavior, including functional communication skills. The clinician uses the RLA during the initial assessment and for follow-up monitoring of the patient. In both the acute-care phase of the patient's recovery and in the rehabilitative phase, the RLA is useful for goal planning and prognostication. Each level of the scale has more detailed behavioral and communicative characteristics associated with it, but in the representation of the scale below, we have included only the general clinical presentation. We refer the reader to http://www.rancho.org/, which is the website of Ranchos Los Amigos National Rehabilitation Center for the fuller version of this scale. We recommend that the clinician continually monitor the patient's progress by using the scale at each bedside or office visit, starting with the initial evaluation session in the hospital. Table 7–5 describes the RLA.

Disability Rating Scale (DRS)

The DRS (Rappaport et al., 1982) provides a very functional picture of the brain-injured patient to those around him or her (Table 7–6). Unlike the RLA, the DRS covers the full range of human activity that must be considered if full recovery is to be addressed. This scale can be used at the early stages of hospitalization through the community reentry phase of recovery. Furthermore, the DRS is a perfect platform upon which to design interdisciplinary goals designed to enhance the patient's functional outcomes.

General Treatment Issues

Early treatment is best, and communicative recovery is optimized with comprehensive cognitive and neurobehavioral therapy (Pegg, Auerbach, & Seel, 2005). One must consider, however, the level of severity when developing a treatment plan for a person with TBI. The patient's awareness of the event and understanding of the deficits is a critical element in their rehabilitation and must always be included in the treatment plan. A psychosocial goal is for the individual to become more aware that they have changed due to their injury. Unfortunately, some patients are severely disoriented and are unable to comprehend the fact that their reality has changed. This type of psychosocial scenario affects not only the *physical* delivery of speech-language pathology services, for example, the patient may never accept that they need services and may try to escape the treatment room; but it also sets up obstacles to optimal recovery that may not be overcome. Therefore, the clinician must reflect on the severity of the patient's impairments when planning treatment and remain pragmatic, realistic, and functionally oriented.

There are some general features common to most patients with TBI, and it is important to discuss and/or address these issues directly or through outside consultations. These include:

■ difficulty sleeping
■ feeling stressed

Table 7–5. The RLA Levels of Cognitive Function Scale with Behavioral Characteristics

Levels of Cognitive Functioning	Clinical Presentation
Level I	*No responses* to pain, touch, sound, or sight. Total assistance required.
Level II	*Generalized response* to any type of stimuli regardless of type or location. Total assistance required.
Level III	*Localized response*; blink to strong light; respond to physical discomfort; inconsistent response to commands. Total assistance required.
Level IV	*Confused and agitated*; alert, active with aggressive and odd behaviors; attention span short; nonpurposeful motor movements; verbalizations inappropriate. Maximal assistance.
Level V	*Confused, inappropriate, nonagitated.* Gross attention to the environment; distractible; constant redirection required; can become overstimulated; inappropriate social interactions. Maximal assistance.
Level VI	*Confused and appropriate*; inconsistently oriented; recent memory and attention are impaired; can follow simple directions; goal-directed with assistance; begin to recall the past; emerging awareness of self. Moderate assistance required.
Level VII	*Automatic and appropriate*; performs daily routines robotically; skills deteriorate in unfamiliar environments; planning is unrealistic; awareness is superficial, but the person cannot attach meaning to it. Minimal assistance for ADLs is required.
Level VIII	*Purposeful and Appropriate*; unclear assessment of their abilities; self-centered; irritable; low tolerance for frustration; able to acknowledge others' feelings with assistance; can execute familiar tasks with minimal assistance. Stand-by assistance is required.
Level IX	*Purposeful and Appropriate*; able to complete familiar tasks independently and shift between tasks independently; they can self-monitor and can anticipate problems with assistance. These patients often use an assistive memory device to recall a schedule. Stand-by assistance on request is required.
Level X	*Purposeful and Appropriate*; can multitask; independently initiate and carry out unfamiliar routines; anticipate impact of their impairments; can think about consequences of decisions; social interactions are consistently appropriate. Modified independent level of assistance is required.

Source: Hagen, C. (1998). *Revised levels of cognitive functioning, rehabilitation of the head injured adult: Comprehensive physical management* (3rd ed.). Downey, CA: Professional Staff Association of Rancho Los Amigos National Rehabilitation Center, http://www.rainbowrehab.com/Education_&_Publications/ranchos-los-amigos.php. Used with permission.

Table 7–6. The Disability Rating Scale

Disability Rating Scale (DRS)			
Category	**Item**	**Instructions**	**Score**
Arousability, Awareness, and Responsivity	Eye Opening	0 = *spontaneous* 1 = *to speech* 2 = *to pain* 3 = *none*	
	Communication Ability	0 = *oriented* 1 = *confused* 2 = *inappropriate* 3 = *incomprehensible* 4 = *none*	
	Motor Response	0 = *obeying* 1 = *localizing* 2 = *withdrawing* 3 = *flexing* 4 = *extending* 5 = *none*	
Cognitive Ability for Self-Care Activities	Feeding	0 = *complete* 1 = *partial* 2 = *minimal* 3 = *none*	
	Toileting	0 = *complete* 1 = *partial* 2 = *minimal* 3 = *none*	
	Grooming	0 = *complete* 1 = *partial* 2 = *minimal* 3 = *none*	
Dependence on Others	Level of Functioning	0 = *completely independent* 1 = *independent in special environment* 2 = *mildly dependent* 3 = *moderately dependent* 4 = *markedly dependent* 5 = *totally dependent*	
Psychosocial Adaptability	Employability	0 = *not restricted* 1 = *selected jobs* 2 = *sheltered workshop (noncompetitive)* 3 = *not employable*	
		Total DRS Score	

Disability Categories: 0 (Total DRS Score) = None (Level of Disability); 1 = Mild; 2–3 = Partial; 4–6 = Moderate; 7–11 = Moderately Severe; 12–16 = Severe; 17–21 = Extremely Severe; 22–24 = Vegetative State; 25–29 = Extreme Vegetative State.

Source: Rappaport, M., Hall, K. M., Hopkins, H. K., Belleza, T., & Cope, D. N. (1982). Disability rating scale for severe head trauma: Coma to community. *Archives of Physical Medicine and Rehabilitation, 63,* 118–123. Copyright Elsevier (1982). Reprinted with permission.

- hyperemotionalality
- forgetfulness
- anger
- depression
- self-consciousness

The goal is to work toward increasing the patient's ability to be aware of an impairment or behavioral change; to identify it when it occurs; and then learn to self-monitor any disruptive behaviors before they can interfere with social interaction, activities of daily living (ADLs), or communication. Knowledge is power, and time is essential (Perri, 2012). Depending on the level of severity, a patient's rehabilitation can range from weeks to years. For mild cases, treatment can focus on *optimization* and perhaps even *rebuilding* the areas of cognitive-linguistic weakness. Executive functions, language functions, and behavior can all be addressed directly and effectively with a patient who has the ability to understand the goals and procedures of treatment. For example, reducing or eliminating tangential output in discourse is more realistic in these patients because they have the ability to comprehend the tasks, materials, and the long-term goal. Choosing to address the patient's ability to manage their own finances by working on their bills with them, makes more sense with a patient who can read, scan, and do simple arithmetic. Every patient has areas of strengths and weaknesses, and it the responsibility of the clinician to identify them and build a treatment plan around them.

In moderately impaired and severely impaired patients, rehabilitation can be prolonged, and rightly so. Once the patient has moved to the rehabilitation level of care, the speech-language pathologist must utilize all of the information obtained from evaluations and reports during the acute care stay, in order to plan treatment in rehab. Rehabilitation stays are more truncated now due to reimbursement issues, so clinicians must work more efficaciously, using solid evidence to guide their treatment methods. In the more severe cases, treatment will focus on developing compensatory strategies to meet the patient's ADL needs. These patients may never be independent; however, as in the more mild cases, the clinician must identify the strengths and weaknesses and design a plan based on those findings. Gener-ally, memory, attention, visuospatial skills, executive functions, problem-solving, and language must all be addressed at some level with the idea that *recovery* (defined as "return to normal functioning") is not likely, but *optimization* of strengths and *compensation* for weaknesses is much more realistic. These patients benefit from the use of scheduling tools, memory logs, address books, and multimodality reminders in order to keep them oriented and connected socially. Today, electronic devices such as smartphones and small computer devices such as iPads are available and very helpful for all of the above.

There are many formal and informal methods to address the deficit areas noted above. One of the latest techniques to address problem solving and reasoning is referred to as SOLVE (Neimeier, Kreutzer, & Taylor, 2005). Here, the clinician trains the patient to use this method in order to facilitate optimal decision making. It has the following components:

- Situation analysis: "What's the problem?"
- Options: "What are some options in this case?"
- Listen: "Ask others for their opinion/solution, and listen to what they have to say."
- Voice: "Tell me what your choice is."
- Evaluate: "How did using your choice work out? Was it an effective solution?"

In this electronic age, e-mail and texting have become the communication methods of choice for social communication, taking the place of the traditional phone call. As a consequence, a patient who is impulsive and unable to make sound judgments regarding social proprieties will need some training in social problem solving. A creative method to teach this is known as "COPS: Caution On Pushing Send" also referred to as "Would you want your grandmother to read this?" It is an easy concept to teach to help the individual with brain injury, who can communicate in writing, to think of what another person may think when reading an e-mail the patient is planning to send. A discussion can then ensue about options and optimal methods to communicate his or her ideas.

According to Sohlberg et al. (2008), the clinician must incorporate mass practice during therapy for individuals with TBI. Modifying tasks into small steps with models before performance is required may facilitate errorless learning. Individualized attention work, that is, intense treatment sessions lasting at least an hour weekly, should take place. Outcome measures taken to record daily and weekly progress will help to determine the efficacy of the treatment. It is also recommended that the clinician incorporate training to improve the patient's awareness of errors, identification of errors, and the ability to self-monitor performance. Furthermore, due to the presence of aberrant behaviors in this clinical population, the clinician must include goals that facilitate self-control of inappropriate, nonproductive, and/or disruptive behaviors. Training often requires practice in various settings if the new skill is to be used appropriately and functionally (Kennedy et al., 2008).

Regardless of the treatment plan, remember to follow these basic steps:

- Consider the patient's needs and available support systems.
- Identify the problems the patient is having in activities of daily living.
- Know the patient's functional levels.
- Know what motivates the patient and use it.
- Be aware of the amount of cueing the patient needs and make it readily available.
- Coordinate care with family and the therapeutic team.
- Fade supports as the patient becomes more self-reliant.
- It is important to provide direct and consistent feedback to patients.
- Repeated stimulus drills are recommended as the SLP attempts to help the patient process information, gain capacity and speed, shift attention, and resist distractions.

Errorless Learning

Errorless learning is a restorative approach, not a compensatory one. The critical element in errorless

learning is the attempt to eliminate errors during the acquisition stage of learning, for example, a new skill, a new behavior, or a task. The stages of errorless learning are:

- Break the task into small steps.
- Model first, then ask for a response.
- Discouraging guessing.
- When an error is made, it is corrected immediately.
- Fade the prompts used for skills acquisition.

This type of intervention is similar to drill work because it requires massed practice in order to achieve accuracy. Errorless learning can be an effective method with the TBI population because it involves direct instruction, teaches specific tasks, is strategy-based instruction, and focuses on self-monitoring. The patient experiences internal rewards as they accomplish the task without error. Research does show that new neuronal growth occurs as a result of the repetition and drill. Also, because this therapeutic approach is effective with specific tasks, one can use it to accomplish very functional goals for ADL If, however, the restorative feature of errorless learning is not effective, the clinician can then turn to the compensatory approach (Halpern & Goldfarb, 2013).

A Note About Generalization in People with TBI

Transfer and maintenance of skills learned in the clinic to real-life situations is not guaranteed in people with TBI. Ylvisaker, Szekeres, and Feeney (2008) suggest that treatment must be "context sensitive, every day, and routine-based" (p. 902) in order for generalization to occur. This is most easily accomplished by selecting goals that reflect the patient's ADL needs and have relevance and personal meaning. Furthermore, this highlights the importance of understanding the premorbid lifestyle of the patient that can be obtained through a thorough case history taken at the time of the initial contact (and may include family members' input). One can also use the Communication History and Interest Form (Klein & Hahn, 2007, pp. 7–11). Simply stated, generalization can occur if the therapeutic goals reflect the patient's premorbid life and interests.

The Brain Injury Association of America has excellent resources and includes a listing of cognitive aids to assist in treatment (http://www.biausa.org) along with outreach for each state. Professionals, patients, family, and friends can interact with experts using live chats, learn through workshops, gain information on how to access benefits, and connect with community resources for optimal care.

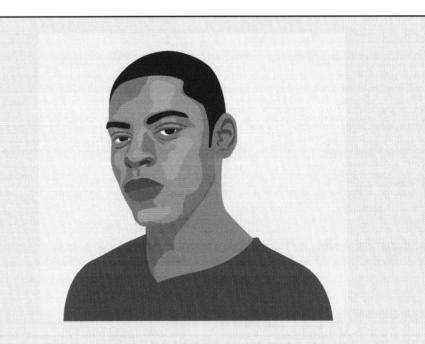

Case Scenario: Samuel

History and Physical (H & P): 22-year-old African American male admitted s/p motor vehicle accident (MVA) versus tree with lateral impact; patient was unrestrained and found partially ejected from the vehicle; combative but conscious on the scene; moving all extremities. Initial CT scan of the head revealed bilateral mandibular fractures and diffuse subarachnoid hemorrhage (SAH) at the vertex; subdural hematoma (SDH) at the falx; GCS in ED: 9/15.

Past Medical History (PMH): No significant past medical history; independent with all ADLs prior to this admission.

Social History: Lives alone; high school graduate with a history of learning disability; works in environmental services for a local hospital.

Surgical History: Unremarkable.

A Functional Analysis of Samuel's TBI

Once Samuel is stabilized in the acute care phase of his recovery, most, if not all, of his rehabilitation will take place in a brain injury unit at a rehabilitation hospital (see Figure 7–3 for Samuel's Diagnostic Profile and Figure 7–4 for his ALD Target Model). Typically, patients like Samuel will be discharged to a free-standing rehabilitation hospital for a short stay and then to home. He will then begin outpatient services including a community reentry program. To return to work and his premorbid social environment, Samuel will need to improve both his communication skills and his behaviors, as deficits in both areas will affect his employability and his ability to establish and maintain social relationships. The clinician must always focus on the three major areas of impairment in people with TBI: the neurologic and physical, the cognitive-linguistic, and the behavioral/emotional. Not every patient will demonstrate equal impairment in all three areas. For example, Sam has cognitive-linguistic impairment as well as behavioral difficulties. Other patients may demonstrate significant cognitive-linguistic deficits yet have fewer behavioral challenges, although this is a rarer scenario in the context of significant cognitive-linguistic deficits.

Treatment for Samuel must address his cognitive deficits and his irritability. He will have more difficulty becoming a contributing member to society if he cannot solve problems, think critically, and have an insightful understanding of his deficit areas. Therefore, helping Samuel develop self-monitoring skills to prevent emotional outbursts is important. Here the SLP can co-treat with a rehabilitation psychologist and other professionals, each focusing on aspects within their own scope of practice. In addition, the SLP can reinforce the self-monitoring techniques that the psychologist taught Samuel to use when necessary. Samuel's memory deficits must be addressed very early during his rehabilitation. Without a functional memory, Samuel will be dependent on others for many ADLs. Finally, family counseling and education must always be an integral part of Samuel's rehabilitation program. The family will need support and information to help them manage and understand the "new Sam," as he charts a challenging course back to functional cognitive-linguistic and behavioral skills.

Critical Thinking/Learning Activity

1. What are some tools that you can use to monitor Samuel's auditory comprehension progress? How would you chart this data?
2. How will you manage Samuel's attentional problems during the evaluation?
3. What are some ways that you can use the family to assist you in Samuel's treatment?
4. Design a family education program based on Samuel's profile.
5. How will you use the DRS in Samuel's case?

Treatment Considerations

Samuel was at Level V (Confused Inappropriate Non-agitated, requiring maximal assistance) on the RLA at the time of evaluation, and his DRS score was 5 (Moderate). His lack of deficit awareness, impaired attention (poor eye contact),

Language Expression

- **Automatic Speech:** WFL for counting, days of the week, alphabet with a verbal prompt to facilitate initiation.
- **Repetition Ability:** WFL for words and sentences.
- **Lexical Retrieval-Naming:** Confrontation naming is WFL when interested in participating.
- **Conversational Ability:** Difficulty maintaining a conversational thread; however, he can respond to simple questions accurately.
- **Pragmatic Skills:** Intermittent turn-taking errors; poor eye contact; flat affect; occasional taboo language noted in response to questioning; spontaneous utterances are WFL.
- **Paraphasias:** None.

Speech

- **Rate:** WFL
- **Intelligibility:** WFL in known and unknown contexts; hypophonia can affect intelligibility.
- **Prosody:** Monotone.
- **Articulation:** WFL
- **Fluency:** WFL

Auditory Comprehension

- **Answering Yes/No Questions:** WFL for simple yes/no questions; perseveration noted on items of increased complexity.
- **Executing Commands:** WFL for simple one-step commands.
- **Understanding Stories & Paragraphs:** Poor auditory comprehension at the paragraph level; patient perseverated on a "yes" response to all questions related to the material in the paragraph.
- **Understanding Conversational Speech:** Poor; has difficulty understanding connected speech.
- **Identifying Objects & Their Functions:** WFL

Reading

- **Word-level Comprehension:** Mildly impaired, worse on multisyllabic and abstract words.
- **Sentence-level Comprehension:** Moderately impaired; however, premorbidly patient read at the 4th–5th grade level and was in learning support throughout high school.
- **Oral Reading:** Reading aloud is slow and labored.
- **Oral Spelling:** WFL for monosyllabic words; spelling polysyllabic words impaired and may be due to memory impairment (may be at premorbid level according to parent).

Written Expression

- **Copying:** Copies basic shapes and letters when attentive.
- **Writing to Dictation:** Unable to comply with directions.
- **Self-generated:** Functional for name, but not his address; legible but disorganized.
- **Written Spelling:** Poor at word level; may be due to premorbid learning disability complicated by current head injury.
- **Drawing:** Scribbles when given pen and paper.

Cognition

- **Attention/Concentration:** Externally distractible and resentful of redirection to task. Selective attention is poor for tasks requiring sustained concentration.
- **Alertness:** Variable, but improved from baseline on admission.
- **Visuospatial Skills:** WFL for ADL needs in hospital environment.
- **Memory:** Short-term memory impaired for semantic and episodic information; better at procedural tasks. Long-term memory is mildly impaired for events from recent past. Retrograde amnesia present.
- **Executive Functions:** Requires daily and frequent orientation to time/place/date. Poor problem-solving for home-based ADL scenarios; perseverated on "I don't know," and "That's a stupid question." Safety awareness is poor for hospital and home-based environments. Unable to sequence a series of daily events to plan his day.

Behavioral Symptoms

- **Deficit Awareness:** Poor; unaware of communication deficits; poor self-monitoring skills.
- **Frustration:** Not noted at the time of assessment.
- **Emotional Lability:** Periodic tearfulness observed during therapy sessions.
- **Current Personality Characteristics:** Emotional outbursts are common; flat affect; irritable.

Figure 7–3. Diagnostic profile for Samuel.

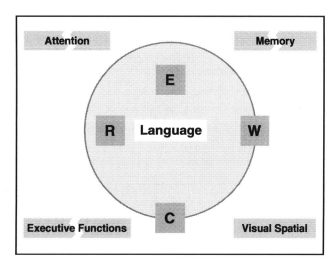

Figure 7–4. Acquired Language Disorders Target Model for Samuel.

and compromised auditory comprehension will create challenges to his ability to participate in therapy, especially in the acute phase of his hospitalization. The team must immediately address Samuel's attentional problems, so that he can participate in therapy and process incoming information. This is critical, especially during his acute care hospitalization, when many staff members are working with him and making requests of him so that they can help him. Daily monitoring of his attentional, executive functions and auditory processing skills is critical for planning the next level of care for Samuel. The RLA and the DRS would be useful in this regard. In the acute care phase of TBI, the major emphasis is on assessment and monitoring progress, for example, via the RLA, the DRS, and serial testing, so that the therapist at the next level of care has the information needed to establish optimal, realistic, and functional rehabilitation goals. The three primary areas that need to be addressed to optimize Samuel's functional communication and prepare him for rehabilitation are:

- Auditory comprehension
- Behavior
- Executive functioning

The following are more detailed treatment considerations for Samuel's case:

- It is important to demonstrate patience. Samuel will need more time to process and respond. You also will need to be aware that as he moves through the RLA levels, his behavior will become more manageable.
- Supplement auditorily presented information with pictures and written words. This will optimize his response by engaging his visual attention system.

- Talk to nursing about the medications that Samuel is prescribed. This will affect his ability to participate and even determine the most optimal time for your session with him.
- Design auditory comprehension tasks that build on Samuel's strengths, for example, start at the one-step command level gradually building to more complexity.
- Reinforce his successful trials to facilitate compliance and engagement in therapy.
- Use objects, sentences, tasks that relate to his current needs. For example, use his toothbrush and comb during a processing task instead of disconnected and abstract commands.
- Reinforce positive and compliant behavior during therapy. Use the reinforcement schedule that is most appropriate for his age and one that will help to ensure generalization of the desired behavior(s).
- Provide continual counseling and education to Samuel's caregivers. Engage them in the therapeutic process, so that they can get firsthand knowledge about his skills and deficit areas. Teach them how to implement the therapeutic program with Samuel.

Therapeutic Options

- Peer group training of pragmatic skills (Wiseman-Hakes, Stewart, Wasserman, & Schuller, 1998)
- Web-based family problem-solving intervention (Wade, Wolfe, Brown, & Pestian, 2005)
- Behavioral interventions for behavior disorders after TBI (Ylvisaker et al., 2007)
- Social skills intervention for adolescents with TBI (Turkstra & Burgess, 2007)
- Intervention for memory disorders after TBI (Avery & Kennedy, 2007)
- Treatment of discourse deficits following TBI (Cannizzaro, Coelho, & Youse, 2007)
- Teaching compensatory strategies: modeling, direct instruction, and functional practice (Ylvisaker et al., 2008)
- The Rivermead Postconcussion Symptoms Questionnaire (King, Crawford, Wenden, & Wade, 1995)

References

Avery, J., & Kennedy, M. R. T. (2007). Intervention for memory disorders after TBI. *Traumatic brain injury: Cognitive communication rehabilitation* (pp. 10–15). Rockville, MD: American Speech-Language-Hearing Association.

Brain Trauma Foundation. (2000a, June). The American Association of Neurological Surgeons: The joint section on neurotrauma and critical care. *Journal of Neurotrauma, 17*(6–7), 573–581.

Brain Trauma Foundation. (2000b, June). The American Association of Neurological Surgeons: The joint section on neurotrauma and critical care. Glasgow Coma Scale score. *Journal of Neurotrauma, 17*(6–7), 563–571.

Brown, A. W., Malec, J. F., McClelland, R. L., Diehl, N. N., Englander, J., & Cifu, D. X. (2005). Clinical elements that predict outcome after traumatic brain injury: A prospective multicenter recursive partitioning (decision-tree) analysis. *Journal of Neurotrauma, 22*(10), 1040–1051.

Bushnik, T., Englander, J., & Duong, T. (2004). Medical and social issues related to posttraumatic seizures in persons with traumatic brain injury. *Journal of Head Trauma Rehabilitation, 19*(4), 296–304.

Cannizzaro, M. S., Coelho, C. A., & Youse, K. (2007). Treatment of discourse deficit following TBI. *Traumatic brain injury: Cognitive communication rehabilitation* (pp. 17–21). Rockville, MD: American Speech-Language-Hearing Association.

Carroll, L. I., Cassidy, J. D., Peloso, P. M., Borg, J., Von Holst, H., Holm, L., . . . World Health Organization Collaborating Centre Task Force on Mild Traumatic Brain Injury. (2004). Prognosis for mild traumatic brain injury: Results of the WHO Collaborating Center Task Force on Mild Traumatic Brain Injury. *Journal of Rehabilitation Medicine, 43*(Suppl.), 84–105.

Dawodu, S. T. (2007). *Traumatic brain injury: Definition, epidemiology, and pathophysiology.* Retrieved from http://www.emedicine.com/pmr/TOPIC212.HTM

Elovic, E., & Zafonte, R. D. (2001). Spasticity management in traumatic brain injury. *Physical Medicine Rehabilitation State of Art Review, 15,* 327–348.

Guy, S. (2012, October 4). Psychological toll of wars in Afghanistan and Iraq mounts as veterans return home. *NBC News.com,* Rock Center with Brian Williams.

Hagen, C. (1998). *Revised levels of cognitive functioning, rehabilitation of the head injured adult: Comprehensive physical management* (3rd ed.). Downey, CA: Professional Staff Association of Rancho Los Amigos National Rehabilitation Center (http://www.rainbowrehab.com/Education_&_Publications/ranchos-los-amigos.php). Used with permission.

Halpern, H., & Goldfarb, R. (2013). *Language and motor speech disorders in adults* (3rd ed.). Burlington, MA: Jones & Bartlett Learning.

Hirtz, D., Thurman, D. J., Gwinn-Hardy, K., Mohamed, M., Chaudhuri, A. R., & Zulusky, R. (2007). How common are the "common" neurological disorders? *Neurology, 68,* 326–377.

Hovda, D. A. (2007). *What is so mild about mild traumatic brain injury?* [Powerpoint slides]. Retrieved from http://www.calbia.org/hovda.pdf

Jennett, B., & Bond, M. (1975). Assessment of outcome after severe brain damage. *Lancet, 1,* 480–484.

Kalinian, H. (2008). *Definition of postconcussive syndrome or concussion.* Retrieved from http://www.neuropsychconsultant.com/postconcussive.html

Kennedy, M. R. T., Coelho, C., Ylvisaker, M., Sohlberg, M. M., Avery, J., Turkstra, L. S., & Yorkston, K. (2008). Intervention for metacognitive and executive dysfunction after TBI. In L. S. Turkstra & J. McCarty (Eds.), *Evidence-based practice in traumatic brain injury* (pp. 31–37). Bethesda, MD: American Speech-Language-Hearing Association Professional Development.

Kesler, S. R., Adams, H. F., Blasey, C. M., & Bigler, E. D. (2003). Premorbid intellectual functioning, education, and brain size in traumatic brain injury: An investigation of the cognitive reserve hypothesis. *Applied Neuropsychology, 10*(3), 153–162.

King, N. S., Crawford, S., Wenden, F. J., Moss, N. E., & Wade, D. T. (1995). The Rivermead post concussion symptoms questionnaire. *Journal of Neurology, 242*(9), 587–592.

Klein, E., & Hahn, S. (2007). *Focus on function II: Gaining essential communication skills* (2nd ed.). Austin, TX: Pro-Ed.

Langlois, J. A., Rutland-Brown, W., & Thomas, K. E. (2006). *Traumatic brain injury in the United States: Emergency department visits, hospitalizations, and deaths.* Atlanta, GA: Centers for Disease Control and Prevention.

Legome, E., & Wu, T. (2006). *Postconcussive syndrome.* Retrieved from http://www.emedicine.com/EMERG/topic865.htm

Neimeier, J. P. (2010). *Evidence-based assessment and interventions for traumatic brain injury.* Franklin, TN: Summit Professional Education.

Neimeier, J. P., Kreutzer, J. S., & Taylor, L. A. (2005). Acute cognitive and neurobehavioral intervention for individuals with acquired brain injury: Preliminary outcome data. *Neuropsychology Rehabilitation, 15,* 129–146.

Niogi, S.N., Mukherjee, P., Ghajar, J., Johnson, J., Kolster, R.L., & Sarkar, R., McCandliss, B.D. (2008). Extent of microstructural white matter injuring in post-concussive syndrome correlates with impaired cognitive reaction time. A 3T diffusion tensor imaging study of mild traumatic brain injury. *American Journal of Neuroradiology, 29,* 967–973.

Northeast Center for Special Care. (2007). *Rancho Los Amigos Cognitive Scale*. Retrieved from http://www.northeastcenter.com/rancho_los_amigos.htm

Numminen, H. J. (2011). The incidence of traumatic brain injury in an adult population—How to classify mild cases? *European Journal of Neurology*, 460–464.

Ozen, L. J., & Fernandes, M. A. (2012). Slowing down after a mild traumatic brain injury: A strategy to improve cognitive task performance. *Archives of Clinical Neuropsychology*, *27*(1), 85–100.

Pangilinan, P. H. (2008). *Classification and complications of traumatic brain injury*. Retrieved from http://www.emedicine.com/pmr/topic213.htm

Parcell, D. L., Ponsford, J. L., Rajaratnam, S. M., & Redman, J. R. (2006). Self-reported changes to nighttime sleep after traumatic brain injury. *Archives of Physical Medicine and Rehabilitation*, *87*(2), 278–285.

Pegg, P. O., Jr., Auerbach, S. M., & Seel, R. T. (2005). The impact of patient-centered information on patients' treatment satisfaction and outcome in traumatic brain injury rehabilitation. *Rehabilitation Psychology*, *50*, 366–374.

Perri, G. (2012). Understanding mild traumatic brain injury. *Brain Injury Association of Kentucky*. Retrieved from http://www.brainline.org

Polito, M. Z., Thompson, J. W. G., & DeFina, P. A. (2010). A review of the international brain research foundation novel approach to mild traumatic brain injury presented at the international conference on behavioral health and traumatic brain injury. *Journal of the American Academy of Nurse Practitioners*, *22*, 504–509.

Ponsford, J., Grant, M., Cameron, P., Fitzgerald, M., Mikocka-Walus, A., & Schonberger, M. (2012). Predictors of postconcussive symptoms 3 months after mild traumatic brain injury. *Neuropsychology*, *26*(3), 304–313.

Rappaport, M., Hall, K. M., Hopkins, H. K., Belleza, T., & Cope, D. N. (1982). Disability rating scale for severe head trauma: Coma to community. *Archives of Physical Medicine and Rehabilitation*, *63*, 118–123.

Sohlberg, M. M., Avery, J., Kennedy, M. R. T., Coelho, C., Turkstra, L. S., Ylvisaker, M., & Yorkston, K. (2008). Attention training after TBI. In L. S. Turkstra & J. McCarty (Eds.), *Evidence-based practice in traumatic brain injury* (pp. 26–31). Bethesda, MD: American Speech-Language-Hearing Association Professional Development.

Sohlberg, M. M., Ehlhardt, L., & Kennedy, M. (2005). Instructional techniques in cognitive rehabilitation: A preliminary report. *Seminars in Speech and Language*, *26*, 268–279.

Springhouse. (2007). *Alarming signs and symptoms: Lippincott manual of nursing practice*. Philadelphia, PA: Lippincott Williams & Wilkins.

Szaflarski, J. (2006, April 6). Study supports theory why brain-injured children often recover. *Science Daily*. Retrieved from http://www.sciencedaily.com/releases/2006/04/060406102527.htm

Teasdale, G., & Jennett, B. (1974). Assessment of coma and impaired consciousness. A practical scale. *Lancet*, *13*(2), 81–84.

Turkstra, L. S., & Burgess, S. (2007). Social skills intervention for adolescents with TBI. *Perspectives on Neurophysiology and Neurogenic Speech and Language Disorders*, *17*(3), 15–20.

Vos, P. E., Alekseenko, Y., Battistin, L., Ehler, E., Gerstenbrand, F., Muresanu, D. F., . . . von Wild, K. (2012). Mild traumatic brain injury. *European Journal of Neurology*, 191–198.

Wade, D. T., King, N. S., Wenden, F. J., Crawford, S., & Caldwell, F. E. (1998). Routine follow-up after head injury: A second randomized controlled trial. *Journal of Neurology, Neurosurgery, and Psychiatry*, *65*, 177–183.

Wade, S. L., Wolfe, C. R., Brown, T. M., & Pestian, J. P. (2005). Can a web-based family problem-solving intervention work for children with traumatic brain injury? *Rehabilitation Psychology*, *50*(4), 337–345.

Webb, W. G., & Adler, R. K. (2008). *Neurology for the speech-language pathologist* (5th ed.). St. Louis, MO: Mosby Elsevier.

Wetzel, C. D., & Squire, L. R. (1982). Cued recall in anterograde amnesia. *Brain and Language*, *51*, 70–81.

Wiseman-Hakes, C., Stewart, M. L., Wasserman, R., & Schuller, R. (1998). Peer group training in pragmatic skills in adolescents with acquired brain injury. *Journal of Head Trauma Rehabilitation*, *13*(6), 23–38.

Ylvisaker, M., Szekeres, S. F., & Feeney, T. (2008). Communication disorders associated with traumatic brain injury. In R. Chapey (Ed.), *Language intervention strategies in aphasia and related neurogenic communication disorders* (5th ed., pp. 917–918). Philadelphia, PA: Lippincott Williams & Wilkins.

Ylvisaker, M., Turkstra, L., Coelho, C., Yorkston, K., Kennedy, M., Sohlberg, M., . . . Avery, J. (2007). Behavioral interventions for children and adults with behavior disorders after TBI: A systematic review of the evidence. *Brain Injury*, *21*(8), 769–805.

Chapter 8
DEMENTIA

Introduction

Dementia is classified as a syndrome in that it is characterized by a constellation of symptoms (Bayles & Tomoeda, 2007). Individuals who are diagnosed with dementia have multiple cognitive deficits. Dementia can result from various etiologies such as cerebrovascular disease, Alzheimer's disease, HIV disease, Parkinson's disease, Huntington's disease, Pick's disease, Creutzfeldt-Jakob disease, head trauma, or other medical conditions including substance-induced dementia. Individuals with a diagnosis of dementia must exhibit memory impairment and may exhibit one or more of the following symptoms: aphasia, agnosia, apraxia, and/or impaired executive functions, significant enough to affect occupational and social functioning (American Psychiatric Association, 2004). The incidences of dementia are increasing. Part of this is due to the fact that people are living longer, and it is estimated that by the year 2050, 14 million Americans will be diagnosed with Alzheimer's dementia. As recently as 30 years ago, dementia was unfamiliar to most Americans, including speech-language pathologists (SLPs) (Bayles & Tomoeda, 2007).

Characteristics

According to the Diagnostic and Statistical Manual of Mental Disorders–5th edition; (American Psychiatric Association, 2013), the incidence of dementia is relatively high in the population and rises with age. In countries with higher-income, the overall prevalence of dementia is 5% to 10% during the seventh decade of life. Approximately 7% of people diagnosed with Alzheimer's disease range between the ages of 65 and 74 years, which rises dramatically to 53% for those between 75 to 84 years of age. Within the DSM-5 (Diagnostic and Statistical Manual of Mental Disorders–5th edition), dementia is included in the section on neurocognitive disorders (NCDs). Core features include an acquired cognitive decline in one or more of six cognitive domains (complex attention, executive function, learning and memory, language, perceptual-motor, and social cognition). Furthermore, agitation is generally present with advanced cognitive impairment across all NCDs. Diagnosis often begins with concern by a knowledgeable informant as well as below expected performance on an objective assessment, both are required for a diagnosis, and the DSM-5 provides more information on cognitive, behavioral, and functional symptoms to further assist with differential diagnosis. NCDs include the following etiological subtypes:

- Alzheimer's disease
- Frontotemporal lobar degeneration
- Lewy body disease
- Vascular disease
- Traumatic brain injury
- Substance/medication induced
- HIV infection
- Prion disease
- Parkinson's disease

- Huntington's disease
- Due to another medical condition such as multiple sclerosis
- Due to multiple etiologies
- Unspecified neurocognitive disorder

Of those listed, Alzheimer's disease, frontotemporal lobar degeneration, and Lewy body disease are considered neurodegenerative. Diagnostic criteria according to DSM-5 are listed below.

For a medical diagnosis of neurocognitive disorder due to Alzheimer's disease (responsible for 60% to 90% of those with dementia according to the DSM-5) there must be an insidious onset and gradual progression in one or more of the cognitive domains. The individual also experiences memory decline and difficulty learning plus decline in one additional cognitive domain (usually executive function). As the disease progresses, visuoconstructional/perceptual motor ability and language are also affected. However, the clinician must keep in mind that cerebrovascular disease, another neurodegenerative disease, substance use or other mental, neurologic, or systemic disease must be ruled out first before a diagnosis of Alzheimer's disease can be made (American Psychiatric Association, 2013).

For a medical diagnosis of frontotemporal neurocognitive disorder, there is an insidious onset and gradual progression with prominent decline in social cognition and/or executive abilities. For the behavioral variant, the person experiences three or more of the following symptoms: behavioral disinhibition, apathy, loss of sympathy/empathy, preservative/ritualistic behavior, or hyperorality/dietary changes. There is also a prominent decline in the person's social cognition and/or executive functions. For the language variant, the person exhibits prominent decline in speech production, word finding/naming objects, grammar, or comprehension of words. Learning, memory and perceptual-motor functions are largely spared. Similar to Alzheimer's disease, cerebrovascular disease, another type of neurodegenerative disease, substance use or other mental, neurologic, or systemic disease must be ruled out before a diagnosis of a frontotemporal NCD can be made.

For a diagnosis of neurocognitive disorder with Lewy bodies, there must be an insidious onset and gradual progression. The core features include fluctuating cognition with variations in attention and alertness levels. The patient often has recurrent and detailed visual hallucinations, spontaneous features of parkinsonism and cognitive decline. Again, cerebrovascular disease, another type of neurodegenerative disease, substance use or other mental, neurologic, or systemic disease must be ruled out before a diagnosis of Lewy body dementia can be made.

Diagnostic Factors

Dementia is usually diagnosed long after its initial onset. The first symptoms are generally memory difficulties and forgetfulness. One diagnostic challenge is to differentiate mild dementia from cognitive decline due to depression (pseudo-dementia). Radiologic imaging such as CT scan, lab tests, and neuropsychological assessment may help differentiate and identify dementia versus other disease processes than can mimic dementia. A more recently developed diagnostic screening test is now available, called the Electrical Alzheimer's Test (Warner, 2003). Electrodes for an electroencephalogram are placed on the head and spine of the patient to detect changes in the brain's electrical functions. It takes about 15 minutes to administer and can be done as an outpatient. The electroencephalogram (EEG) measures a person's P300 latency (event-related evoked potentials) to determine if it is normal. The P300 latency reflects information processing of cognitive events. As Alzheimer's disease begins as a slowing of the brain's processing speed, this test has been found useful in detecting signs of cognitive decline before they are manifested clinically. There is some speculation that this is generated in the frontal, temporal, and parietal lobes. In people with early stage dementia, P300 latency is in excess of 400 msec, although a prolonged P300 latency does occur with normal aging. According to Barclay (2003), P300 may be one test subtle enough to identify changes in the brain before documentation of memory loss. Whereas age, memory, and mental status impairment have been well established, it is not consistently accepted that the neurodevelopment patterns of the P300 component are an electrophysiological memory marker.

Neuropsychologists, speech-language pathologists, and other clinicians must evaluate individuals with suspected dementia. A case history including an interview with significant other(s) is advised due to familiarity with the patient. They can report any memory problems or word finding difficulties that they observe. Premorbid intelligence is another important factor to consider, so that the clinician can compare the patient's current functioning with his or her premorbid status. Hearing loss, impaired vision, depression, and medication usage are just a few additional pieces of information that must be taken into consideration when assessing a person's mental status (Hopper & Bayles, 2008). According to Hopper and Bayles (2008), a comprehensive battery of tests to assess communicative functions must be administered. Cognitive abilities including memory must be assessed. Below is a summary of selected assessment measures for dementia:

- Arizona Battery for Communication Disorders of Dementia (ABCD), Story Retelling Subtest for screening purposes (Bayles & Tomoeda, 1993)
- FAS Verbal Fluency Test (Borkowski, Benton, & Spreen, 1967)
- Mini-Mental State Examination (Folstein, Folstein, & McHugh, 1975) to screen attention, concentration, language, and memory
- Boston Naming Test (Kaplan, Goodglass, & Weintraub, 1983)
- Boston Diagnostic Aphasia Examination-3 (Goodglass, Kaplan, & Barresi, 2000)
- The Functional Linguistic Communication Inventory (Bayles & Tomoeda, 1994)
- Western Aphasia Battery-Revised (Kertesz, 2006)
- Clinical Dementia Rating Scale (Hughes, Berg, Danziger, Coben, & Martin, 1982)
- Global Deterioration Scale (Reisberg, Ferris, de Leon, & Crook, 1982)
- Addenbrooke's Cognitive Examination (Mioshi, Dawson, Mitchell, Arnold, & Hodges, 2006

For a comprehensive list of various assessment scales used in dementia, see http://www.ncbi.nlm.nih.gov/pmc/articles/PMC3487532/

Dementia has both irreversible and reversible etiologies. The most familiar causes of irreversible dementia include Alzheimer's disease, Huntington's disease, vascular disease, and Parkinson's disease, fronto-temporal-parietal dementia, Creutzfeldt-Jakob disease, and Lewy body disease. For a more extensive review of the dementias see Bayles and Tomoeda (2007). Fifty percent of those with dementia have Alzheimer's type, and 20% have vascular dementia due to multiple infracts and vascular disease. The average life expectancy for a patient with Alzheimer's disease is typically 8 years, although it can progress for 12 years or more from awareness of symptoms and diagnosis to death. However, rapid decline is linked to three characteristics: early age onset, delusions or hallucinations, or extrapyramidal signs. In these patients, small, lacunar infarcts are chronic, closing down the microvessels in the cortical and subcortical arterial system, thereby compromising function in the areas of respective distribution. The causes of reversible dementia include, but are not limited to, drug toxicity, vitamin deficiency, infections and tumors, normal pressure hydrocephalus, renal failure, congestive heart failure, and thyroid disease.

Stages of Dementia

There are typically three stages in dementia classification: early, middle, and late. Abilities change in the areas of cognition and memory, self-care, communication, and physical and sensory abilities as dementia progresses. In most instances, the individual's decline is gradual and insidious, occurring over a 6-year period of time before there is any clinical evidence (Collie & Maruff, 2000).

Early Stage Dementia

In early stages of dementia (generally referring to Alzheimer's dementia), the person's ability to communicate depends on their recent memory. As a consequence, they can define words and describe pictures but may have difficulty following a line of conversation. However, they still may have the ability to follow a three-step command (Figure 8–1). Some of their sentences remain incomplete, and they may repeat themselves. Comprehension of longer

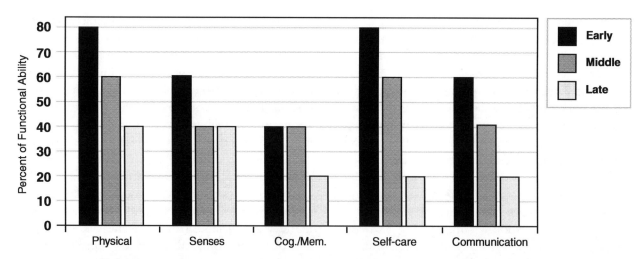

Figure 8–1. Abilities and stages of dementia. From *The Source for Alzheimer's and Dementia* by Pam Reese © 2000. Reprinted with permission of LinguiSystems, Inc.

material may be reduced. Reading and writing at this stage are often spared, but spelling errors are common. Syntax is normal. Decreases in psychomotor speed, perceptual speed, abstract reasoning, visuospatial performance, and episodic memory are typically seen in early stages (Bayles, 2004). From a functional standpoint, the person with early stage dementia often has minimal difficulty with activities of daily living; however, one may observe a decline in the following areas:

- Difficulty handling finances
- Disoriented to time and place
- Episodic and working memory difficulties including recalling personal information
- Difficulty with complex tasks
- Decreased awareness of recent events
- Disjointed conversation (cohesion and content)
- Mild semantic dysnomia (apple for pear, pen for pencil, etc.)
- Mini-Mental State Exam (score 16–24 of 30).

Middle Stage Dementia

In middle stage dementia, people may be disoriented to time and place. The individual can usually name items when given confrontation naming tasks but has difficulty engaging in conversation. Verbal output tends to have less meaning. Syntax remains intact, but sentence fragments are common. Comprehension for two-step commands is generally accomplished, but three steps tend to be difficult. Writing words to dictation is often intact; however, writing any lengthy material is difficult (Bayles, 2004). The individual may still be able to read, but they often forget what they read. The following symptoms may be present:

- Disoriented for time and place
- Restlessness and distractibility are common
- Poor episodic memory with lack of awareness for recent events
- Encoding and retrieval deficits
- Poor semantic memory
- Poor attention and focus
- Visual perception and constructional deficits
- Cognitive deficits
- Forgetfulness for common information
- Greater knowledge about remote past than present
- Assistance is needed with ADLs (activities of daily living)
- Verbal output is fluent but slower and less informative with word-finding problems
- Agitation and anxiety may be present

- Reading and writing are impaired
- Mini-Mental State Exam Scores (8–15 of 30).

Late Stage Dementia

In the late stage of dementia, there is extensive memory loss. The individual is disoriented for time, place, and factors relating to self. Problem-solving abilities are very limited. Minimal functional vocabulary may remain. Most remaining language consists of either common social phrases or nonsense. Some people become mute. However, many can still follow a simple one-step command and read a basic word (Bayles, 2004). At this point, they often become incontinent, and they have difficulty walking. The following characteristics are typically seen at this late stage:

- Disoriented for person, place, and time
- Very severe cognitive deficits
- In very late stage, person may be nonambulatory
- Severe impairment in working and declarative memory
- Verbal output is diminished and communication is out of context, but grammar is generally intact
- All verbal abilities may be lost (especially in patients who are bladder and bowel incontinent), and person may be mute
- For those who are only bladder incontinent, they may be able to respond to greetings, recognize their written name, recognize common drawn objects, and follow single-step directions (Bayles, Tomoeda, Cruz, & Mahendra, 2000)
- Common language deficits are reflected in being mute, perseverative, echolalic, and palilalic (excessive repetitive utterances)
- Scores on Mini-Mental State Exam (0–9 of 30).

Memory Systems and Dementia

To understand the nature of dementia and its effects on the lives of patients and their families, it is help-ful to become familiar with the memory systems at work in normal and impaired cognition. Memory has been defined as representations that are stored through a process of encoding, consolidation, and retrieval for acquisition and manipulation of knowledge (Baddeley, 1999). The discussion below describes the relationships among the three primary areas of memory: sensory memory, working memory, and long-term memory.

Sensations come into the peripheral nervous system and may enter consciousness. Sensory memory lasts from less than 1 second to a maximum of 2 seconds. If sensory information enters conscious awareness, sensation is attended to and can then be interpreted. Previous experiences assist in the interpretation and meaning of the stimuli.

Multiple systems are involved in memory. Short-term memory, also referred to as working memory, requires attention and concentration to remember or retain information. Baddeley (2002) reviewed his model of a limited capacity system for temporary storage of information and expanded it to include the episodic buffer. In his system, the visuospatial sketchpad holds visual images while the phonological loop temporarily stores verbal information. The central executive manages these subsystems by apportioning attention to them. Therefore, a person can hold a concept, word, picture, or idea in memory and manipulate it to solve problems (Baddeley, 1983; Fockert, Rees, Frith, & Lavie, 2001). The system serves as a link between working memory and long-term memory, so that new information can be stored as an episode and later retrieved (Baddeley, 2002).

Long-term memory involves declarative knowledge of factual information (also known as declarative or explicit memory) and nondeclarative memory (also known as implicit memory), which refers to motor memories and conditioned responses (Squire, 1992). Working memory processes information from long-term memory. Diseases that affect cortical areas generally affect declarative memory. Diseases that affect subcortical structures (i.e., basal ganglia) generally produce nondeclarative memory deficits (Hopper & Bayles, 2008). Table 8–1 presents a breakdown of memory deficits.

Table 8–1. Declarative and Nondeclarative Memory Systems

Declarative Memory (Explicit)	Nondeclarative Memory (Implicit)
Semantic (Concepts) • Involves conceptual knowledge and understanding of constructs from which people organize their world and experiences.	Procedural (Motor Skills) • Involves learned skills that become automatic with practice and repetition (riding a bike).
Episodic (Events) • This ability is most affected early on in dementia. This autobiographic system receives and stores information about events that people experience.	Procedural (Verbal and Cognitive Skills) • Involves learned skills that occur without conscious awareness, such as knowing how to get information to someone through the mail.
Lexical (Words) • Memory for words, their meanings, spelling, and pronunciation. These are the linguistic representations of concepts.	Priming • Associations are made so that earlier experiences trigger words, thoughts, and memories of similar experience.
	Conditioned Responses • A reaction to a previous similar stimulus occurs due to a chain of associated triggers. Habits are often developed because of associations for events that are repeated.

Types of Dementia

Vascular Dementia (VaD)

Vascular dementia is the second most common cause of dementia. People with hypertension, atherosclerosis, and a history of previous strokes are all at risk for acquiring this type of dementia. Vascular dementia is usually caused by ischemia or a restriction of blood flow in the vessels of the brain. Those patients who demonstrate symptoms consistent with dementia after sustaining multiple deep, lacunar strokes, are usually diagnosed with multiinfarct dementia (MID). It is possible to develop a vascular dementia secondary to large cerebral infracts, ischemic events, and/or microvascular disease, that is, the occlusion of the fine capillaries within the cortex. Approximately one-fourth to one-third of patients who have had one or more ischemic stroke develops vascular dementia within 3 months (Pohjasvaara et al., 1998).

Dementia of the Alzheimer's Type (DAT)

Dementia of the Alzheimer's type (DAT), more commonly known as Alzheimer's disease, this is by far the most common type of dementia observed in the population. It was also known as presenile dementia, as its onset can be seen in the fifth decade, unlike senile dementia which is associated with normal aging. The cognitive-linguistic, affective, and behavioral aspects of each type are similar, however. On autopsy, the brain of the person with DAT will show changes in the association areas of the parietal, temporal, and frontal lobes, as well as in the hippocampus, a major structure for memory. DAT tends to begin in the hippocampal area, which is essential to forming episodic memories. This is why individuals in early stages have difficulty recalling recent events. As the disease progresses to the frontal region and tempero-parietal regions of the brain, declarative memory is affected for semantic and lexical memories, and the person will have difficulty organizing information and recalling words and concepts. The basal ganglia and motor cortex are not impacted throughout most of the disease's progression and, therefore, procedural memory often remains intact (Bayles, 2004). Autopsied brains also reveal neuronal plaques, neurofibrillary tangles, and granulovascular degeneration, which are all abnormal tissue changes. Although tangles and plaques lead to cell death and impact intercellular transmission, subcortical structures and the motor strip remain unaffected. Therefore, the speech of individuals with DAT generally is spared (Bayles, 2004). The brain's biochemistry also degenerates in these patients, in that there is a reduction in the function of the cholinergic and noradrenergic systems that disrupt nerve transmission. Unfortunately, the etiology of DAT is not certain. Some educated guesses include aluminum toxicity, immune dysfunction, and viral infection. More commonly, age, family history, and genetics are implicated According to research from the Alzheimer's Association (2013), individuals who have a parent or sibling with Alzheimer's are more likely to develop the disease. The gene with the strongest risk impact is APOE-e4. While everyone inherits a copy of APOE from their mother and father, those who inherit APOE-e4 are at increased risk for developing Alzheimer's (20%–25% of cases). After the age of 65, the risk doubles every five years. After age 85, approximately 50% of individuals are at risk for DAT.

Parkinson's Dementia

The dementia associated with Parkinson's disease (PD) is not observed until the very late stages of the disease process. Parkinson's disease is a neurodegenerative disease with complex motor disturbances due to a loss of striatal dopaminergic neurons in the substantia nigra. Typical features of the motoric aspect of this disease are slow movements (bradykinesia), rigidity, pin wheeling, tremor, a masked-like face, and disturbances in gait (festinating), posture, and balance. Treatments for PD include dopamine to restore that neurotransmitter to optimal levels and deep brain stimulation (DBT). According to Bayles (2004), individuals with PD have motor speech difficulties due to damage of the basal ganglia and striatal-cortical circuits as well as deficits in memory, attention, and executive functioning. However, knowledge for language, including sentence comprehension and confrontation naming, tends to be preserved.

Individuals at the end stage of PD can manifest with cognitive changes consistent with dementia, although the best estimate indicates that approximately 29% of all patients develop it (Marttila & Rinne, 1976). The etiology of the dementia in PD

is still debated. Some researchers believe that it is due to cortical degeneration and others to subcortical degeneration that impairs the neurologic control of attention (Brown & Marsden, 1988). Rinne et al. (2000) reported that there was reduced fluorodopa uptake in PD individuals in the caudate nucleus and the frontal cortex. They stated that this impairs performance on any tests that require executive functions. Regardless of etiology, PD patients who do develop dementia have problems communicating due to deficits in memory, attention, and the higher level executive functions (Bayles, 2004).

Fronto-Temporal-Parietal Dementias (FTP)

Frontal lobe dementias are rare (fewer than 10% of all diagnosed cases of dementia). Fronto-Temporal-parietal dementia (FTP) typically has a very early onset, usually in the fourth or fifth decade of a person's life. It is primarily associated with personality changes, reduced language abilities, and difficulty executing complex tasks. People with this type of dementia will become moody, self-centered, and unable to be empathic. They may appear unfeeling. A true diagnosis can only be made upon autopsy. Under those conditions, the brain will reveal significant cell loss in the frontal and temporal cortices.

With fronto-temporal dementia (FTD) as the second most common cause of dementia in younger individuals, there is progressive atrophy of frontal and/or anterior temporal regions of the brain resulting in progressive language impairments that are common in semantic dementia (SD) and progressive nonfluent aphasia (PNFA). PNFA with more of an agrammatism but spared semantics than SD, was detected later and found to have a more rapid decline (Leyton, Hornberger, Mioshi, & Hodges, 2010). A third type of dementia has more recently been identified as logopenic/phonological aphasia in which the individual has limited speech and severe word finding deficits. Grammar is spared, but sentence repetition and sentence comprehension are impaired (Gorno-Tempini et al., 2008).

Pick's disease is a type of frontal lobe dementia, with characteristics that set it apart from the more general type described above. Neary et al. (1988)

suggest that Pick's disease is a variant form of FTP dementia (Neary et al., 1988). It is also rare, seen predominantly in women, with an incidence of one tenth as much as that of DAT. The etiology of Pick's dementia is due to the loss of neurons, gliosis, and neuronal inclusions called Pick's bodies. The pattern of degeneration in these patients is different from that of FTP or DAT. In the case of the Pick's patient, the neuronal deterioration is primarily frontal but includes the inferior motor area and the anterior temporal lobes. Pick's disease and DAT both share one similar structural feature: the deterioration of the hippocampus and the amygdaloid nucleus.

The FTP dementias, including Pick's, have characteristic cognitive, behavioral, and language features. Behaviorally, these patients will demonstrate reduced spontaneity, reduced insight, and reduced executive functions. Their language abnormalities will be noted early in the process, unlike DAT. These patients will have reduced initiation, palilalia, echolalia, and logorrhea (more so in Pick's). Mutism can also be observed in middle to late stage Pick's disease.

Creutzfeldt-Jakob Disease

Creutzfeldt-Jakob disease is caused by the presence of prions. Prions are unconventional, transmissible agents (not a virus or a bacterium). They are a special type of protein that can be transmitted from one animal to another. They can cause a group of degenerative diseases of the nervous system. These diseases can be manifest as sporadic, infectious, or inherited disorders. Only about 15% of cases have a genetic link. Creutzfeldt-Jakob disease (CJD) is defined by the American Medical Association as:

> A rare transmissible encephalopathy most prevalent between the ages of 50 and 70 years. Affected individuals may present with sleep disturbances, personality changes, ataxia, aphasia, visual loss, weakness, muscle atrophy, myoclonus, progressive dementia, and death within one year of disease onset.

A familial form exhibiting autosomal dominant inheritance and a new variant (potentially associated with encephalopathy, bovine spongiform) have been described. Pathologic features include prominent cerebellar and cerebral cortical spongiform degeneration and the presence of prions (Johnson & Gibbs, 1998). The prognosis for these patients is not favorable. They usually die within 1 year of the diagnosis. As noted in the AMA definition above, these patients will have symptoms consistent with aphasia.

Huntington's Disease

Huntington's disease (HD), also known as Huntington's chorea, is a progressive and fatal neurodegenerative disease. It is a genetic disease (autosomal dominant), characterized by choreoathetoid movements and dementia. The incidence of HD in the population is approximately five per 100,000 and affects people of northern European descent. The age of onset is in one's 30s or 40s. The initial symptoms are personality changes and sometimes frank psychosis, with depression being a very common feature. This neurodegenerative disease is classified as a hyperkinetic movement disorder, hence the choreoathetoid movements.

Communication and cognitive functions are both affected by HD. Early after onset, the patient begins to manifest characteristics of a hyperkinetic dysarthria, and HD patients are often nonverbal during the end stage of the disease process. Language deficits associated with HD include difficulty initiating conversational speech, language formulation problems, word finding problems, poor auditory processing for complex material, and slow response time. They also can demonstrate reading and writing problems. Cognitively, they have difficulty learning new information and new tasks, exhibit reduced executive functions, and poor attention and concentration (Klasner, n.d.).

All of these difficulties can be and usually are present in one individual. They often begin in a mild form and become more severe as the disease progresses. Abilities are often unpredictable, because deficits occur randomly during the general progression of the disease. This unpredictability creates more coping difficulties for the Huntington's disease patient, because he or she cannot rely on having or maintaining various skills at any given time. For example, the Huntington's disease patient could make a request clearly at one moment, but then have significant difficulty articulating that same request a moment later.

Overview of Research on Treatment for Dementia

As of 2010, there were an estimated 5.1 million Americans with Alzheimer's disease and other dementias (Hopper et al., 2013). Speech-language pathologists are often called on to support the patient with dementia and their family. In a 2011 caseload review survey by the American Speech-Language-Hearing Association (ASHA), SLPs ranked working with individuals with dementia and communication-related disorders as the third most common treatment they provided in health care settings (dysphagia and aphasia were first and second, respectively). It is estimated that by the year 2050, approximately 13.5 million Americans over 65 years old will have dementia (Alzheimer's Association, 2012). Although medication can help slow the disease process, it cannot prevent its progression and ultimate decline.

Previous practice guidelines include computer-assisted cognitive interventions, spaced-retrieval training, Montessori-based interventions, reminiscence therapy, simulated-presence therapy, caregiver-administered cognitive stimulation, and caregiver education for more successful communication. The current focus, according to ASHA, is on direct cognitive interventions with individualized goals, specific to the patient's needs and family requests.

In an attempt to review more current literature, Hopper et al. (2013) reviewed 43 studies with a total of 556 participants who met inclusion criteria for cognitive intervention with dementia. Most of the information about treatment effects came from 11 single-subject, multiple–baseline designs and looked at verbal instruction strategies to assist individuals

with dementia complete their ADLs. According to Hopper et al. (2013), results indicated that Spaced Retrieval Training had positive outcomes for individuals' abilities to recall facts and perform tasks. Most frequently, treatment tasks involved recalling names of people and objects. Interventions using memory aids were helpful when they included caregiver education and memory books or memory wallets (Egan, Berube, Racine, Leonard, & Rochon, 2010). Other noted treatments included Errorless Learning for learning facts. Some procedures appeared to have the best results when effort was expended during learning trials for novel stimuli (Dunn & Clare, 2007), as an add-on to errorless learning strategies. Verbal instruction cueing had positive outcomes for ADLs especially when electronic memory aids were added (Lancioni et al., 2010).

Overall results indicated that learning occurred best in individuals with mild and mild-moderate dementia. Spaced Retrieval Training was found to be promising in helping individuals recall facts and procedures. Errorless Learning and Vanishing Cues also had positive results. Although generalization is desirable, it presented greater challenges as dementia progressed. Regardless of the training type, it was suggested that intervention focus on functional tasks and ADLs to improve the quality of the person's life at any given point in time.

The WHO-ICF framework can be used to individualize cognitive-communication treatment for a person with dementia (see Appendix F). The broader areas within the ICF specifically related to dementia are: focusing on repetitive verbalizations, language referring to body functions and ADL needs, and word-finding difficulties. These are the problems most often cited by the family of the patient with dementia (Byrne & Orange, 2005). Therefore, speech-language pathologists working with these individuals should support the patient's language abilities by providing objects, pictures, words, gestures, or any other means as needed to improve the reception and expression of functional language (World Health Organization, 2001).

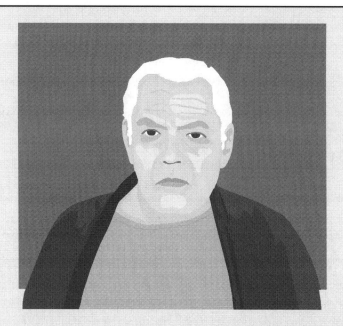

Case Scenario: Max

History and Physical (H & P): Max, a 76-year-old male presented to a neurologist on consult from his primary physician as an outpatient. The patient was brought in by his wife who reported problems with simple calculations, telling time, and home repair tasks, which were normally simple and routine for him to do.

Past Medical History (PMH): Cardiomyopathy; cortical atrophy noted on last MRI with enlarged sulci; hypercholesterolemia; family reported difficulty with numbers and time for approximately 6 months prior to this admission (PTA).

Social History: Self-employed in a trucking business; married with two grown children in the area. Some postsecondary education (Associate's Degree); naval officer during WWII. Family reported that patient is "less moody" over the past few months.

Surgical History: Hernia repair.

A Functional Analysis of Max's Dementia

Max's ability to understand and use language is intact for his ADL needs (see Figure 8–2 for Max's Diagnostic Profile and Figure 8–3 for his ALD Target Model). However, he has difficulty formulating language to discuss recent events and facts, dates and time, facts of general knowledge related to his personal history, and political and social history of the times. His semantic memory is also beginning to show signs of decline, manifested by semantic paraphasias. There are concomitant word-finding problems. Max's procedural memory is still intact, so he can perform basic meal preparation, gardening, and minor home repairs.

Language Expression

Automatic Speech: WFL	**Repetition Ability:** WFL
Lexical Retrieval-Naming: Naming difficulties noted, specifically names of people and locations; poor confrontation naming.	**Conversational Ability:** Common social phrases were used appropriately; able to express his wants and needs at the sentence level; able to engage in a one-on-one dialogue that was concrete, and context driven (contextualized language); narrative discourse focused on two topics: lack of income and returning to work; patient could be redirected with verbal cue.
Pragmatic Skills: WFL	**Paraphasias:** Semantic paraphasias noted in conversation.

Speech

Rate: WFL	**Intelligibility:** WFL	**Prosody:** WFL	**Articulation:** WFL	**Fluency:** WFL

Auditory Comprehension

Answering Yes/No Questions: Answers to abstract yes/no questions were mildly impaired.	**Executing Commands:** WFL executing one-step commands was WFL; following complex multistep questions was mild-moderately impaired.
Understanding Stories & Paragraphs: WFL for short paragraphs up to 5 sentences in length. Errors increase as paragraph increases.	**Understanding Conversational Speech:** Sentence comprehension was WFL; comprehension at the conversational level was variable depending on the number of people involved and the complexity of the information.
Identifying Objects & Their Functions: WFL	

Reading

Word-level Comprehension: WFL	**Sentence-level Comprehension:** Good for simple declarative sentences; moderately impaired as the semantic and syntactic complexity increased, e.g., connectives and clausal relationships.
Oral Reading: WFL for simple, commonly used high frequency words and simple declarative sentences.	**Oral Spelling:** Moderately impaired for irregularly spelled words and polysyllabic words.

Written Expression

Copying: Able to copy words and sentences.	**Writing to Dictation:** Able to write sentences to dictation.
Self-generated: Writes functionally at the phrase level to express his needs if necessary.	**Written Spelling:** Moderately impaired for irregularly spelled words and polysyllabic words characterized by missing letters.
Drawing: Not functional for communication purposes and often ended up in perseverative "doodles."	

Cognition

Attention/Concentration: Mild-moderately impaired raising the issue of safety at home and in public.	**Visuospatial Skills:** Patient was unable to consistently recognize family members and thought they were impostors.
Memory: Semantic memory is moderately impaired; moderately-severely impaired episodic memory for recent events; procedural memory is functional for overlearned tasks, e.g., gardening, minor home repairs, meal preparation.	**Executive Functions:** Relied on family members to make appointments; unable to plan and organize a daily task independently; poor judgment for home safety scenarios.

Behavioral Symptoms

Alertness: Level of alertness during daytime hours was WFL; sometimes awakens fully alert and agitated in the middle of the night asking to go to his adult day-care program.	**Deficit Awareness:** "There is something wrong with my brain. It's like there's a hole in it."
Frustration: Agitation and anxiety noted; more agitated at night.	**Emotional Lability:** Not noted.
Current Personality Characteristics: Premorbidly rigid, confident, assertive and rule-bound (ex-military officer); currently, more dependent, frightened, still inflexible.	

Figure 8–2. Diagnostic profile for Max.

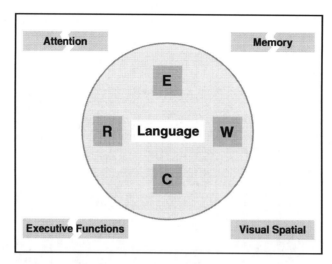

Figure 8–3. Acquired Language Disorders Target Model for Max.

However, due to his attentional deficits, his safety at home and in public can be compromised. This can lead to dangerous errors while executing activities of daily living.

Max is able to write sentences to dictation but can only use writing functionally at the phrase level to express his needs if necessary. His reading comprehension is good for sentences, but is moderately impaired at the more complex paragraph level. This may limit his ability to read and understand detailed or lengthy written instructions. Training the family to give Max written instructions at the short phrase level, supplemented by pictures and/or symbols, is suggested. For example, a written note placed above the sink, "Rinse dishes" paired with a picture or drawing of a dish being washed, may facilitate clean-up. Because Max has a progressive and degenerative disease, the family is advised to manipulate the environment for his comfort and ease. Communication with Max is best when it is about the here and now, supplemented by tangible objects relevant to the context. Max's wife, the primary caretaker, is encouraged to reduce her rate of speech and allow time for him to process and respond. It is also recommended that she not call attention to his difficulties because he does not have the ability to readily repair his errors. She must also be instructed to reduce the number of people participating in a conversation if Max is to be included. In general, indirect therapy is most appropriate for Max at this stage of his dementia with a focus on counseling and education of his family regarding the goals and procedures of this therapeutic approach. The clinician can also consider the FOCUSED Caregiver Training Program by Ripich, Ziol, Fritsch, and Durand (1999) for more formal intervention. Finally, Max's wife may benefit from a support group for families dealing with dementia.

Critical Thinking/Learning Activity

- What information indicates that this is a person with dementia?
- With progression of the disorder, how would this patient's prosopagnosia impact communicative effectiveness with his family members?
- What are the family counseling and education issues in this case, and how would you address them?
- What can you do to facilitate communication when Max is part of a group of people having a conversation?
- Write a SOAP note on this patient. Assume that you are seeing the patient for the first time after the evaluation session. Include three short-term therapeutic objectives in your note.

Treatment Considerations

Max was diagnosed with dementia of the Alzheimer's type. He tries to participate in conversations but demonstrates frustration when he is unable to do so effectively. As a consequence, he withdraws into silence. His language is composed primarily of idioms, common social phrases, and stereotypic utterances. Because of his memory impairments and inability to drive safely, Max is very dependent on his wife for transportation to appointments. He often wakes his wife during the night thinking that it is, "time to leave." Max has some awareness of his deficits and told his daughter, "There's something wrong in my head." When out in the community, he often become impatient and has difficulty staying in one place for more than 15 minutes. Max is most affected by his cognitive rather than linguistic problems. He can still communicate with his family and friends effectively enough to have his daily wants and needs met. As a consequence, Max's therapy must focus primarily on compensations for his cognitive deficits and secondarily on his minor linguistic impairments. However, the clinician must keep in mind that dementia is a progressive disease process, so Max's therapy must change as he does, with different accommodations set according to his needs. There are various treatment programs and therapeutic techniques specific to dementia that the clinician can employ, which are highlighted below.

Some Therapeutic Options

We suggest that the speech-language pathologist consider the following selected programs when planning therapy for people with dementia:

- Spaced-Retrieval Training (SRT; Camp & Schaller, 1989; Hopper et al., 2005). SRT uses a verbally mediated technique to help with safety and activities of daily living. The patient rehearses a specific response or action to a stimulus across repeated trials. The time between the presentation of the stimulus and the request from the clinician for the response is gradually increased. The patient eventually learns the new behavior. For example, greeting someone who enters the room requires certain steps to accomplish the act. The SLP would use SRT to facilitate the learning of these steps (Camp, Foss, O'Hanlon, & Stevens, 1996).

■ FOCUSED Caregiver Training Program (Ripich et al., 1999). Family/ caregiver counseling and education is a cornerstone of treatment for people with dementia. The clinician must educate the family/ caregivers about the disease process itself, the goals and procedures of therapy, and their role in the treatment plan. The SLP must also provide counseling about issues of living with a person with dementia and its progressive nature. One program specific to family and/or caregiver training, supporting functional communication is FOCUSED (Ripich, 1994). In this approach, the suggestions for communication enrichment follow the acronym. The F is for *Face-to-Face* communication; O reminds the communication partner to *Orient* the patient to the topic; C refers to keeping the continuity of the topic *Concrete*; U helps remind the conversational partner to help *Unstick* any communication blocks; S refers to *Structure* in using yes or no and direct choice questions; E is to support and encourage an *Exchange* in conversation; and D refers to the importance of using *Direct*, short, and simple sentences when speaking to the person with dementia.

■ Stimulus generalization (Thompson, 1989). The clinician can use a stimulus generalization approach to treat persons with dementia. In this approach, a trained response acquired during the treatment session is generalized to a new context where there may be different people, materials, or places. For example, the person with dementia may learn to ask for clarification when he or she does not understand what is said during the therapy session. This therapy approach teaches the patient to transfer this new behavior to a new context, that is, at home, the physician's office (Thompson, 1989).

■ External memory aids (Reese, 2000). *Memory books and daily logs* can be used to optimize the patient's ability to perform his or her activities of daily living. The clinician facilitates the patient's completion of the daily log and discusses the content. The use of photographs from the patient's life may also enhance quality of life and augment communication due to the familiarity of the contextual references. Any of these activities can be used to address semantic and word retrieval goals. Traditional therapeutic approaches can be used to address cognitive-communicative impairment (Helm-Estabrooks, 1995). The use of technology and apps may also be used during therapy for a variety of goals, since they are so numerous. (See https://sites.google.com/site/ipadforelderlypeople/ipad-dementia)

- Strength-based communication and programming (Eisner, 2001).
- Validation therapy (Feil, 1991). Validate through words and gestures to review what the person says, regardless of fact (Toseland et al., 1997).
- Graphic and written cues (Hoerster, Hickey, & Bourgeois, 2001). Provide written information and photos to support recognition memory; use a memory wallet, book, or daily log.
- Montessori-based interventions (Orsulic-Jeras, Schneider, & Camp, 2000).

References

Alzheimer's Association. (2012). *Alzheimer's disease facts and figures.* Chicago, IL: Author. Retrieved from http://www.alz.org/national/documents/Facts _Figures_2011.pdf

Alzheimer's Association. (2013). *What we know today about Alzheimer's disease.* Chicago, IL: Author. Retrieved from http://www.alz.org/research/science/ Alzheimer'ss_disease_causes.asp

American Psychiatric Association. (2013). *Diagnostic and statistical manual of mental disorders* (5th ed.). Arlington, VA: Author.

Baddeley, A. D. (1983). Working memory. *Philosophical transactions of the Royal Society of London. Series B, Biological Sciences, 302*(1110), 311–324.

Baddeley, A. D. (1999). *Essentials of human memory.* Hove, East Sussex, UK: Psychology Press.

Baddeley, A. D. (2002). Is working memory still working? *European Psychologist, 7*(2), 85–97.

Barclay, L. (2003). P300 latency accurately predicts memory impairment. *Clinical Electroencephalography, 34,* 124–139.

Bayles, K. (2004). Dementia. In R. Kent (Ed.), *The MIT encyclopedia of communication disorders.* Cambridge, MA: A Bradford Book.

Bayles, K. A., & Tomoeda, C. K. (1993). *Arizona battery for communication disorders of dementia.* Austin, TX: Pro-Ed.

Bayles, K. A., & Tomoeda, C. K. (1994). *The functional linguistic communication inventory.* Austin, TX: Pro-Ed.

Bayles, K. A., & Tomoeda, C. K. (2007). *Cognitive-communication disorders of dementia.* San Diego, CA: Plural.

Bayles, K. A., Tomoeda, C., Cruz, R., & Mahendra, N. (2000). Communication abilities of individuals with late-stage Alzheimer's disease. *Alzheimer's Disease and Associated Disorders, 14*(3), 176–181.

Borkowski, J. G., Benton, A. L., & Spreen, O. (1967). Word fluency and brain damage. *Neuropsychologia, 5,* 135–140.

Brown, R. G., & Marsden, C. D. (1988). Internal and external cues and the control of attention in Parkinson's disease. *Brain, 111,* 323–345.

Byrne, K., & Orange, J. B. (2005). Conceptualizing communication enhancement in dementia for family caregivers using the WHO-*ICF* framework. *Advances in Speech-Language Pathology, 7,* 187–202.

Camp, C. J., Foss, J. W, O'Hanlon, A. M., & Stevens, A. B. (1996). Memory intervention for persons with dementia. *Applied Cognitive Psychology, 10,* 193–210.

Camp, C. J., & Schaller, J. (1989). Epilogue: Spaced-retrieval memory training in an adult day-care center. *Educational Gerontology, 15*(6), 641–648.

Collie, A., & Maruff, P. (2000). The neuropsychology of preclinical Alzheimer's disease and mild cognitive impairment. *Neuroscience and Biobehavioral Reviews, 24*(3), 365–374.

Dunn, J., & Clare, L. (2007). Learning face-name associations in early-stage dementia: Comparing the effects of errorless learning and effortful processing. *Neuropsychological Rehabilitation, 17,* 735–754.

Egan, M., Berube, D., Racine, G., Leonard, C., & Rochon, E. (2010). Methods to enhance communication between individuals with Alzheimer's disease and their caregivers: A systematic review. *International Journal of Alzheimer's Disease, 2012,* 1–12.

Eisner, E. (2001). *Can do activities for adults with Alzheimer's disease.* Austin, TX: Pro-Ed.

Feil, N. (1991). Validation therapy. In P. K. H. Kim (Ed.), *Serving the elderly: Skills for practice* (pp. 89–116). Edison, NJ: Aldine Transaction.

Fockert, J. W., Rees, G., Frith, C. D., & Lavie, N. (2001). The role of working memory in visual selective attention. *Science, 291*, 1803–1806.

Folstein, M. F., Folstein, S. E., & McHugh, P. R. (1975). "Mini-Mental State." A practical method for grading the cognitive state of patients for the clinician. *Journal of Psychiatric Research, 12*(3), 189–198.

Goodglass, H., Kaplan, E., & Barresi, B. (2000). *Boston Diagnostic Aphasia Examination* (3rd ed.). Philadelphia, PA: Lippincott Williams & Wilkins.

Gorno-Tempini, M.L,, Brambati, S.M., Ginex, V., Ogar, J., Dronkers, N.F., Marcone, A., . . . Miller, B. L. (2008). The logopenic/phonological variant of primary progressive aphasia. *Neurology, 71*, 1227–1234.

Helm-Estabrooks, N. (1995). *Cognitive-linguistic task book*. Sandwich, MA: Cape Cod Institute.

Hoerster, L., Hickey, E., & Bourgeois, M. (2001). Effects of memory aids on conversations between nursing home residents with dementia and nursing assistants. *Neuropsychological Rehabilitation, 11*(3–4), 399–427.

Hopper, T., & Bayles, K. A. (2008). Management of neurogenic communication disorders associated with dementia. In R. Chapey (Ed.), *Language intervention strategies in aphasia and related neurogenic communication disorders* (5th ed.). Philadelphia, PA: Lippincott Williams & Wilkins.

Hopper, T., Bourgeois, M., Pimentel, J., Qualls, C. D., Hickey, E., Prymark, T., & Schooling, T. (2013). An evidence-based systematic review on cognitive interventions for individuals with dementia. *American Journal of Speech-Language Pathology, 22*, 126–145.

Hopper, T., Mahendra, N., Kim, E., Azuma, T., Bayles, K. A., Cleary, S, & Tomoeda, C. K. (2005). Evidence-based practice recommendations for working with individuals working with dementia: Spaced retrieval training. *Journal of Medical Speech-Language Pathology, 13*, 27–34.

Hughes, C., Berg, L., Danzinger, W., Coben, L., & Martin, R. (1982). *Clinical Dementia Rating Scale*. Hagerstown, MD: Lippincott Williams & Wilkins.

Johnson, R. T., & Gibbs, C. J. (1998). Creutzfeldt-Jakob disease and related transmissible spongiform encephalopathies. *New England Journal of Medicine, 339*(27), 1994–2004.

Kaplan, E., Goodglass, H., & Weintraub, S. (1983) *Boston Naming Test*. Philadelphia, PA: Lippincott Williams & Wilkins.

Kertesz, A. (2006). *Western Aphasia Battery-Revised*. Austin, TX: Pro-Ed.

Klasner, E. (n.d.) *Huntington's disease, Fact Sheet 9, communication skills*. Retrieved from http://members.aol.com/hdanwlancs/Fsheet9.html

Lancioni, G. E., Singh, N. N., O'Reilly, M. F., Sigafoos, J., Tatulli, E., Rigante, V., . . . Minervini, M. (2010). Technology-aided verbal instructions to help persons with mild to moderate Alzheimer's disease perform daily activities. *Research in Developmental Disabilities, 31*, 1240–1250.

Leyton, C. E., Hornberger, N. M., Mioshi, E., & Hodges, J. R. (2010). Application of Addenbrooke's Cognitive Examination to diagnosis and monitoring of progressive primary aphasia. *Dementia and Geriatric Cognitive Disorders, 29*, 504–509.

Marttila, R. J., & Rinne, U. K. (1976). Dementia in Parkinson's disease. *Acta Neurologica Scandanavica, 54*, 431–441.

Mioshi, E., Dawson, K., Mitchell, J., Arnold, R., & Hodges, J. R. (2006). The Addenbrooke's Cognitive Examination Revised (ACE-R): A brief cognitive test battery for dementia screening. *International Journal of Geriatric Psychiatry, 21*, 1078–1085.

Neary, D., Snowden, J. S., Northen, B., & Goulding, P. (1988). Dementia of frontal lobe type. *Journal of Neurosurgery and Psychology, 51*, 353–361.

Orsulic-Jeras, S., Schneider, N. M., & Camp, C. J. (2000). Montessori-based activities for long-term care residents with dementia: Outcomes and implications for geriatric rehabilitation. *Topics in Geriatric Rehabilitation, 16*, 78–91.

Pohjasvaara, T., Erkinjuntti, T., Ylikoski, R., Hietanen, M., Varaja, R., & Kaste, M. (1998). Clinical determinants of post stroke dementia. *Stroke, 29*, 75–81.

Reese, P. B. (2000). *The source for Alzheimer's and dementia* (p. 12). East Moline, IL: LinguaSystems.

Reisberg, B., Ferris, S. H., de Leon, M. J., & Crook, T. (1982). The global deterioration scale for assessment of primary degenerative dementia. *American Journal of Psychiatry, 139*, 1136–1139.

Rinne, J. O., Portin, R., Ruottinen, H., Nurmi, E., Bergman, J., Haaparanta, M., & Solin, O. . . . (2000). Cognitive impairment and the brain dopaminergic system in Parkinson's disease: Fluorodopa positron emission tomographic study. *Archives of Neurology, 57*, 470–475.

Ripich, D. N. (1994). Functional communication training with AD patients: A caregiver training program. *Alzheimer's Disease and Associated Disorders, 8*(3), 95–109.

Ripich, D. N., Ziol, E., Fritsch, T., & Durand, E. J. (1999). Training Alzheimer's disease caregivers for successful communication. *Clinical Gerontologist, 21*(1), 37–56.

Squire, L. R. (1992). Priming and multiple memory systems: Perceptual mechanisms of implicit memory. *Journal of Cognitive Neuroscience, 4,* 244–256.

Thompson, C. K. (1989). Generalization in the treatment of aphasia. In L. V. McReynolds & J. Spradlin (Eds.), *Generalization strategies in the treatment of communication disorders.* Lewiston, NY: BC Decker.

Toseland, R., Diehl, M., Freeman, K., Manzanares, T., Naleppa, M., & McCallion, P. (1997). The impact of validation group therapy on nursing home residents with dementia. *Journal of Applied Gerontology, 16*(1), 31–50.

Warner, J. (2003). Current research on diagnosing dementia. *Journal of Neurology, Neurosurgery and Psychiatry, 74,* 413–414.

World Health Organization. (2001). *The World Health Report: Mental health: new understanding, new hope.* Retrieved from http://www.who.int/whr/2001/en/whr01_en.pdf

Chapter 9

ENCEPHALOPATHY

Introduction

Encephalopathy is a nonspecific term that describes a disease or disorder of the brain. The disease alters the brain's functions and/or structure of both the left and the right hemispheres. Encephalopathies may be caused by an infection due to bacteria, virus, or prion. The presenting feature of encephalopathy is a subtle change in a person's personality, behavior, cognitive functioning, level of alertness, level of attentiveness, lethargy, and distractibility. The most common neurobehavioral symptom seen in hospitals is an acute alteration of mental state. According to Shulman and Romano (1999), the highest percentage of patients with encephalopathy are found in geriatric wards. Approximately 5% to 15% are on medical-surgical floors, and 20% to 30% of individuals with encephalopathy are on surgical intensive care units.

Cerebral dysfunction associated with encephalopathy is often due to one of the following: dehydration, hypoglycemia, diabetic keto-acidosis, drug intoxication, uremia, meningitis, and more. This is certainly not a comprehensive accounting of all possible etiologies leading to encephalopathy, but those listed are among the most frequently encountered in a clinical setting (Table 9–1).

Characteristics

Encephalopathy causes a change in mental state as a result of organ failure due to metabolic dysfunction, mitochondrial dysfunction, brain tumor with

Table 9–1. Examples of Encephalopathies

Organ Affected	Causes
Liver damage	Hepatic encephalopathy
Kidney damage/failure	Uremic encephalopathy
Cardiorespiratory arrest	Hypoxic/Anoxic encephalopathy
Hypertension	Hypertensive encephalopathy
Hypotension	Hypoxic encephalopathy
Cushing's syndrome	Endocrine encephalopathy
Addison's disease	Endocrine encephalopathy
Thyroid disease	Endocrine encephalopathy
Thiamine deficiency	Wernicke's encephalopathy

an increase of pressure in the skull, toxic exposure over time, chronic trauma, poor nutrition, or lack of oxygen and blood to the brain (National Institute of Neurological Disorders and Stroke, 2007). Unfortunately, in the early stage of this process, the patient lacks the insight and judgment to fully recognize the symptoms. One of its most salient features is confusion. Alterations in memory, cognition, and attentional abilities are also prevalent. Myoclonus or involuntary twitching and nystagmus (rapid involuntary eye movements), tremor, seizures, dementia, and difficulty speaking and swallowing may also be evident (National Institute of Neurological Disorders and Stroke, 2007). The patient may progress from chronic confusion and hypersomnolence to delirium, and possibly even coma. If the patient becomes delirious, there may be visual delusions or hallucinations that are often unpleasant in nature.

Organ disease is the etiology of metabolic encephalopathy. If the metabolic byproducts produced by the organs are not removed or properly processed, an imbalance of magnesium, calcium, phosphorous, sodium, and glucose levels, may occur and affect brain function. To determine the cause of an encephalopathy, the blood and spinal fluid are examined, and electroencephalograms and imaging studies are conducted (National Institute of Neurological Disorders and Stroke, 2007

Drug and Alcohol Intoxication

Drug intoxication causes an acute change of mental status and can occur whenever there is an excess of a drug in the bloodstream. This can be due to addiction, recreational use, or even iatrogenic causes (medically induced). It is typically associated with drugs that have an anticholinergic effect, that is, drugs that block the uptake of acetylcholine at the synapse. The drugs most commonly associated with drug intoxication are:

- Over-the-counter cold preparations
- Antihistamines
- Antidepressants
- Neuroleptics
- Anti-Parkinson's medication
- Narcotics
- High-dose steroids
- Sedatives/tranquilizers
- Amphetamines
- Cocaine
- Hallucinogens
- Alcohol.

Chronic alcoholism is responsible for many hospital admissions. Therefore, the speech-language pathologist must become familiar with the clinical and cognitive manifestations of alcohol-related illness. The National Survey of Drug Use and Health found that approximately 19 million Americans were dependent on or abused alcohol in 2005. Of these, three million were dependent on or abused an illicit drug. Fifty-six percent of the 19 million were seen in ambulatory care settings (hospitals and clinics; Substance Abuse and Mental Health Services Administration, Office of Applied Studies, 2006).

The person admitted to the hospital with alcohol-related illness may be in a state of delirium tremens (DT). The patient experiencing DTs is subject to perceptual hallucinations, anxiety, acute mental disorder, and sweating (diaphoresis). Typically, the patient will be placed on a thiamine IV (intravenous) drip before glucose is administered. These patients are often dehydrated and electrolyte-depleted, so IV fluids are also ordered by the medical staff. Furthermore, this type of patient may have low sodium (hyponatremic), but if sodium is replaced too rapidly, there can be central pontine destruction of the myelin sheath (myelinolysis), which may result in changes to cranial nerve V (trigeminal nerve), cranial nerve VI (abducens), cranial nerve VII (facial), and cranial nerve VIII (acoustic) nerve. To prevent severe withdrawal symptoms and seizures, benzodiazepines (valium or xanax) are usually given. The speech-language pathologist may be consulted to assess the patient's cognitive-linguistic status once the patient is stabilized and transferred to a medical floor.

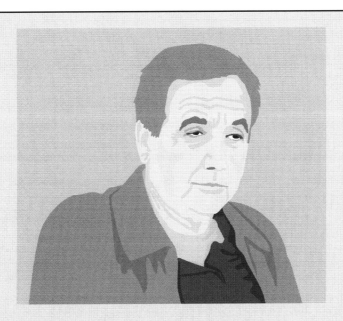

Case Scenario: Tommy

History & Physical (H & P): Tommy is a 57-year-old white male, admitted to the emergency department (ED) via EMS status post (s/p) being found down (breathing but unconscious at the scene) outside of a bar in his neighborhood. His BP was 86/34 with a HR of 130; intubated prophylactically by EMS; vital signs stabilized in ED; diagnosed with alcohol poisoning.

Past Medical History (PMH): Severe alcoholism; hypertension (HTN); Hepatitis B and C; insulin dependent diabetes mellitus (IDDM); pancreatitis; multiple hospitalizations for alcohol-related illnesses and injuries; undocumented history of cocaine abuse (per wife's report patient did use the drug "about two years ago, then went back to drinking heavily").

Social History: Former truck driver but hasn't worked since the age of 50 due to revocation of his CDL (commercial driver's license). Patient has five children, ages 21 to 35, all in the area. Lives with wife in first-floor apartment, five steps to enter. Wife works full-time in a factory. Smokes two to three packs of cigarettes per day. The patient completed 11th grade. Patient's interests include "anything about 'Nam" according to wife. Patient was a Vietnam War veteran and was active in his VFW post.

Surgical History: s/p cholecycstectomy (removal of gall bladder)

A Functional Analysis of Tommy

At the time of the assessment, Tommy's ability to understand language was intact for grammatically simple utterances at the conversational level (see Figure 9–1 for Tommy's Diagnostic Profile and Figure 9–2 for his ALD Target Model).

Language Expression					
Automatic Speech: WFL	**Repetition Ability:** WFL	**Lexical Retrieval-Naming:** WFL	**Conversational Ability:** Able to express his wants and needs at the sentence level; able to engage in one-on-one dialogue; narrative discourse was not focused due to tangential speech.	**Pragmatic Skills:** Poor topic maintenance; tangential output causes interrupted discourse; inappropriate pauses; turn-taking impaired; frequently interrupts speaker	**Paraphasias:** None.

Speech				
Rate: WFL	**Intelligibility:** WFL in known and unknown contexts; however, moderate-severe vocal hoarseness noted.	**Prosody:** WFL	**Articulation:** No articulation errors	**Fluency:** WFL

Auditory Comprehension				
Answering Yes/No Questions: WFL for concrete and personal yes/no questions; moderate-severe impairment at the abstract level.	**Executing Commands:** Execution of one-step commands was WFL. Following complex, multistep directions was moderately impaired.	**Understanding Stories & Paragraphs:** Moderately impaired for stories composed of three or more events.	**Understanding Conversational Speech:** Variable depending on complexity of information.	**Identifying Objects & Their Functions:** WFL

Reading			
Word-level Comprehension: WFL	**Sentence-level Comprehension:** Able to read the daily newspaper and understand its basic contents.	**Oral Reading:** WFL for his premorbid educational level.	**Oral Spelling:** WFL for regularly spelled words.

Written Expression				
Copying: Able to copy words and sentences.	**Writing to Dictation:** WFL up to sentence level.	**Self-generated:** Able to generate a list of shopping items and write basic sentences.	**Written Spelling:** WFL for ADL needs.	**Drawing:** Patient refused to complete this task.

Cognition			
Attention/Concentration: Variable; better when interested in topic, e.g., the War in Vietnam.	**Visuospatial Skills:** Geographic disorientation and unable to find his way back to his room independently.	**Memory:** Procedural memory intact for ADLs including minor home repairs and self-care; moderately impaired episodic memory requiring mnemonic devices.	**Executive Functions:** Judgment and reasoning for home and public safety are compromised making him unsafe to live independently. Requires 24-hour supervision. Unable to plan his daily routine.

Behavioral Symptoms				
Alertness: Reduced level of alertness interferes with response accuracy.	**Deficit Awareness:** Poor; anosagnosia; "There's nothing wrong with me, it's you people."	**Frustration:** Agitated and aggressive; requires wrist restraints when out of bed (OOB) to chair.	**Emotional Lability:** Cries out of context.	**Current Personality Characteristics:** Impulsive; angry at times due to dependency on others.

Figure 9–1. Diagnostic profile for Tommy.

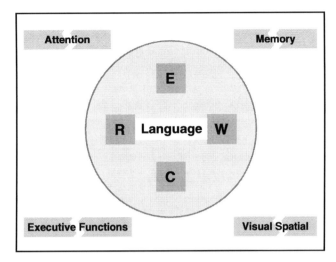

Figure 9–2. Acquired Language Disorders Target Model for Tommy.

As sentence complexity increased, his comprehension diminished. This affected Tommy's ability to participate in the social milieu of his environment. His expressive language, however, was functional for his activities of daily living (ADL) needs, although his ability to create a cohesive narrative discourse was inhibited. This was further complicated by Tommy's difficulty with turn-taking, impulsive responding characterized by interrupting the speaker, and inappropriate pause times. For example, if Tommy wanted to describe a special event he attended or relate information about his vacation experiences, the listener would need patience and understanding of Tommy's expressive language difficulties. Tommy's family and caregivers could use the training that they received from the speech-language pathologist (SLP) during his hospital stay to alert listeners to Tommy's expressive problems and cue him during his discourse and social interactions. Fortunately, Tommy demonstrated no lexical retrieval problems or paraphasias subsequent to his brain insult, which is a good prognosticator for his eventual community re-entry. Tommy's speech intelligibility was 100% in known and unknown contexts, and this was certainly to his benefit socially.

Tommy's procedural memory was intact for doing simple chores around the house and engaging in basic self-grooming tasks. However, his impaired episodic memory caused frustration, and the family will need to use memory logs and daily personal logs to optimize Tommy's ability to function in his home and neighborhood environment. Tommy is not safe to be left alone at this time. His judgment and reasoning for home and public safety scenarios were compromised. As a consequence, Tommy needs 24-hour supervision at home until he begins to show progress in executive functioning. His anosagnosia (lack of deficit awareness) also complicates the home and public safety situation. Tommy believed that he had no difficulty managing his daily routines and saw no need for close monitoring.

The SLP should recommend continued therapy at home once Tommy is discharged form the hospital. The SLP who treats Tommy at home, should continue to focus on deficit awareness, memory, family/counseling and education, and thought organization. Independent reentry into the community may not be possible for Tommy; however, he can build upon the strengths that he has to optimize the areas that are impaired.

Critical Thinking/Learning Activity

- What is the speech-language pathologist's role in the evaluation of this type of patient?
- Based on Tommy's PMH is this an acute onset type or a progressive type of encephalopathy, and what would be its etiology?
- How would this patient's lack of deficit awareness affect his ability to return to the social fabric of his environment?
- What are the family counseling and education issues in this case? How would you address them?
- As an SLP, what characteristics would you look for to help differentiate the person with dementia and the person with a toxic-metabolic encephalopathy?
- What referrals would you make after evaluating this case? Why?

Treatment Considerations

Tommy's medical diagnosis was alcohol poisoning. Testing conducted over three sessions (due to patient's medical condition) revealed moderate cognitive-linguistic deficits. Tommy's receptive skills were within functional limits (WFL) for simple, concrete information at the time of testing. His difficulty with more complex information presented auditorily requires some environmental adjustments, for example, limiting the ambient noise and having only one person speak to him at a time. His family will need ongoing communication counseling while he is an inpatient and during his rehab stay because his impaired auditory comprehension will affect his social interactions with them and others Furthermore, his lack of deficit awareness, should it persist and become chronic, will complicate matters. Tommy's expressive language is functional for his ADL needs. His more significant impairments are in the cognitive areas of memory, thought organization, judgment, and reasoning. As a consequence, Tommy will need to be supervised at home for compliance with his medications, appointments, and daily activities requiring organizational skills until he demonstrates the ability to manage these tasks independently and in sobriety. Drug and alcohol treatment is recommended for Tommy and his family.

It is important to remember the role that level of severity plays in the treatment planning and implementation for patients with encephalopathy. Furthermore, intervention is always provided within a functional/compensatory framework in these cases, and not one of remediation. The speech-language pathologist should consider the following treatment approaches when planning therapy for people with encephalopathy of any of the above-mentioned types:

- When working with this type of patient, it is important to provide family/caregiver counseling and education, which are critical elements to the rehabilitation of the patient with encephalopathy. The family/caregivers need to understand: the cause of the encephalopathy, the results of the cognitive-linguistic evaluation, the goals of therapeutic intervention, and how to communicate effectively with this type of patient. For example, it is best not to expect the patient to do things that they cannot understand or execute successfully, and calling attention to their deficits is often unproductive. Instead, instruct the family/caregivers to support the patient by implementing at home the compensatory strategies that you developed during the patient's stay at the hospital or rehab facility. Providing them with written information as well will help to reinforce your objectives, eliminate any misinterpretation of your auditory presentation, and allow the family to refer to your recommendations in the future.
- Memory books and daily logs can be used to optimize the patient's ability to perform the patient's ADL. The clinician facilitates the patient's completion of the daily log and discusses the content. Developing activities to facilitate spatial and temporal orientation are also helpful with these patients.
- Cotreating with occupational therapy and/or therapeutic recreation personnel provides the ability to integrate aspects of the patient's premorbid life into his or her life post-injury. Furthermore, it provides a context within which to optimize the patient's social language and to incorporate the patient's behavioral goals as well. Working in a group promotes generalization of skills developed during individual therapy.
- The clinician should consider consulting the Office of Vocational Rehabilitation (OVR) in their state to determine if the patient's skill set post therapy would support employment. The speech-language pathologist can then work with the OVR representative to enhance and/or reinforce the skills needed for a particular job.

Some Therapeutic Options

- Therapeutic approaches addressing cognitive-communicative impairment (Helm-Estabrooks, 1995).
- Graphic and written cues. Provide written information and photos to support recognition memory; use a memory wallet, book, or daily log (Hoerster, Hickey, & Bourgeois, 2001).

- ■ Montessori-based interventions. Create structured and stimulating activities for engagement and social interaction (Orsulic-Jeras, Schneider, Camp, Nicholson, & Helbig, 2001).
- ■ Spaced Retrieval Training (SRT) is a verbally mediated technique that may be used to help with safety and activities of daily living. The patient rehearses a specific response or action to a stimulus across repeated trials. The time between the presentation of the stimulus and the request from the clinician for the response are gradually increased. The patient eventually learns the new behavior. For example, writing one's name requires certain steps to accomplish the act. The SLP may use SRT to facilitate the learning of these steps (Camp, Foss, O'Hanlon, & Stevens, 1996).
- ■ Memory books and daily logs can assist with spatial and temporal orientation as well as planning, organizing, and implementation. Use of board games and card games to develop attentional skills and expand focus and concentration.

References

Camp, C. J., Foss, J. W., O'Hanlon, A. M., & Stevens, A. B. (1996). Memory intervention for persons with dementia. *Applied Cognitive Psychology, 10,* 193–210.

Helm-Estabrooks, N. (1995). *Cognitive-linguistic task book.* Sandwich, MA: Cape Cod Institute Publishing Division.

Hoerster, L., Hickey, E., & Bourgeois, M. (2001). Effects of memory aids on conversations between nursing home residents with dementia and nursing assistants. *Neuropsychological Rehabilitation, 11*(3 & 4), 399–427.

National Institute of Neurological Disorders and Stroke. (2007). *NINDS Encephalopathy Information Page.* Retrieved from http://www.ninds.nih.gov/disorders/encephalopathy/encephalopathy.htm

Orsulic-Jeras, S., Schneider, N. M., Camp, C. J., Nicholson, P., & Helbig, M. (2001). Montessori-based dementia activities in long-term care: Training and implementation. *Activities, Adaptation, and Aging, 25,* 107–120.

Shulman, L. M., & Romano, J. G. (1999). Neurologic emergencies. In W. J. Weiner & C. G. Goetz (Eds.), *Neurology for the non-neurologist* (4th ed.). Philadelphia, PA: Lippincott Williams and Wilkins.

Substance Abuse and Mental Health Services Administration, Office of Applied Studies. (2006). *Results from the 2005 national survey on drug use health: National findings* (NSDUH Series H-30, DHHS Publication No. SMA–06–4194). Rockville, MD: Table G.29.

Chapter 10

PAST, PRESENT, AND FUTURE CONSIDERATIONS IN ACQUIRED LANGUAGE DISORDERS

Historical Overview of Efficacy and Evidence in the Treatment of Acquired Language Disorders (ALD) in Adults

Any discussion regarding the treatment efficacy in acquired language disorders in adults, and specifically, aphasia rehabilitation, must begin with Darley's (1972) paper on the topic. Although our book has discussed various acquired language disorders in adults, we believe that using Darley as a platform to discuss treatment efficacy is an appropriate starting place due to his generalizable reasoning. Darley found 10 "reports" that were mostly descriptive analyses and retrospective in nature. He concluded that the data were not robust and that any clinician must be cautious when making statements about treatment efficacy. Darley's article is seminal, and the reader is directed to Wertz and Irwin's thorough, clear, and concise synopsis of it (Wertz & Irvin, 2001).

Darley proposed three general questions that the clinician must confront and answer in order to determine if the treatment protocols used in aphasia rehabilitation are effective (Darley, 1972, pp. 4–5):

1. Does language rehabilitation accomplish measureable gains in language function beyond what can be expected to occur as a result of spontaneous recovery?
2. Are the language gains attributable to therapy worth the necessary investment of time, effort, and money?
3. What are the relative degrees of effectiveness of various modes of treatment of aphasia?

Furthermore, Darley also offered four "fundamental considerations" that one must address in the design of any efficacy studies of treatment in aphasia (Darley, 1972):

1. The patients in a study of treatment in aphasia must be aphasic. Darley was not convinced that the descriptions of the aphasic syndromes existing at the time of his writing were accurate. Furthermore, he admonished researchers to recognize and thoroughly describe any concomitant conditions, for example, apraxia of speech, confusion, and so forth.
2. There must be a clear differentiation between improvement based on therapeutic intervention and spontaneous recovery, which requires control subjects who are not included in the therapy program. This raises the ethical question of denying treatment to those in need, but for a study to be rigorous and valid, this is the best experimental scenario.

3. In order to monitor change, the clinician must gather quantitative data that are reliable and objective. More interesting, in today's context of functionality, is Darley's interest in monitoring changes in the patient's behavior and quality of life by measuring psychological and psychosocial status before and after therapy. He even suggested using evoked potentials to make these measurements.

4. The clinician must clearly define and describe the procedures followed, the rationale and the materials employed, and that therapy must be delivered by "trained professionals" (Darley, 1972, p. 14).

As noted above, Darley considered that the data at his time of writing was sparse and unconvincing. Returning to his three questions, the following information has emerged:

1. Does language rehabilitation accomplish measureable gains in language function beyond what can be expected to occur as a result of spontaneous recovery?

It apparently does. Robey (1998) conducted a meta-analysis of efficacy studies in aphasia treatment and found that those patients who received treatment had better long-term outcomes than those who were not treated. This included patients at all stages of their recovery. Robey's work in this area is an important follow-up to Darley's, and the clinician should become familiar with it. The reader is directed to Robey (1994) and Robey (1998).

2. Are the language gains attributable to therapy worth the necessary investment of time, effort, and money?

There are no current data to answer this question. Researchers, however, have addressed the issue of cost versus benefit, but arrived at no firm conclusions (Brookshire, 1994; Shewan & Kertesz, 1984; Wertz et al., 1986). How does one measure the cost of treatment versus non-treatment in a realistic way? The researchers above attempted to do so by calculating the cost per increase in scores on a language test or percentile rank. However, a truer cost/benefit analysis must measure changes in *functionality*. Is the patient now able to communicate effectively in a social context? Has the patient's quality of life improved as a result of language rehabilitation? Has there been a reduction in the language deficits subsequent to language intervention? Wertz and Irwin (2001) suggest that perhaps we should be measuring whether the patient's improvement can be noticed by a "naive observer" (p. 244). Obviously, this is a critical question requiring a serious answer from the discipline as it has therapeutic and sociopolitical implications.

3. What are the relative degrees of effectiveness of various modes of treatment of aphasia?

The current answer to this question is that there does not seem to be any significant differences between the different treatment approaches used in aphasia. Wertz et al. (1981) did report that there was a small but significant difference in the outcomes of patients who were treated individually versus those treated in a group setting. However, more recent work with adults in groups within the LPAA context has shown efficacy (Elman & Bernstein-Ellis, 1999).

Randomized Controlled Trials (RCTs) and Aphasia Treatment

Greener, Enderby, and Whurr (1999) stimulated vigorous discussion among speech-language pathologists when they concluded that aphasia treatment had not been shown to be "clearly effective or clearly ineffective within a randomized controlled trial (RCT)" (p. 1). In typical experiments, subjects are assigned to groups randomly. However, in the case of studies conducted with aphasic individuals, presence in a group is determined by the presence and type of aphasia and are considered quasi experiments (Douglas, Brown, & Barry, 2002). Robey (1998) identified 479 studies and found 55 quasi experiments in his meta-analysis. One of the interesting findings Robey reported was that there was actually a decrease in the number of RCTs conducted since the 1980s. Despite this, he did report the following findings from his meta-analysis:

1. The patients who were treated had better outcomes than those who did not have treatment in all stages of recovery across time postonset.
2. The patient outcome was better when treatment was started in the acute phase of recovery.
3. Patients who received greater than 2 hours of therapy per week had better outcomes than those who received less.
4. The most commonly reported form of treatment was individual.
5. The largest gains were seen in those patients who were rated as severe and moderately severe. No study in his analysis was designed to measure treatment effects in the mildly impaired patient population.
6. There were not enough studies examining the differential effects for the different types of aphasia therapy, for example, Melodic Intonation Therapy versus Stimulation-Facilitation Therapy.

Although the results on efficacy in this analysis were not as powerful as one would hope, the support for intervention at all levels of recovery is worth noting. Of the 12 studies reported on by Greener et al. (1999), only one used an RCT design. It appears that this move away from RCTs is related to the emergence of the single subject design that motivated Robey, Schultz, Crawford, and Sinner (1999) to conduct a meta-analysis of research on the efficacy of single-subject experiments in aphasia treatment. Unfortunately, only 12 out of 63 single-subject studies that Robey and his colleagues reported on provided quantifiable results (Robey, 1999). The authors found this unsatisfactory concluding that single-subject designs were not able to produce evidence that supported the effectiveness of any given treatment (Robey, 1998).

The obvious challenges for researchers interested in using RCTs in aphasiology or any brain disorder are the issues of patient variability, selection criteria, well-described treatment protocols, objective and quantifiable results, and ethical considerations. As can be seen from the above discussion, RCTs in communication sciences and disorders have not been forthcoming. If, however, the single-subject design is the preferred methodology for testing the efficacy of treatment in communication sciences and disorders, then there needs to be rigorous protocols in place that allow for replication, multiple baselines, and the production of results for functional outcomes. That is, future research into treatment efficacy must find a way to measure quality of life issues in the aphasic population as well as changes in test results, and so forth, posttreatment. Thus, this is a call for single-subject and, for that matter, any group designs, to include both quantitative and qualitative measures so that efficacy can be determined in functional and objective domains.

We believe that Darley (1972) "hit the nail on the head." His questions have not been satisfactorily answered, and his "fundamental considerations" are powerfully relevant today. If we keep his mandate in mind as we continue to critically examine our practice, we believe that we will eventually arrive at the desired outcome: finding the best cost/time effective approaches that hold the welfare of the patient paramount while providing functional benefits to the patient within his social milieu.

Treatment Approaches and Future Trends

Research in the treatment of adults with acquired language disorders is advancing. Recent reviews have focused on three exciting avenues of intervention. These interventions reflect advances in biological/pharmacologic knowledge, research about intensity of treatment, and changes based on computer-assisted technologies that are cost-effective and time efficient. All of these point to a future of growth for us as clinicians and enhanced outcomes for our patients. We address each of these briefly below.

Biological and Pharmacologic Interventions

The advent of pharmacologic interventions to increase blood flow in the acute phase of stroke, combined with new discoveries about neuroplasticity in the adult and the possibility of infusing the brain with new tissue, all contribute to a future of great promise for the rehabilitation of the stroke patient with a language disorder. Wineburgh and Small (2004) propose that the treatment of aphasia in the adult is at a crossroads where all three of the above-mentioned variables can come together to improve language rehabilitation outcomes. However, these biological aspects of intervention must be supplemented with and complemented by behavioral therapy, that is, speech-language therapies in order for the person with aphasia to integrate the benefits of the biological changes into their daily behaviors.

The current practices in treatment of aphasia have been shown to be effective (Robey, 1998). However, looking toward the future, Wineburgh and Small (2004) believe that in cases where biological intervention occurs, for example, stem cell infusion or neuronal implantation, the speech-language pathologist will be required to determine if his intervention is "harmful" or "beneficial" to the patient after the procedure. As we know very little about the biology of language processes, the clinician will need to understand if the speech-language intervention *postprocedure* will facilitate recovery or inhibit it. This requires a shift in thinking from "effective" therapy to "beneficial" therapy (Wineburgh & Small, 2004). Our current practice does not include biological intervention; however, with the emergence of stem cell technology and more refined knowledge of cortical neurophysiology poststroke, the speech-language pathologist can look forward to a very exciting future in which he or she will play a major role in the functional rehabilitation of the adult with an acquired language disorder.

There is a long history of using pharmacologic agents in the treatment of aphasia, starting with Alexander Luria, the Soviet neurologist, who used galanthamine (an anticholinesterase agent) to improve speech, language, cognitive, and motor functions in people with stroke (Webb & Adler, 2008). Other drugs used in the treatment of aphasia include bromocriptine (dopaminergic), amphetamines, cholinergic agents, GABAergic agents, and serotoninergic agents. Berthier (2005) reported that pharmacologic agents that act on the catecholamine system, for example, bromocriptine, have demonstrated variable results in the treatment of

people with aphasia in placebo-controlled studies. The findings on bromocriptine, however, show very selective effectiveness. It appears that it is most effective in acute and chronic aphasia of the nonfluent type and in cases of reduced verbal initiation, for example, transcortical motor aphasia (Berthier, 2005). Donepizil, a drug acting on the cholinergic system, showed more promise in chronic aphasias and was well tolerated by the patients, and its efficacy was maintained over the long term (Berthier, 2005). Although Wineburgh and Small (2004) report that pharmacotherapy "has never been shown to have any effectiveness" in the treatment of aphasia, Webb and Adler (2008) point out that pharmacologic intervention seem to be useful complements to traditional treatment approaches to aphasia. The controversy continues, but as biochemical technology advances and the pathophysiology of stroke continues to be refined, expect to see more agents coming onto the market for the treatment of aphasia.

Intensity of Treatment

Current fiscal constraints, imposed by CMS (for Center for Medicare and Medicaid Services) and private insurers on rehabilitation services, restrict the duration of speech-language pathology services available to people with aphasia. Therefore, it makes good clinical and fiscal sense, within the context of health care today, to provide the best service and to obtain the best outcome in the shortest amount of time. In a meta-analysis conducted by Robey (1998), he concluded that providing at least 2 hours of therapy per week facilitated gains in patients and recommended that 2 hours per week should constitute a minimum of therapeutic services for people with aphasia. Bhogal, Teasell, and Speechley (2003) also conducted a meta-analysis of studies investigating aphasia therapy and found that a significant treatment effect followed 8.8 hours of therapy per week for 11.2 weeks versus studies that provided only 2 hours of therapy per week for 22.9 weeks. They concluded that speech outcomes are clearly improved if an intensive schedule of therapy is used in patients with aphasia.

The Rehabilitation Institute of Chicago (RIC) is leading the way in the area of intensive therapy for people with aphasia. Their program—The RIC Intensive Therapy Aphasia Program—provides daily, individual therapy for 2 hours per day; 1 hour of computer-based treatment; 2 hours of group therapy targeting reading, writing, and conversational skills; 1 hour of more specialized treatment with programs such as PACE or alternative and augmentative communication (AAC) devices; and caregiver workshops and support. This offers the patient a total of approximately 30 hours of therapy per week for 4 weeks. These programs were developed at RIC; in order to be eligible, a patient must be at least 18 years old, medically stable, must be able to tolerate the intensity of the therapy, and be either independent in mobility and self-care or be accompanied by a caregiver at all times. For more detailed information on the RIC Intensive Aphasia Therapy Program and how to enroll a patient go to: http://www.ric.org/conditions/stroke-treatment/intensive-aphasia-program/

Computer-Assisted Technology and Treatment of Aphasia

Katz (2008) defines computerized aphasia treatment as the "systematic use of computers and software to improve communication skills in people with aphasia" (p. 852). The straightforwardness of the definition, however, cloaks the complexity of the issue. Katz states that there are three roles that computer-only treatment (COT) and computer-assisted treatment (CAT) play in aphasia therapy:

1. COT programs allow the patient to practice independent of the clinician, family, and/or caregiver once the clinician has designed the treatment program for that patient. This type of software program usually consists of drills. According to Jokel, Cupit, Rochon, and Leonard (2009), MossTalk Words (see Appendix E), may be a beneficial and worthwhile therapy approach for people with primary progressive aphasia (PPA) without cognitive impairment. Using a multiple baseline design, two participants improved their naming skills with this

program and were able to maintain these gains 4 weeks after treatment ended. The patients were seen two to three times per week for therapy. The first patient achieved 80% naming ability on three-word lists after only four sessions per list; whereas the second patient took 12 sessions for each of three-word lists to achieve 80% accuracy. Although these therapeutic gains appear variable, the findings do indicate that in patients with a neurodegenerative process like PPA could still benefit from using MossTalk Words (see Appendix D). Clinicians should consider the fact that treatment must be individualized. Furthermore, every treatment program should be evaluated for its effects, effectiveness, and efficiency, that is, its efficacy, for continued use with that patient.

2. CAT software programs allow the patient and the clinician to work side-by-side. The role of the computer is to present the material, whereas the role of the patient and clinician was a dynamic and interactive one using the software program as the therapy material.

3. AAC in aphasia therapy refers to computers that can utilize icons, digitized speech, and animation, and are used to facilitate functional communication for the person with aphasia.

The clinician is not accustomed to working within a therapeutic context that does not necessarily include the familiar framework of delivering the treatment, measuring the patient's performance, modifying the treatment, and then treating it with the modified version. Yet, within the CAT, COT, and AAC paradigm, this more conventional approach to rehabilitation is not always possible, nor appropriate. As a consequence, Katz (2008) summarizes three models of rehabilitation that are applicable when using computers in aphasia therapy.

Brain-Behavior Relationships

Essentially, this model adheres to the philosophy that language rehabilitation can happen through retraining and works on the premise that the patient can regain lost skills through reorganizing the brain functions that have been damaged.

Behavior Modification

Operant conditioning achieves behavior modification by systematically applying consequences after a stimulus is given. The organism can learn a new behavior or lose an old one. Computer programs can provide a stimulus and reinforce the patient for a correct response, through feedback.

Educational Models

These programs can create *microworlds* within which the patient can operate and learn to solve problems associated with their daily communication needs. The type of learning in this case is not didactic but more inductive. The patient can discover the answers as opposed to being told the answers. Games designed to facilitate rehabilitation of functional language skills certainly have a place in the repertoire of any clinician using CAT and COT methodology.

Within any of these models, the clinician can decide to use stimulation, simulation, drills, or tutorials as treatment protocols because all four of these are available and possible with computer software programs today (Katz, 2008).

Lee and Cherney (2008) describe an interactive computer software program called AphasiaScripts, developed at RIC, which provides both intensive therapy and computer-assisted approaches to treatment. The program is designed to allow the patient to gain practice in conversation. In this approach, an avatar acts as the virtual clinician, that is, conversational partner. The authors describe the program as user-friendly for the patient, but it still requires the expertise of a speech-language pathologist to facilitate the patient's ability to interact with the program. For example, the patient, with the assistance of the clinician, learns how to use cueing to optimize performance, so that he can practice the conversations intensively without a clinician present. AphasiaScripts incorporates both intensity of treatment and the use of computer-assisted technology in order to optimize patient outcomes.

The crucial link in the therapeutic chain between the patient and any CAT, COT, or AAC methods is the speech-language pathologist. It is the clinician who evaluates the patient, designs the treatment objectives, determines which tasks are to be used to implement those objectives, and then trains the patient to use the device or program. That is, there is an "intelligent division of labor between computers and clinician," and the boundaries are clear (Katz, 2008, p. 869). The fine nuances of human interaction cannot be overstated, especially within the context of a therapeutic interaction. CAT and COT technology promises to broaden a clinician's treatment options and optimize patient progress.

AAC for Adults with ALD: Aphasia, Primary Progressive Aphasia, TBI, and Dementia

AAC systems are commonplace technologies in speech-language pathology today. In the earliest stages of use, they were used primarily with pediatric populations, and more specifically, those children with severely disabling conditions, for example, cerebral palsy and autism, among others. The technology improved and so did the applicability of these devices in the adult populations with communication disorders, such as amyotrophic lateral sclerosis (ALS). However, further refinement of computer-based treatment saw the advent of AAC systems being used with people with aphasia, apraxia, TBI, and early-mid stage dementias.

Beukelman, Fager, Ball, and Dietz (2007) reviewed common issues associated with AAC devices in the adult population and chose four to review. They are:

1. AAC acceptance and use
2. AAC use patterns
3. Limitations of the AAC system
4. Future needs of adults who rely on AAC systems.

They included many types of neurological impairment in their discussion, but we restrict our discussion to the four that are covered in this book: aphasia, PPA, TBI, and dementia. AAC systems are broadly divided into two broad categories: low-technology and high-technology. *Low-technology*

AAC systems such as communication books, drawings, photography, written words, and phrases, lack the ability to convey intimate feelings, social etiquette, or even transmit new information. These systems work well in the acute-care setting where the concerns are immediate and are health and medical status-based. *High-Technology AAC* systems, such as Lingraphica and Talking Screen, are available and in use with the adult neurological population. The software in Lingraphica allows the user to manipulate icons, some of which are animated, in order to build utterances. The communicative effectiveness of this device has been measured by using standard pre- and posttest types of assessments. However, the clinician must be aware that although the patient may *perform* well on the device, that may not translate into *functional competence* in the social setting.

There are two fiscally related problems that can occur over the course of treatment. First, the insurer sets limits on the duration of therapeutic intervention, and second, the patient's performance can sometimes plateau at a certain point in therapy, which does not present a sound case to the insurance companies for continued coverage (Fink, Brecher, Sobel, & Schwartz, 2005). As such, computer-based programs such as MossTalk Words and Lingraphica that seek to extend the course of rehabilitation to the home setting (once patient and caregivers are properly trained) seem like appropriate solutions to the above-noted problems. Another reason to use computer-based programs in the course of intervention is to supplement traditional therapy activities. Fink, Brecher, Schwartz, and Robey (2002) concluded that people with chronic aphasia who demonstrate significant phonologically based deficits can derive benefit from a computerized cued-naming methodology during treatment.

AAC Acceptance and Use with People with Aphasia, TBI, PPA, and Dementia

The person with aphasia may not have the symbolic functions necessary to support the use of an AAC system, for example, recognizing words, icons, and assembling these into meaningful sentences.

As a consequence, their use of an AAC system can be restrictive or even nonfunctional. Beukelman et al. (2007) report that people with severe, chronic aphasia do not easily accept an AAC device. They feel that it may interfere with their ability to regain natural language. Their families also are hoping for the same, so they also are not as willing to accept their use. The question as to who actually generates the messages, that is, the patient or someone else, is raised in the literature (Lasker & Beukelman, 1999).

People with a TBI demonstrated a higher level of acceptance and use of AAC devices when compared with people with aphasia. Those who did rely on AAC devices preferred the letter-by-letter spelling method for communicating messages. This is considered a "low-technology" system, and 63% of those using it were still doing so 3 years later. Their cognitive status was not supportive for message formulation using icons or other methods for encoding.

Most clinicians will find that the low-technology options such as communication books, photos, icons, and memento-type materials are typically the preferred approach and the most functional with patients diagnosed with PPA Beukelman et al. (2007) suggest that future research focus on the type of system, effectiveness, and the timing of intervention with AAC devices. They also welcome case studies and "small reports" that investigate AAC acceptance and use among this population.

The overarching goals of AAC use with the person with dementia are: (1) optimization of their current functions and maintaining social engagement; (2) maintain communicative effectiveness for as long as possible; and (3) increase the quality of life for the patient and caregivers. Using AAC systems with this population is emerging and gaining popularity, especially with the introduction of iPads into the therapy room. Using low-technology methods (pictures, mementos, memory books) and complementing those with a higher-level technology like iPads, can extend the patient's social engagement. Beukelman et al. (2007) suggest that focusing research funding on technology that can enhance communication and involvement into the social fabric is critically important.

The Use of Applications (Apps) in the Rehabilitation of the ALD Patient

One of the primary issues is how to determine if an app can be beneficial and which one(s) are best for a specific patient (Holland, Weinberg, & Dittelman, 2012). Because of the increasing availability and types of apps, the clinician needs to develop a strategy for choosing the appropriate one that will be user-friendly and client specific. The authors categorized apps into four main groups. These include:

1. Apps used to improve speech and language through practice drill and exercises
2. Apps to help communicate messages to others in spoken, written, or visual form such as AAC
3. Apps to help a person with aphasia track information including medical needs
4. Apps with built-in features such as images to help manage aphasia.

Searching an app site (such as *iTunes*) on a regular basis can provide clinicians with information on the latest available. Holland et al. (2012) suggest searching under category titles for *education, medical, productivity, hanging with friends,* and *games.* The authors have found that a buy-in is often needed from patients and their families. Many of the patients that we treat with an ALD are not familiar or comfortable with this type of technology. McCall (2012) has found the following four steps helpful in promoting a patient's success with technology. The process includes: (1) determining the patient's strongest communication modality; (2) matching the patient's preferences with his or her strengths; (3) determining the patient's personal goals for using technology; and (4) choosing and training the patient to use technologies to help achieve personal goals.

Therefore, insuring that the patient is comfortable with using devices such as iPads or iTouches is an important element to the treatment plan. Also, the patient and/or caregivers may need access to Wi-Fi in order to take advantage of apps. Another concern is the issue of portability and ability to use various keyboards. Patients and significant others often benefit from demonstrations of the app. As a consequence, there are several questions to help determine possible app buy-in and use.

1. Is the client a candidate for using an app?
2. Will the patient benefit from an app?
3. How do you expect to see your client use the app?
4. Is the patient's living arrangement amenable to app use?
5. Can the patient learn the basic device operations such as tapping, pinching, and swiping?
6. Can the patient learn to use the app independently? One of the most-liked apps has been *Talking Tom,* as even the most impaired individuals can get *Talking Tom* to mimic them.
7. Can the patient use e-mail with assistance to initiate usage with a device?
8. Can the patient benefit from using an app as a training tool to help reestablish language skills? *Tactus Therapy Solutions* has many apps geared to various severity levels. *Lingraphica Small Talk* focuses on language therapy for ALD providing videos and captions for sounds, words, and phrases. *Locabulary Lite* is designed for demonstrations to determine if a patient can use it to communicate in settings such as McDonald's and Starbucks. In addition, the apps *iConverse, Pictello,* or *Visually Assisted Speech Technology* can help patients develop scripts to produce their own messages. Also, *Aphasia Corner* provides an app consisting of National Public Radio Stories that can be regulated for speed and includes written text as information is spoken.

In helping to decide if an app will be successful for patients with an ALD to achieve their goals, Holland et al. (2012) remind us of three necessities: (1) families and friends or staff must be involved; (2) patients must always carry their devices with them to use regularly; and (3) a specific amount of time and commitment must be made to practice. The authors also present a table with 30 apps worth investigating, and Sutton (2012), writing about mobile devices that offer new treatments for people with ALD, presents more than 25 apps worthy of consideration.

The Use of Video Games in the Rehabilitation of the ALD Patient

Physical and occupational therapists have been using video gaming to assist with the arm and hand rehabilitation of their patients (Adriaenssens, Eggermont, Pyck, Boeckx, & Gilles, 1988; King, 1993; Szer, 1983). Although computerized programs are used in the rehabilitation of adults with communication disorders, there is no mention in the literature about the use of video gaming as a possible tool for rehabilitation. We believe that the clinician may want to consider this approach for patients presenting with cognitive impairment. More specifically, gaming matches perfectly the needs of patients like Debra—those with right hemispheric impairments and TBI patients like Samuel. As a consequence, we suggest that the clinician may want to consider video gaming to facilitate growth in the following areas:

- Memory
- Thought organization
- Planning
- Visuospatial skills
- Visual scanning
- Attention to task.

Patients with aphasia also may benefit. For example, using the game as a platform for building a narrative, lexical retrieval, and for sentence building are possible uses. We suggest that the clinician supplements more traditional programs that do have proven efficacy with gaming, because there are no efficacy studies for this approach. Games would need to be selected based on the type of disorder, severity of the disorder, age of the client, content, and applicability, which are essentially the same criteria the clinician would use to assess more traditional programs for his or her patient. For example, there are a number of simulation games that use animals, people, towns, and more. These games allow the user to create life events, stories, and engage in problem-solving behavior with outcomes that affect their characters. One example of this type of game is *The Sims* (http://www.thesims3.com).

It is important to remember that returning the patient to a functional communication status is always the ultimate goal of any treatment approach in ALD. In today's health care environment, with the constraints on reimbursement and number of visits permitted by insurers, the clinician must think creatively and innovatively to meet the long-term goal of functional communication.

For a review of Selected Treatment Programs and Approaches, see Appendix E.

References

Adriaenssens, E., Eggermont, E., Pyck, K., Boeckx, W., & Gilles, B. (1988). The video invasion of rehabilitation. *Burns, 14*, 417–419.

Berthier, M. L. (2005). Poststroke aphasia: Epidemiology, pathophysiology and treatment. *Drugs and Aging, 22*(2), 163–182.

Beukelman, D. R., Fager, S., Ball, L., & Dietz, A. (2007). AAC for adults with acquired neurological conditions: A review. *Alternative and Augmentative Communication, 23*, 230–242.

Bhogal, S. K., Teasell, R., & Speechley, M. (2003). Intensity of aphasia therapy, impact on recovery. *Stroke, 34*, 987.

Brookshire, R. H. (1994). Group studies of treatment for adults with aphasia: Efficacy, effectiveness and believability. *ASHA Special Interest Divisions: Neurophysiology and Neurogenic Speech and Language Disorders, 4*, 5–13.

Darley, F. L. (1972). The efficacy of language rehabilitation in aphasia. *Journal of Speech and Hearing Research, 37*, 3–21.

Douglas, J., Brown, L., & Barry, S. (2002). Is aphasia therapy effective? Exploring the evidence in systematic reviews. *Brain Impairment, 3*(1), 17–27.

Elman, R., & Bernstein-Ellis, E. (1999). The efficacy of group communication treatment in adults with chronic aphasia. *Journal of Speech, Language, and Hearing Research, 42*, 411–419.

Fink, R. B., Brecher, A., Schwartz, M. F., & Robey, R. R. (2002). A computer-implemented protocol for treatment of naming disorders: Evaluation of clinician-guided and partially self-guided instruction. *Aphasiology, 16*, 1061–1086.

Fink, R. B., Brecher, A., Sobel, P., & Schwartz, M. F. (2005) Computer-assisted treatment of word retrieval deficits in aphasia. *Aphasiology, 19*, 943–954.

Flaster, M. (2102). Breakthroughs in stroke recovery. *Bottom Line Health*, 7–9.

Greener, J., Enderby, P., & Whurr, R. (1999, December). Speech and language therapy for aphasia following stroke (Cochrane Review). In *The Cochrane Library* (Issue 4). Oxford: BMJ Books/Update Software.

Holland, A. L., Weinberg, P., & Dittelman, J. (2012). How to use apps clinically in the treatment of aphasia. *Seminars in Speech and Language, 33*, 223–233.

Jokel, R., Cupit, J., Rochon, E., & Leonard, C. (2009). Relearning lost vocabulary in nonfluent progressive aphasia with MossTalk Words®. *Aphasiology, 23*(2), 175–191.

Katz, R. (2008). Computer applications in aphasia treatment. In R. Chapey (Ed.), *Language intervention strategies in aphasia and related neurogenic communication disorders* (5th ed., pp. 852–876). Philadelphia, PA: Lippincott Williams & Wilkins.

King, T. (1993). Hand strengthening with a computer for purposeful activity. *American Journal of Occupational Therapy, 47*, 635–637.

Lasker, J., & Beukelman, D. R. (1999). Peers' perceptions of storytelling by an adult with aphasia. *Aphasiology, 13*, 857–869.

Lee, J. B., & Cherney, L. R. (2008). The changing "face" of aphasia. *Perspectives on Neurophysiology and Neurogenic Speech and Language Disorders, 18*, 15–23.

McCall, D. (2012). Steps to success with technology for individuals with aphasia. *Seminars in Speech and Language, 33*, 234–242.

Robey, R. R. (1994). The efficacy of treatment of aphasic persons: A meta-analysis. *Brain and Language, 47*, 582–608.

Robey, R. R. (1998). A metanalysis of clinical outcomes in the treatment of aphasia. *Journal of Speech and Hearing Research, 41*, 172–187.

Robey, R., Schultz, M., Crawford, A., & Sinner, C. (1999). Single-subject clinical outcome research: Design, data, effect sizes, and analyses. *Aphasiology, 13*, 445–473.

Shewan, C., & Kertesz, A. (1984). Effects of speech language treatment in recovery from aphasia. *Brain and Language, 23*, 272–299.

Sutton, M. (2012, June 05). App-titude: Apps to aid aphasia. *ASHA Leader.*

Szer, J. (1983). Video games as physiotherapy. *Medical Journal of Australia, 1*, 401–402.

Webb, W. G., & Adler, R. K. (2008). *Neurology for the speech-language pathologist.* Philadelphia, PA: Elsevier.

Wertz, R. T., Collins, M. J., Weiss, D., Kurtzke, J. F., Friden, T., & Brookshire, R. H. (1981). Veterans Administration cooperative study on aphasia: A comparison of individual and group treatment. *Journal of Speech and Hearing Research, 24*, 580–594.

Wertz, R. T., & Irwin, W. H. (2001). Darley and the efficacy of language rehabilitation in aphasia. *Aphasiology, 15*(3), 231–247.

Wertz, R. T., Weiss, D. G., Aten, J. L., Brookshire, R. H., Garcia-Bunuel, L., & Holland, A. L. (1986). Comparison of clinic, home, and deferred language treatment for aphasia. A Veterans Administration Cooperative study. *Archives of Neurology, 43*, 653–658.

Wineburgh, L. F., & Small, S. L. (2004, April 27). Aphasia treatment and the crossroads: A biological perspective. *ASHA Leader, 18*, 6–7.

Appendix A
CASE HISTORY FORM

Date of Evaluation: _____

Client's Name: _____

Gender: _____ Age: _____ Date of Birth: _____

Street Address: _____

City: _____ State: _____ Zip: _____

E-mail Address: _____

Preferred Phone Number: _____

Name/Address/Phone of Referral Source:

_____

Has the client ever been examined in this center before? _____

If so, when? _____

Background Information

Date of Onset of Current Illness/Condition: _____

Please describe any communication difficulties.

Health and Medical History

Please list the patient's/client's past medical history:
Do you have any of the following?

Hearing Loss	YES	NO
Vision Problems	YES	NO
Swallowing Problems	YES	NO
Heart Problems	YES	NO
Asthma	YES	NO
Allergies	YES	NO
COPD	YES	NO
Headaches	YES	NO
Seizure Disorder	YES	NO
Neuromuscular Problems	YES	NO
GI problems	YES	NO
History of Drug Abuse	YES	NO
History of Alcohol Abuse	YES	NO
History of Mental Illness	YES	NO

Other: _____

Please list your current medications:

Please list any surgeries and their dates below:

If you ever had a prior speech, language, or cognitive evaluation examination please specify where, when, and type of assessment below:

Educational History

Describe your educational status:
(Highest grade achieved, ever enrolled in a special class, grades repeated, special problems in school, if any, etc.)

Psychosocial and Family History

Please indicate your current marital status:

Single _____   Married _____

Civil Union _____   Separated _____

Divorced _____   Widowed _____

What is your previous or current occupation?

List any children (names and ages):

Do you live alone or do you live with others? Please describe.

What are your hobbies and interests?

Information furnished by: _____

Relationship to client: _____

Appendix B

SKILLS ASSESSMENT INVENTORY

The Skills Assessment Inventory (SAI) is to be used by the clinician and the client's family to help identify functional therapeutic activities prior to treatment.

How to Use the SAI

To assess each skill, observe the client, ask for his or her input when possible, and obtain information from family members or close friends to determine those skills that you will target in treatment. Circle the number from 0 to 5 that best corresponds with the client's perceived ability to perform each task. Items scored in the middle ability range (3s and 4s) should be targeted first because they will allow the client to experience some success. Those that are rated as difficult (0s and 1s) should be avoided initially; they may present frustration. Once you have targeted a few important skills that are in the middle ability level, turn to the corresponding activity pages in this manual and follow the specified directions. Monitor progress on an ongoing basis. We suggest you revisit the client's SAI on a monthly basis.

Note: It is not essential that the client work on all activities in this manual. Select those that relate to the client's life and personal needs. From Klein, E. R., & Hahn, S. E. (2007). *Focus on function: Gaining essential communication* (2nd ed.). Pro-Ed. Reprinted with permission.

0 = Not Applicable 2 = Much Difficulty in Performing Task 4 = Usually Independent

1 = Unable to Perform 3 = Performs Task with Assistance 5 = Normal Functioning

PART I: Basic Living Skills

Chapter 1 Basic Communications						
1. Expressing Needs and Desires	0	1	2	3	4	5
2. Starting Conversations	0	1	2	3	4	5
3. Responding to Emergency and Safety Situations	0	1	2	3	4	5
4. Understanding Common Phrases	0	1	2	3	4	5
5. Talking to Service Personnel	0	1	2	3	4	5
Chapter 2 Using a Telephone						
6. Using a Phone	0	1	2	3	4	5
7. Using a Telephone Directory	0	1	2	3	4	5
8. Using a Phone to Call for Assistance	0	1	2	3	4	5
9. Making Appointments	0	1	2	3	4	5
10. Using the Phone to Get Information	0	1	2	3	4	5
11. Taking Phone Messages	0	1	2	3	4	5
Chapter 3 Managing and Understanding Time						
12. Understanding Measurements of Time	0	1	2	3	4	5
13. Setting a Clock and Telling Time	0	1	2	3	4	5
14. Designing a Daily Schedule	0	1	2	3	4	5
15. Designing a Weekly Schedule	0	1	2	3	4	5
16. Following Calendar Dates and Appointments	0	1	2	3	4	5
17. Recording Events and Keeping a Log	0	1	2	3	4	5
Chapter 4 Managing and Understanding Finances						
18. Understanding Basic Measurements of Money	0	1	2	3	4	5
19. Understanding Bills	0	1	2	3	4	5
20. Writing Checks and Balancing a Checkbook	0	1	2	3	4	5
21. Using an Automated Teller Machine (ATM)	0	1	2	3	4	5
22. Understanding Bank Statements	0	1	2	3	4	5
23. Understanding Graphs and Charts	0	1	2	3	4	5

Chapter 5 Shopping						
24. Working with Money to Purchase Items	0	1	2	3	4	5
25. Using Coupons and Calculating Discounts	0	1	2	3	4	5
Chapter 6 Meals and Cooking						
26. Understanding Basic Measurements and Quantity	0	1	2	3	4	5
27. Planning Menus and Writing Shopping Lists	0	1	2	3	4	5
28. Using a Microwave Oven	0	1	2	3	4	5
29. Cooking with Recipes	0	1	2	3	4	5
Chapter 7 Getting Around						
30. Reading Signs and Symbols	0	1	2	3	4	5
31. Reading Maps	0	1	2	3	4	5
32. Giving Directions to Places	0	1	2	3	4	5
Chapter 8 Activities Around the House						
33. Understanding Measurements of Distance	0	1	2	3	4	5
34. Sequencing Daily Events	0	1	2	3	4	5
35. Reading Directions to Accomplish Tasks	0	1	2	3	4	5
36. Giving Directions to Complete Tasks	0	1	2	3	4	5
37. Using Math to Solve Common Problems	0	1	2	3	4	5
38. Filling in Order Forms	0	1	2	3	4	5
39. Ordering from a Catalog	0	1	2	3	4	5
40. Reading Automobile Classified Advertisements	0	1	2	3	4	5
41. Writing Classified Advertisements	0	1	2	3	4	5
42. Writing Letters	0	1	2	3	4	5
43. Addressing Envelopes	0	1	2	3	4	5

PART II: Social, Leisure, and Work Activities

Chapter 9 Social Participation						
44. Understanding Stories in a Social Setting	0	1	2	3	4	5
45. Retelling Stories	0	1	2	3	4	5
46. Describing and Discussing Photos	0	1	2	3	4	5
47. Using Situational Speech in Dialogue	0	1	2	3	4	5

0 = Not Applicable   2 = Much Difficulty in Performing Task   4 = Usually Independent

1 = Unable to Perform   3 = Performs Task with Assistance   5 = Normal Functioning

48. Performing Social Exchange	0	1	2	3	4	5
49. Expressing Opinions through Dialogue	0	1	2	3	4	5
50. Discussing Feelings and Recognizing Emotions	0	1	2	3	4	5
51. Answering Questions Involving Quantity	0	1	2	3	4	5
52. Role Playing	0	1	2	3	4	5
53. Understanding Body Language and Facial Expression	0	1	2	3	4	5
54. Drawing Inferences from Photos	0	1	2	3	4	5
55. Understanding Idioms	0	1	2	3	4	5
Chapter 10 Leisure						
56. Finding Page Numbers	0	1	2	3	4	5
57. Reading Television and Cable Listings	0	1	2	3	4	5
58. Reading a Table of Contents	0	1	2	3	4	5
59. Understanding News Articles	0	1	2	3	4	5
60. Using a Dictionary	0	1	2	3	4	5
61. Understanding Restaurant Checks	0	1	2	3	4	5
62. Reading a Menu	0	1	2	3	4	5
63. Understanding Directions	0	1	2	3	4	5
64. Playing Games	0	1	2	3	4	5
65. Using the Internet	0	1	2	3	4	5
66. Communicating via e-mail	0	1	2	3	4	5
Chapter 11 Work						
67. Reading Help-Wanted Classified Advertisements	0	1	2	3	4	5
68. Completing Applications	0	1	2	3	4	5
69. Writing a Basic Résumé	0	1	2	3	4	5
70. Writing a Job Application Cover Letter	0	1	2	3	4	5
71. Creating a List of Professional and Personal References	0	1	2	3	4	5
72. Responding to Interview Questions	0	1	2	3	4	5
73. Solving Problems Through Dialogue	0	1	2	3	4	5

Appendix C

COGNITIVE-LINGUISTIC EVALUATION

Name: _____ Age: _____ Date: _____

Primary Care Physician: _____

Medical Diagnosis: _____

Date of Incident: _____

Condition Prior to Incident: _____

Date of CT Scan/MRI: _____ Findings: _____

Relevant Medical History: _____

_____

_____

Medications: _____

Examiner: _____

Instructions: Administer selected sections or all sections as appropriate for the client. Specific instructions are provided under each subheading. Make additional observations in the right-hand column. The client will need a pen or pencil to complete the writing portion of the evaluation.

From Shipley, K. G., & McAfee, J. G. (2004). *Assessment in speech-language pathology: A resource manual* (3rd ed.). Clifton Park, NY: Delmar Learning, a part of Cengage Learning. Reproduced with permission.

Orientation and Awareness

Ask the client the following questions. Score a plus (+) or minus (–) for correct or incorrect responses.

Comments

_____ What day is it?_____

_____ What month is it? _____

_____ What year is it? _____

_____ What season is it?_____

_____ Approximately what time do you think it is? _____

_____ What state are we in?_____

_____ What city are we in?_____

_____ What county are we in?_____

_____ Where do you live?_____

_____ What is the name of this building? _____

_____ Why are you in the hospital? _____

_____ How long have you been here? _____

_____ When did you have your accident? _____

_____ What kind of problems do you have because of your accident?_____

_____ What is my name? _____

_____ What is my profession? _____

_____ Who is your doctor?_____

_____ About how much time has passed since we started talking together today?

Memory

Immediate Memory. Ask the client to repeat the following sequences or sentences. Score a plus (+) or minus (–) for correct or incorrect responses.

Comments

_____ 0, 7, 4, 2 _____

_____ 8, 6, 0, 1, 3 _____

_____ 2, 9, 1, 4, 6, 5_____

_____ car, duck, ring, shoe_____

Comments

____ rain, desk, ladder, horse, cake _____

____ The keys were found under the table. _____

____ He always reads the newspaper before he has breakfast. _____

____ After their victory, the baseball team had pizza and watched a movie._____

Ask the client to retell this story:

____ Helen had a birthday party at the petting zoo. Ten of her friends came. All
the children laughed when a goat was found eating the cake and ice cream. _____

Recent Memory. Ask the client the following questions. Score a plus (+) or minus (–) for correct or incorrect responses.

Comments

____ What did you have for breakfast? _____

____ What did you do after dinner last night? _____

____ What did you do after breakfast this morning? _____

____ What else have you done today? _____

____ Have you had any visitors today or yesterday?_____

____ What other therapies do you receive? _____

____ Who is your doctor?_____

____ How long have you been a resident here? _____

Long-Term Memory. Ask the client the following questions. Score a plus (+) or a minus (–) for correct or incorrect responses.

Comments

____ Where were you born? _____

____ When is your birthday? _____

____ What is your husband's/wife's name?_____

____ How many children do you have?_____

____ How many grandchildren do you have?_____

____ Where did you used to work? _____

____ How much school did you complete? _____

____ Where did you grow up?_____

____ How many brothers and sisters do you have? _____

Auditory Processing and Comprehension

Ask the client the following questions. Score a plus (+) or minus (−) for correct or incorrect responses.

Comments

____ Is your last name Williams? _____

____ Is my name Jim? _____

____ Are you wearing glasses? _____

____ Do you live on the moon? _____

____ Have you had dinner yet? _____

____ Do cows eat grass? _____

____ Do fish swim? _____

____ Do four quarters equal one dollar? _____

____ Are there forty-eight hours in a day? _____

____ Is Alaska part of the United States? _____

Problem Solving

Ask the client the following questions. Score a plus (+) or minus (−) for correct or incorrect responses.

Comments

____ What would you do if you locked your keys in your house? _____

____ What would you do if your newspaper did not get delivered? _____

____ What would you do if you could not find your doctor's phone number? _____

____ What would you do if your TV stopped working? _____

____ What would you do if you forgot to put the milk
away when you got home from the grocery store? _____

Logic, Reasoning, Inference

Ask the client what is wrong with these sentences. Score a plus (+) or minus (−) for correct or incorrect responses.

Comments

____ He put salt and pepper in his coffee. _____

____ Six plus one is eight. _____

Comments

____ I put my socks on over my shoes._____

____ Hang up when the phone rings. _____

____ The dog had four kittens. _____

Ask the client what these expressions mean. Score a plus (+) or minus (−) for correct or incorrect responses.

Comments

____ Haste makes waste. _____

____ An apple a day keeps the doctor away. _____

____ When it rains it pours._____

____ He's a chip off the old block._____

____ Beauty is only skin deep. _____

Ask the client the following questions. Score a plus (+) or minus (−) for correct or incorrect responses.

Comments

____ What is worn on your feet, knit, and used to keep you warm?_____

____ What has a busy tail, climbs trees, and stores nuts? _____

____ What is thin and lightweight, used to wipe tears, and used during a cold? _____

____ How are a sweater, pants, and a blouse alike? _____

____ How are orange juice, soda, and milk alike?_____

Thought Organization

Ask the client to answer the following questions or tasks. Score a plus (+) or minus (−) for correct or incorrect responses.

Comments

____ What does the word "affectionate" mean? _____

____ What does the word "deliver" mean? _____

____ What are the steps you follow to wash your hair?_____

____ What are the steps you follow to make your bed?_____

____ How would you plan a meal for two dinner guests?_____

Calculation

Ask the client to answer the following questions. Score a plus (+) or minus (–) for correct or incorrect responses.

Comments

____ If you went to the mall and spent $8.00 in one store
and $7.50 in another store, how much did you spend? _____

____ If tomatoes cost $1.50 per pound and you bought
2 pounds, how much did you spend on tomatoes? _____

____ If you went to the store with $3.00 and returned
home with $1.75, how much did you spend? _____

____ If toothbrushes cost $3.00 each and you have
$10.00, how many toothbrushes can you buy? _____

____ If you have a doctor's appointment at 10:30 and it takes
you 30 minutes to get there, what time should you leave? _____

Reading and Visual Processing

Ask the client to read the six words in each row and cross out the one that does not belong. Score a plus (+) or minus (–) for correct or incorrect responses.

____ Cow   Apple   Carrot   Cheese   Banana   Oatmeal

____ Desk   Chair   Blue   Bed   Couch   Table

Ask the client to read the following sentences and do what they say. Score a plus (+) or minus (–) for correct or incorrect responses.

Comments

____ Look at the ceiling. _____

____ Point to the door, then blink your eyes. _____

____ Sing Happy Birthday. _____

Ask the client to read the following paragraph out loud and answer the questions about it. Score a plus (+) or minus (–) for correct or incorrect responses.

Mark and Rick are brothers. They both entered a tennis tournament, hoping to win the $1,000 grand prize. Mark won his first two matches, but was eliminated after losing the third match. Rick made it all the way to the semi-finals. He lost, but was awarded a can of tennis balls as a consolation prize.

Comments

____ Are Mark and Rick cousins? _____

____ What sport did they play? _____

Comments

____ What was the grand prize? _____

____ Did one of them win the grand prize? _____

____ Which one did the best in the tournament? _____

Show the client these two clocks and ask them what time the clocks say. Score a plus (+) or minus (−) for correct or incorrect responses.

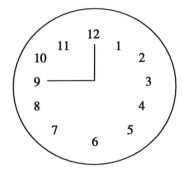
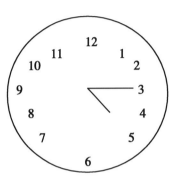

Now ask the client to copy the clocks below. Note accuracy of construction.

Ask the client to put an "X" through all the circles on this page. Note the client's attention to the left half of the page.

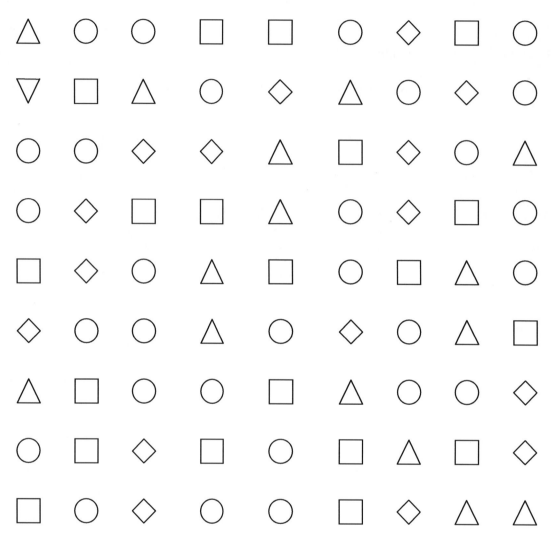

Write your name. Write today's date.

Write a short description of what you have done today in speech therapy.

Writing

Ask the client to complete the writing tasks presented on the opposite page. Observe accuracy of response, completeness, and organization of response, legibility, and observance of left visual field. Make comments in the right margin.

Write your name. Write today's date. Write a short description of what you have done today in speech therapy.

_____

_____

Pragmatics and Affect

Check all behaviors observed during your assessment.

Comments

_____ Inappropriate physical proximity _____

_____ Inappropriate physical contacts_____

_____ Left visual field neglect _____

_____ Poor eye contact _____

_____ Lack of facial expression _____

_____ Gestures (inappropriate, absent)_____

_____ Lack of prosodic features of speech (intensity, pitch, rhythm) _____

_____ Poor topic maintenance _____

_____ Lack of appropriate turn taking _____

_____ Perseveration _____

_____ Presupposition (too much, too little) _____

_____ Inappropriately verbose _____

_____ Lack of initiation _____

_____ Easily distracted _____

_____ Frequent interruptions _____

_____ Impulsive _____

_____ Poor organization _____

_____ Incompleteness_____

Appendix D

SELECTED TREATMENT PROGRAMS AND APPROACHES

Outline

A Treatment Sequence for Phonological Alexia/Agraphia

Overview

Phonological alexia and agraphia often result from damage to the left perisylvian cortex. For individuals with this damage, reading and spelling of real words is usually more difficult than for nonwords. The ability to segment sounds and identify sound-symbol correspondence becomes impaired. Therefore, treating alexia and agraphia involves strengthening phonological processing and the orthographic representation of words. Beeson, Rising, Kim, and Rapcsak (2010) presented two people with aphasia and written language and phonological processing deficits who received treatment that resulted in improved reading and spelling. Treatment included sublexical skills training for phonological awareness, segmentation, sound blending, and manipulation of syllables in words and nonwords, thereby strengthening the link between sounds and letters. Therapy targeted 20 consonants in the initial position of words and 12 vowels in the medial position. Participants wrote a letter that corresponded to a spoken sound and also said the sound that corresponded to the visually presented letter. Four tasks were provided during treatment to retrain phoneme-grapheme correspondence for consonants. The following example explains the treatment sequence:

Task	Response
1. Write the letter that makes the sound	/p/
2. Think of a key word for /p/ and try to write that word;	"pig"
3. Look at this picture. Your key word for /p/ is pig. Write pig and then underline the /p/ sound in the word pig.	
4. Your key word is pig. Copy pig and underline the /p/ in the word pig.	

Vowel training followed the same process, with the exception that some vowel sounds have more than one corresponding letter. Treatment involved segmenting nonwords into their sounds and converting speech sounds to letters for written words. Syllable segmentation, writing, and saying the component sounds in each syllable were required. Spelling was supported by blending sounds into whole words. To help with spelling problems, treatment included three basic steps: (1) generate possible spelling using phonological knowledge; (2) evaluate spelling via orthographic knowledge of letters; and (3) compensate for spelling difficulties via technology to check and correct errors. Over 3 months of therapy, both participants improved their phonological and written language skills and indicated that they were satisfied with treatment outcomes.

Anagram, Copy, and Recall Therapy (ACRT)

Background

ACRT, originally known as Anagram and Copy Treatment (ACT), trains the written modality as a compensatory strategy for communicating basic wants and needs (Beeson, Hirsch, & Rewega, 2002). The primary focus is the accurate spelling of single words for effective and functional communication. This therapy is suitable for aphasic patients who display limitations in both written and verbal output. Specifically, ACRT is appropriate for two groups of individuals: (1) those with poor verbal outputs who have severe aphasia and must rely on written expressions to communicate; and (2) those with good verbal output, who have mild aphasia with underlying spelling deficits. Such deficits may interfere with the activities of daily living, such as e-mailing, creating to-do lists, and taking telephone messages. For both groups of patients, individual words are trained. For the purposes of functional communication, it is recommended that the chosen words in ACRT be specific and relevant to the patient.

The authors used a cuing hierarchy that involved anagram letters and the act of copying single words repeatedly. It's based on "a cognitive model of single word writing referred to as the lexical-semantic route" (Helm-Estabrooks & Albert, 2004), which is explained below.

The Process of Writing Single Words

1. First, a person perceives and recognizes the visual stimulus. For example, the image of a "fish" is shown. The following systems and tasks are then engaged.
   a. *Semantic System:* Within a person's semantic system, there exists a conceptual representation of the word "fish." For example, *edible, fins, salt water, swims, gills.*
   b. *Graphemic Output Lexicon:* People store the learned ability to spell in long-term storage, also known as the graphemic output lexicon.
   c. *Graphemic Output Buffer:* The specific "spatially ordered lettered strings" (Helm-Estabrooks & Albert, 2004, p. 293) that accompany each learned word are stored in the graphemic output buffer, which is held in short-term memory.
   d. *Allographic Conversion:* Learned spellings are converted to actual, physical letter forms.
   e. *Graphomotor Program:* Finally, target words are physically written, "fish." This is the last step to be activated (Helm-Estabrooks & Albert, 2004, p. 293).

Methodology

ACRT is best suited for patients with intact semantic, visual recognition, and graphomotor skills, but with remaining deficits in written naming skills. Graphomotor skills are defined as the process of converting graphemes to letters and then writing those letters (Helm-Estabrooks & Albert, 2004). The following pretests are given to determine appropriate candidates (Helm-Estabrooks & Albert, 2004).

Test of Graphomotor Skills

Ask patient to copy the following sentence:

THE QUICK BROWN FOX JUMPS OVER THE LAZY DOG.

Test of Single-Word Reading Comprehension

Can the patient match a printed word to the visual representation of that word? The Boston Diagnostic Aphasia Examination (BDAE) (Goodglass & Kaplan, 1983) contains a reading subtest with a picture-word matching task. It is recommended that the patient scores with at least 75% accuracy.

Test of Written Confrontation Naming

Helm-Estabrooks and Albert (2004) suggest that specific pictures from the Boston Naming Test (BNT); Kaplan, Goodglass, & Weintraub, 2000) be used to determine single-word spelling ability. These pictures are as follows:

1. Bed
2. Tree
3. Pencil
4. House
5. Comb
6. Saw
7. Broom
8. Camel
9. Bench
10. Dart
11. Canoe
12. Wreath
13. Igloo
14. Cactus
15. Pyramid

The clinician is instructed to present one picture at a time and have the patient write the name of the picture on an unlined 8.5 × 11 piece of paper, using a black marker. The patient should demonstrate some understanding of the word form, that is, at least some letterforms should be present in the written production. For example, if a client is presented with the word "bench," and he or she is able to write "be" or "ben," this patient would be an appropriate candidate. These 15 words also may be used post treatment to demonstrate improvement. Therefore, these words should not be used in the course of treatment.

Test of Visual Memory

Helm-Estabrooks and Albert (2004) suggest the following two subtests to assess visual memory:

1. The Visual Memory Span subtest of the Wechsler Memory Scale–3rd edition (Wechsler, 1997).
2. The Design Memory subtest of the Cognitive-Linguistic Quick Test (CLQT); (Helm-Estabrooks, 2001).

Scoring Spelling Responses from the 15-Word List (from the Written Confrontation Naming Subtest)

Helm-Estabrooks and Albert (2004) developed a 0 to 5 scoring system. This ensures that if a patient partially spells a word right, he or she earns credit. This system is also appropriate for measuring change over the therapeutic course.

Note: Some patients will make several attempts at the correct spelling of a word. Only count their final attempt when scoring. The scoring system is unique to Helm-Estabrooks and Albert (2004) and follows below:

0 = Totally incorrect, illegible, all letters wrong, substitution of a drawing

1 = Less than half correct or all right letters in the wrong order

2 = Half correct, or half letters in wrong order

3 = If more than half is correct, but not fully correct, or if two letters are reversed or letters are added to correct a word, score as:

4 = Self-corrected

5 = Fully correct on first attempt

Example: Possible scoring scenarios with the word "wreath":

5 points = "wreath"

4 points = "wreth" then "wreath" (patient self-corrected)

3 points = "wraeth"

1 point = "wr"

0 points = "siss"

The authors provide a formula for determining the patient's percentage correct and hence a relative level of severity. To determine the percentage correct, follow these steps:

15 (total words) × 5 (highest possible score) = 75 possible points

Example: A patient earns a total of 46 points out of 75:

46/75 = .61 × 100 = 61% of possible points.

The following scoring criteria are from Helm-Estabrooks and Albert (2004).

1. Do not penalize for a combination of uppercase and lowercase letters (e.g., bED).
2. For scoring spelling of words written:
   a. When the target word contains an odd number of letters, a partial score is either 3 or 1, but not a score of 2 (half correct).
   b. When a letter or two are added before or after the correct word, give 3 points.
      Example:
      "hos" for house = 3 points

"hoh" for house = 1 point
"broomer" for broom = 3 points

   c. When the phonetic spelling is used, score as usual and describe the phonetic spelling.
      Example:
      "kom" for comb = 3 points (note use of phonetic spelling)
   d. When an acceptable semantic substitute is used, score it as a correct word.
      Example:
      "home" for house = 5 points
   e. Always score nonsense words as 0.
      Example:
      "meem" for igloo = 0 points

How to Prepare for an ACRT Session

It is advisable that a discussion be held with the patient's family to formulate a list of words that will prove most beneficial to the patient. This may include objects, actions, or feelings relevant to the patient's life and activities of daily living (ADL) needs. Check with the family periodically to verify that these target words remain important, or if any new ones should be added to the list of treatment words.

ACRT follows a hierarchy, beginning with words that are monosyllabic, regularly spelled, and easily visualized. When these are mastered, the clinician may gradually add more complex and irregularly spelled words. Once the target word list has been compiled and organized, these words may be pictorially represented through simple line drawings, personal photographs, and/or photographs clipped form magazines and newspapers.

Measuring Patient Response and Improvement with ACRT

The guidelines below will help the clinician determine if ACRT is effective for the patient:

1. ACRT is directly responsible for the patient's improvement in correctly spelling target words.
   a. A multiple baseline design may be used to determine if improvement is a direct result of

ACRT. (Refer to Beeson, 1999; Beason et al., 2002; and Helm-Estabrooks & Albert, 2004 for more details.)

2. "The effects of treatment are generalizing to the pre- and posttest BNT items" (Helm-Estabrooks & Albert, 2004, p. 299).

   a. Administer the 15 pictured items from the BNT to the patient after every 6 sessions of ACRT and at the end of treatment. Use the 0 to 5 scoring system.

3. The patient is improving their writing skills for functional communication purposes.

   a. Together with family members or caretakers, look at the patient's communication in the form of written notes, grocery lists, to-do lists, e-mails, and conversational exchanges.

Copy and Recall Treatment (CART)/ Oral Reading Treatment (ORT): Concurrent Treatment for Reading and Spelling in Aphasia

People with aphasia who have spoken and written language deficits generally have left perisylvian damage (Benson & Ardilia, 1996). In these individuals, reading is often better preserved than writing. Orjada and Beeson (2005) adapted *Oral Reading for Language in Aphasia* (ORLA; Cherney, 1995) calling it *Oral Reading Treatment* (ORT). Similar to ORLA, ORT is a clinician-guided treatment approach for oral reading. Reading accuracy and comprehension can improve along with overall language skills using ORT in combination with *Copy and Recall Treatment* (CART; Beeson, Rising, & Volk, 2003), Orjada and Beeson (2005) discussed retraining orthographic representations for targeted words with repeated copying and recall. Treating phonological awareness and sound-letter correspondence improved spelling, whereas scripted language improved connected discourse. ORT and CART were provided over 19 total treatment sessions to one individual with aphasia. The authors hypothesized that by combining these two approaches, there would be an increase in reading accuracy rate and spelling skills with a possible positive influence on spoken language performance. The patient assisted in developing personally relevant scripts that were paired with pictures and recorded for practice. The patient and clinician engaged in choral reading followed by the patient reading aloud by himself, which was at a slower than normal rate. Targeted words were also highlighted in the text to make them more salient for the patient. As a result, reading rate and accuracy improved and was maintained for the scripts. Written spelling also improved with repetition. As a result of the ORT and CART concurrent treatment for reading and spelling, the patient's verbal output also improved. After readministration with the *Western Aphasia Battery* (WAB), clinically significant expressive language gains were found. For example, mean length of utterance (MLU) increased from 3.62 to 7.4 morphemes on picture description tasks and to 9.47 during conversation. ORT and CART are composed of the following procedures.

ORT

ORT uses printed text for each sentence. These sentences are recorded in a talking photo album, and these sentences are used to improve reading accuracy. The protocol is below:

1. The clinician reads each sentence of the script, pointing to every word.
2. The clinician and the client read the same sentence in unison while the clinician points to each word.
3. The client reads the sentence alone while pointing to each word.
4. The clinician calls attention to any errors the client makes.
5. The client then self-corrects.
6. The client repeats the oral reading until they reach 100% accuracy.
7. ORT Home Program

   a. Every day the client uses the talking pictures photo album in lieu of the clinician.
   b. The client plays the recording and reads along silently.
   c. The client then reads in unison with the recorded sentence.
   d. The client then reads the sentence without the support of the audio recording.

CART

1. The client selects 5 to 10 words from each of their three scripts.
2. The client then makes a list of the selected words.
3. The client then copies each target word 3 to 5 times, until they can recall it from memory.
4. The client then writes the word from memory and checks the spelling, correcting any errors.
5. The procedure is repeated for each of the targeted words.

Constraint-Induced Language Therapy (CILT)

Background

Constraint-induced therapy, developed from animal research, is modeled after treatment used in physical therapy (Cherney, Patterson, Raymer, Frymark, & Schooling, 2008). This technique was introduced in 2001 and is primarily used with patients with nonfluent aphasia (Cherney et al., 2008). It is based on the following principles: brain plasticity, massed practice, constraint induction, and behavioral relevance (Pulvermuller et al., 2001). The mechanism responsible for the success of this therapy is currently unknown. However, the mechanism seems to be related to the way motor constraint overcomes learned nonuse (Pulvermuller et al., 2001).

Rationale

The basic principle of this approach is forcing the use of spoken language with massed practice to generate verbal responses that are shaped into longer utterances. Treatment generally involves up to 3 hours per day, 5 days per week. With this extensive amount of treatment, the brain is thought to adapt and compensate for the injury or damage.

Program Features

Because of the fact that CILT requires forced use of verbal language, all responses during treatment must be spoken. Gestures or other nonverbal communication are not permitted. Massed practice and the high intensity of treatment also add to its effectiveness. CILT therapy is usually implemented 6 to 12 months after onset, once the aphasia is considered chronic in nature. However, CILT has also been found to be effective in improving naming and sentence construction with acute stroke patients (1 to 2 months post-stroke).

Using CILT, the goal is toward increasing the quantity and quality of spoken language. As a result, patients indicated positive feedback. Another encouraging feature is that the recommended hierarchy of language is based on relevance to the patient (Kirmess & Maher, 2010). Although the patient's interest plays a part in the choice of words, other factors that appear to impact the outcomes of CILT include the patient's age, physical activity, and motivation. In general, the hierarchy of CILT stimuli involves four levels of increasing complexity:

1. Single word naming and accurately answering yes or no questions.
2. Addressing another person by name and using an interrogative phrase while naming the object presented.
3. Maintaining Level 2 and adding appropriate adjectives and/or adverbs to the verbal output.
4. Engaging in all aspects previously mastered including appropriate descriptors for quantity and/or amount.

Research Findings on CILT

An overall increase in spoken nouns and increased informativeness was found for all three post-CILT cases in a study by Kirmess and Lind (2011). The authors found a generalization effect of greater word production in connected speech when the pre-post language analysis was transcribed from dialogical interviews of patients in the study. CILT appears to be a promising treatment technique in helping people with nonfluent aphasia use verbal language following a stroke.

There have been positive effects from this treatment approach particularly due to its high intensity. Unlike traditional approaches in aphasia therapy that focus on compensatory strategies such as drawing and writing, this approach requires only attempts at verbal communication, which is the *induced constraint*. In this approach, the therapist presents the patient with tasks that require him or her to name objects pictured on cards, such as a card picturing a muffin. The patient is required to name the item using the correct noun, and as they progress, the clinician adds a modifier, for example, two muffins. As they became more advanced, they must put that phrase into a syntactic frame, using the name of the person they are addressing, for example, "Mrs. Jones, can I please have two muffins?" Research indicates that patients who received CILT had a 30% increase in the amount of daily verbal communication used, as reported on their Communication Activity Logs (CAL) (Pulvermuller et al., 2001). It is speculated that there may be cortical reorganization from massed practice that promotes language rehabilitation. Cherney et al. (2008) found that regardless of treatment type, more treatment appears to produce better results when delivered over a restricted time period. Regardless of the treatment approach used, clinicians must make treatment decisions based on clinical experience, the patient's individualized needs, and sound evidence of treatment efficacy.

Systematic reviews found that CILT had a positive effect on individuals with nonfluent aphasia. The high intensity of treatment was considered a major benefit. Using CILT, gains were maintained over a period of 1 to 3 months with language increases maintained at 6-month follow-up (Cherney et al., 2008). Forcing spoken language was thought to be a major factor in the treatment's success. Meinzer, Djundja, Barthel, Elbert, and Rockstroh (2005) also found improvements in the amount of words, naming, repetition ability, and overall quality of communication.

Cueing Strategies

Linebaugh , Pryor, and Margulies (1983) stated that there are three basic principles of cueing hierarchies:

- Cues that elicit a response from the patient with the least amount of help from the clinician are the most desirable. They are the least powerful in the hierarchy.
- Cues should become less powerful as therapy continues.
- The patient must be trained to use self-cueing or *internal facilitators.*

All cueing hierarchies must be client-specific. The ultimate goal is that the patient will require less powerful cues and will have learned to use that cue in response to other stimulus categories. For example, the client will self-cue with the first sound of a word across all semantic categories, not just the category used to train the technique in therapy. The clinician can use semantic cueing to facilitate the client's word retrieval, for example, by providing a descriptive cue for a word, or a sentence completion cue. Those cues are less powerful than having the client imitate the desired word. Therefore, they are higher up in the cueing hierarchy. One can also provide phonological cues, starting with the least powerful cue—providing a target word and phonological foils—proceeding to the most powerful cue, imitation. In between the two, one can cue the patient using a nonreal rhyming word, or an articulatory cue. Linebaugh and Lehner (1977) presented a modified cueing hierarchy by mixing types of cues. For example, they suggested giving the client the written representation of the first letter of the work along with an articulatory cue for the first phoneme. He also added gestural prompting to the hierarchy.

Divergent Word Retrieval

Background

Divergent Word Retrieval is a cognitive stimulation approach. Divergent word retrieval (naming) requires that a person generate as many possible answers in relation to a given topic, such as a named category. For example, given the word "farm," how many different and appropriate farm animals can a person name? Or, given the topic "fishing," how many different words associated with this sport can a person name? As Davis (2000) noted, "In a divergent mode, we generate a quantity and variety of responses" (p. 87). Additionally, divergent naming tasks are open-ended (Chapey, 2001). As a consequence, successful divergent naming involves the ability to generate many logical connections and cognitive flexibility (Guilford, 1967). For example, when provided the word farm, one must have the ability to change from very obvious associations with the word (animals, crops) to more indirect ones, for example, "grain," "bales," and so forth. In a study by Grossman (1981), adults were asked to generate word lists for 10 categories, including furniture, tools, clothing, and sports. Adults without aphasia produced an average of 14.66 words for each category. Adults with fluent aphasia produced 6.71 words, whereas adults with nonfluent aphasia produced 5.29 words (Davis, 2000).

Rationale

Addressing this skill in the evaluation and treatment of patients with aphasia was indicated by Chapey, Rigrodsky, and Morrison (1977). These researchers suggested that in addition to convergent tasks requiring one correct answer (such as with confrontation naming), divergent naming tasks were also needed to assess a "full range of word-finding conditions" (Davis, 2000, p. 87). Therefore, this task requires a patient to access memory in a broad sense of the term for stored semantic concepts, in order to offer a variety of appropriate or alternative responses (Chapey et al., 1977). Wepman (1972, 1976) supported the cognitive stimulation aspect to aphasia therapy. He believed that the use of discussions with a central topic and expanding on ideas within that topic should be focal points of aphasia treatment. It has been suggested that cognitive rehabilitation should go beyond the mere task of asking patients to recall a spoken word, which Lindfors (1987) describes as a lower level cognitive process. Instead, the clinician should aim to stimulate higher level cognitive processes. They should facilitate inferencing, thought organization, and problem solving in the patient, and that divergent thinking should be one of the domains of cognition targeted for stimulation for the purpose of improving communication skills (Chapey, 1994).

Measurement

When assessing a patient's divergent naming skills, responses can be divided into two categories: (1) fluency (the number of responses a patient is able to generate); and (2) flexibility (the variety of the patient's responses; Chapey, 1994). In some cases, it may be appropriate to look at the amount of unusual responses a patient is able to generate and the amount of important details a patient provides about a relevant topic. Guilford (1967) refers to this as the creativity and the elaboration of the patient's responses on a naming task.

Using the Chapey Speech and Language Checklist (Chapey, 1994, pp. 113–114), the patient is instructed to produce numerous logical possibilities/perspectives/ideas where appropriate. Chapey presents the following tasks as a means to measure a patient's ability to produce divergent naming:

1. List words beginning with a specified letter such as /s/ or /p/
2. Name objects within a group
3. List uses for a common object
4. List problems inherent in a common situation
5. Supply multiple possible solutions to problems
6. Suggest ways to improve a product
7. Specify details in planning an event, making a decision, or describing a procedure
8. Specify numerous episodes or substeps in a story
9. Elaborate

Chapey et al. (1977) and Chapey (1994) offer an example of how to score a patient's response when asked to name "objects that can roll," with the patient's responses as follows:

1. baseball
2. football
3. basketball
4. nickel
5. dime
6. quarter
7. car
8. truck

Fluency score = 8

Flexibility score = 3 (patient included 3 categories: balls, money, and transportation).

Additionally, if the above patient was to produce any words that were not relevant to the category of "objects that can roll," those words would not be counted. The following list offers additional ideas for eliciting divergent naming (Chapey, 1994):

1. Common Situations: List problems that are inherent in a common situation.
2. Brick Uses: List many different uses for a common object.
3. Improve Product: Suggest ways to improve a particular object.
4. Consequences: List the effect of a new and unusual event.
5. Object Naming: List objects that belong to a broad class of objects.
6. Differences: Suggest ways in which two objects are different.
7. Similarities: Produce ways in which two objects are alike.
8. Word Fluency: List words that contain a specified word or letter.
9. Elaboration: List detailed steps needed to make a briefly outlined plan work.

Life Participation Approach to Aphasia (LPAA)

Background

The long-term goal for any patient being treated using the LPAA approach is to reduce the barriers to the patient's participation in daily life activities and social relationships. In this approach, patients assume an active role in recovery. Patient participation occurs along a continuum that is ever changing and reflects status at the time of treatment. This continuum evolves by first addressing immediate goals, such as asking nursing staff to use the bathroom, and later progresses to long-term goals, such as returning to a previous place of employment. LPAA targets any activities in the individual's daily life that are affected by aphasia, even if these activities do not involve communication.

LPAA is based on functional and pragmatic therapy approaches for patients with aphasia. Although it is important for a patient to regain the ability to communicate their basic wants and needs, LPAA goes a step further in that it emphasizes the importance of *living* with aphasia by getting the patient to engage in life despite the communication impairments (Chapey et al., 2008). Although some aphasia therapies address life enhancement only after language deficits have been remedied, this approach identifies this goal from the beginning of treatment (Chapey et al., 2008).

Methodology

The primary focus of this treatment approach is reengagement in life from the moment therapy begins. The patient is heavily involved in helping design a treatment plan that encompasses his or her goals of participation in daily life, thus creating a sense of empowerment. Two components are essential for re-engagement in daily life activities: a support system (family and friends) and patient motivation. Five core values are central to LPAA and should be integrated into assessment and intervention (Chapey et al., 2008. They are as follows:

Core Value #1

Enhancement of life participation.

The clinician and patient work to improve short-term and long-term participation in life. Together, the patient and clinician consider the following:

a. To what extent can the patient with aphasia achieve life participation goals?
b. To what extent does the aphasia interfere with achieving these goals?

Core Value #2

All those affected by aphasia are entitled to service.

Aphasia affects more than just the patient; it also affects family members, colleagues, and friends. Therefore, LPAA aims to support those in close association, which may potentially facilitate improved quality of life for the patient. Examples of supportive services include:

a. Training others how to support and facilitate communication (e.g., Kagan & Gailey, 1993; Lyon et al., 1997)
b. Counseling regarding communication, life participation, and how to live life to the fullest with aphasia (e.g., Holland, 1999; Ireland & Wootten, 1996)
c. Couples therapy—work on communication and relationship together (e.g., Boles, 1998)
d. Group training in supported communication (e.g., training work colleagues, training health care practitioners; Elman, 2000).

Core Value #3

The measures of success include documented life enhancement changes.

Outcome measures are a requirement of this treatment. The clinician is to assess:

a. quality of life
b. degree to which life participation goals have been met.

Core Value #4

Personal and environmental factors are targets of intervention.

For those with aphasia, daily life can be disrupted in two areas:

a. personal, or internal (includes physical, emotional, and psychological changes related to aphasia)
b. environmental, or external (includes social and physical structures that impede ability to function in everyday life activities).

To determine target goals, these two areas must be continuously prioritized and assessed throughout therapy.

Core Value #5

Emphasis is on availability of services as needed throughout all stages of aphasia therapy.

Services are available from the onset and end only when the patient and clinician agree that life participation goals have been met.

Lingraphica

Lingraphica (http://www.lingraphica.com) was developed at the Boston VA Hospital nearly 30 years ago. Researchers first produced a program known as the Visual Communication System (VIC). Simple drawings that depicted categories of people, actions, and objects were produced on index cards. The patients then selected cards from these categories and laid them out to produce phrases and sentences as an alternative means of communication. In 1980, this system was adapted to the computer, and became known as Computer-Assisted Visual Communication (C-ViC; Helm-Estabrooks & Albert, 2004; Shelton, Weinrich, McCall, & Cox, 1996; Steele, Kleczewska, Carlson, & Weinrich, 1992; Steele, Weinrich, Wertz, Kleczewska, & Carlson, 1989; Weinrich, Steele, Carlson, et al., 1989; Weinrich, Steele, Kleczewska, et al., 1989). This program was then adapted into what is known today as Lingraphica, a speech-generating device for use with patients with aphasia. Lingraphica was approved by Medicare in 2002. The cost of this device is reimbursed by most private insurance plans and many state Medicaid programs, including Medicare Part B, The Veterans Administration, Federal Supply Contract V797P–4886a, Aetna, and the Department of Health and Human Services.

Lingraphica provides patients with the ability to access a group of icons, pictures, and symbols that are compiled to represent words, phrases, and sentences. The patient first chooses specific icons and symbols and puts them together in logical order, in either phrase or sentence formats. As such, a patient is able to functionally communicate personal needs, wants, and interests.

Lingraphica Program Features

Lingraphica is a speech-generating computer software program that builds graphic symbols and pictures into phrases and sentences, which are then spoken aloud by a computer-generated and natural-sounding human voice. Essentially, the program integrates the visual and auditory modalities. It is flexible in that it provides multiple opportunities for extensive practice and is appropriate for patients with varying levels of ability and who are at varying stages of recovery. The program is customizable in that it may be individualized to the patient based on his or her specific abilities, needs, and interests. Equipped with a wide variety of vocabulary, patients may select specific words and build phrases and sentences to communicate basic wants and needs. Such phrases and sentences may then be saved and easily retrieved for later use. Lingraphica also comes pre-equipped with standard phrases that may be used when eating in a restaurant or during doctors' visits.

Lingraphica contains 240 exercises ranging in difficulty from "easy" to "hard." It "offers unlimited speech practice, both at home and in therapy, through rehearsal and repetition of icons and phrases that use natural human voices" (http://www.Lingraphica.com). The program is to be administered by a trained and ASHA-certified speech-language pathologist. The following information provides a review of methods for individualizing the program to the patient:

1. Small or large icons may be used, and this choice is based upon the patient's eyesight.
2. A patient may create their own icons. a. Example: Icons of grandchildren
   a. "My granddaughters Mary and Megan" would have two standard icons for "my" and "granddaughters," and two customized icons for "Mary" and "Megan."
3. Two built-in cameras are included:
   a. Still camera: Patient may create still photos for personalized icons.
   b. Video camera: Patient may record video clips.

Other Features Included in Lingraphica

1. Practice Videos
   a. Example: A patient may click on a video demonstration of production of the syllable "pa." When the patient clicks on this icon, a video reveals an up-close demonstration of a woman's lips producing "pa" two times. The idea is for the patient to then imitate this production.
   b. Other videos include additional practice phonemes and standard phrases.
2. Training Videos
   a. These are offered to the patients, to provide user-friendly video tutorials. The video depicts a person walking the patient step-by-step through all program features, and this option is easily accessible through the "Help Menu."
3. Free Technical Support
   a. This is available toll-free, from 9 AM to 5 PM. A patient or caregiver may even e-mail a question and will receive a response within 24 hours.

The website also offers downloadable manuals and reference guides. There is live Internet support and even Web-based training over the Internet.

Lingraphica is user-friendly, with easy-to-understand drop-down menu items. A Spanish version is also included within the program for Spanish-speaking patients. Patients may even qualify for a free and no-obligation trial of Lingraphica. To determine eligibility, the following steps are recommended.

1. The speech-language pathologist (SLP) working with the patient provides the patient's insurance information to Lingraphica staff.
2. Lingraphica staff runs a benefits check to make sure the device will be covered by the patient's personal insurance company. Determination of eligibility is made within 24 hours.
3. If determined eligible, a loaner device is shipped out to the patient. (No paperwork is required.)
4. The SLP receives over-the-phone training, which takes approximately one hour.
5. The trial typically takes 4 weeks to complete, with 2 devoted to the SLP providing the training, and 2 devoted to practice.
   a. During the 4-week trial period, the patient is evaluated and introduced to the basic operations of the device by the speech-language pathologist. Then the patient works independently with the device while also continuing

therapy sessions. The patient and the clinician then decide if the device is appropriate for his or her communication needs (http://www.Lingraphica.com). This decision is aided by a built-in "Clinical Consultant" who also trains the SLP on the device.

6. If after the trial period it is determined that the program is appropriate, Lingraphica will send a Certificate of Medical Necessity form to the patient and will simultaneously gather a physician-written prescription as well as insurance company authorization.

7. The loaner device is shipped back to Lingraphica, free of charge.

8. After all the necessary paperwork has been processed, a customized Lingraphica device is sent to the patient. This device will incorporate information specific to the patient, such as family member names and individual needs and interests.

9. SLP's will receive 2.4 ASHA CEU's after completing the 4-week trial.

The Evidence for Lingraphica

"The Lingraphica has been proven effective in clinical studies, and is based on decades of aphasia research and technology development" (http://www.Lingraphica.com). This information has been documented in a number of publications and presentations, and can be obtained from the following link: http://www.lingraphica.com/slp/research.aspx

Mapping Treatment

Mapping treatment aims to improve the link between meaning and structure at the sentence level. The underlying premise of this therapeutic approach is that the patient has lost the ability to convey meaning using noun-verb relationships, again indicating a problem with thematic roles. Therapy is focused on sentence production using probing questions: What is the verb? Who is doing the *verb-ing*? Who or what is the *verb-ing*? This sentence query approach

becomes more specific over a 3-month period. The patient is asked to:

1. Identify the verb.
2. Identify the agent or actor by using a "who" query before the verb.
3. Identify the patient/theme role by using a "what" query after the verb.
4. Identify the locative by using the "where" query.
5. Ask questions about "when," "why," and "how."
6. Different sentence types are targeted ranging from simple subject + object Noun Phrase (NPs). (*Susan drinks the soda*) to complex subject + object NPs (*The girl from the office was helping Mary's daughter*; Figure D–1).

Melodic Intonation Therapy (MIT)

Background

Goldstein (1942) found that patients with severe aphasia were able to correctly speak words through the activity of singing. Clinicians then searched for therapy options that used melody and rhythm to stimulate speech production. Melodic Intonation Therapy (MIT) became the designated name for a therapy that capitalized on an intact right hemisphere and its role in processing intonation patterns. In 1994, the Therapeutics and Technology Assessment Subcommittee of the American Academy of Neurology identified MIT as an "effective" treatment approach to language therapy. MIT uses rhythmic intonations of phrases and sentences as the tool of language rehabilitation. The program is fully described in Helm-Estabrooks and Albert (2004). MIT is best used with nonfluent aphasics who have poorly articulated output, and moderately preserved auditory comprehension. They also must have good motivation and attention spans, and be emotionally stable. Patients who respond well to this approach have an intact right hemisphere, with a unilateral left hemispheric stroke. Most interesting, patients who have poor repetition skills even for single words also respond well to MIT.

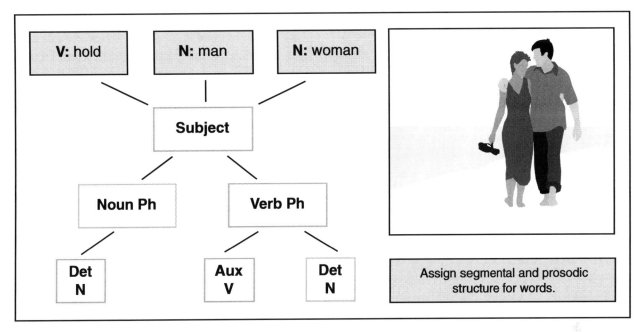

Figure D–1. An example of mapping treatment.

Methodology

MIT follows a hierarchy of 3 levels, using the following target stimuli:

1. Multisyllabic words
2. Short, high-probability phrases
3. Increasing phonologically complex sentences

The first 2 levels are musically intoned. The third level is first intoned, then given exaggerated speech prosody, and, finally, spoken with normal speech prosody.

Preparation

1. Consider the communication needs of the patient and the family.
2. Preselect stimulus items with associated pictures.
3. Stimulus items should be high-probability syllables, phrases, or sentences. The Sentence Production Program for Aphasia (SPPA) provides appropriate hierarchies of syntactic difficulty.
4. Include MIT score sheet.

5. Sit across from the patient using a tabletop surface.
6. Begin with imperative sentences and sounds that are most visible, such as bilabials.
7. Rotate a wide variety of words, phrases, and sentences.

Presentation

1. Intone target stimulus slowly.
2. Use continuous voicing.
3. Include high and low tones associated with normal speech prosody (pitch).
4. Incorporate the rhythm and stress patterns found in normal speech.
5. Face the patient so they may have visual access to your mouth.
6. Use right hand to hold the patient's left hand, tapping it on the table for each syllable.
7. Use left hand to signal to the patient when to listen and when to intone.
8. Progress consecutively through all steps of each level; no step may be skipped.
9. Allow 4 attempts of each step.

Scoring

For specific scoring procedures, refer to *Manual of Aphasia and Aphasia Therapy* (Helm-Estabrooks & Albert, 2004). Essentially, a patient's score will determine progression to a more advanced level, discontinuation of therapy, or a complete discharge. Progression from one level to the next is dependent on the patient achieving a score of 90% or higher, using an assortment of target stimuli, during 5 consecutive therapy sessions. The levels are described below.

Level 1. Pictures and environmental cues associated with the target stimuli are incorporated throughout. Hand tapping is used for all target stimuli productions.

1. Humming—The melody pattern of the stimulus item is hummed while a picture or environmental cue is provided. The patient's hand is tapped accordingly. Proceed to sing the stimulus item twice. No patient response is required.
2. Unison intoning—Intone stimulus item in unison. Hand tapping continues. If the patient is unsuccessful after 4 repetitions, return to Step 1 and introduce a new stimulus item.
3. Unison intoning with fading—Begin in unison, intoning and hand tapping. Halfway through stimulus item, fade voice. The patient must complete the rest of the stimulus item independently.
4. Immediate repetition—Target stimulus is intoned and tapped as the patient listens. The patient independently repeats the target stimulus while hand tapping continues.
5. Response to probe question—Without hand tapping, quickly intone a probe question. For example, "What did you say?" The patient must then respond. Hand tapping may be provided only as the patient answers the question.

After all 5 steps are completed in succession, proceed back to Step 1 and introduce a new stimulus item.

Level 2. Delays between the target stimulus and the required response are introduced at this level. Pictures and environmental cues associated with the target stimuli, as well as hand tapping, are included.

If the patient is unable to complete a step with a delay, the individual is allowed to back up to a previous step. This will affect the patient's overall score. If the patient is unsuccessful even with this, the clinician introduces a new target stimulus.

1. Introduction of target phrase—Using hand tapping, target phrase is intoned and repeated twice. No response is required.
2. Unison with fading—Begin in unison; tone and tap. Halfway through target phrase, fade voice as the patient continues independently. Repeat target phrase twice in this format, even if the patient is successful.
3. Delayed repetition—Intone target phrase and tap.
4. Provide a 6-second delay between Steps 3 and 4. Request repetition and hand tap as the patient repeats, but do not provide verbal assistance. If the patient fails, back up to Step 2: Unison with fading. If this proves successful, attempt Step 3 again. If the patient still fails, return to Step 1 and introduce new stimulus item.
5. Response to probe question—Without hand tapping, quickly intone a probe question. For example, "What did you say?" The patient must then respond. Hand tapping may be provided simultaneously as the patient answers the question. If the patient is unsuccessful in providing a response, back up to Step 3. If the patient proves successful at Step 3, wait 6 seconds before attempting the probe question once again. If the patient fails to answer this time, return to Step 1 and introduce a new stimulus item.

Level 3. This stage involves more complex utterances, with the aim of introducing normal prosody back into the patient's speech. A transitional step known as *sprechgesang* (speech song) is first introduced to achieve the return to normal prosody and is thought to sound similar to choral reading. The rhythm and stress of the target stimuli are emphasized. The previous intoning of stimuli is now replaced by the rising and falling pitches found in normal speech. Backing up to previous steps is also allowed in Level 3, but will affect the patient's overall score.

1. Delayed repetition—Intone the target phrase while hand tapping, and pause for 6 seconds. The patient repeats once. Provide hand tapping, should the patient require it. If the patient fails, back up one level to Step 2: Unison with fading. If successful, attempt Delayed repetition in Level 3 again. If the patient fails, introduce new stimulus item.

2. Introducing "Sprechgesang"—Introduce the target phrase twice. Do not sing; instead, exaggerate the rhythm and stress, doing so in a slow manner. Incorporate hand tapping. No response is required.

3. "Sprechgesang" (with fading)—Using sprechgesang, begin the target phrase in unison with the patient. Fade voice while the patient completes the phrase independently. If the patient fails, repeat utterance in unison, but do not fade voice. Successful performance of this results in attempting Step 3 again. If the patient fails after backing up, return to Step 1 with a new stimulus item.

4. Delayed spoken repetition—The target phrase is spoken to the patient using normal prosody, without hand tapping. Allow for a 6-second delay. The patient must repeat with normal prosody. If successful, move to Step 5 after a 6-second delay. If the patient is unsuccessful, attempt Step 4 again. If the patient continues to be unsuccessful, return to Step 1 and present a new stimulus item. Important: Include a 6-second delay in between Step 4 and 5.

5. Response to a probe question—Ask a question using normal prosody. The patient should respond, also using normal prosody. If the patient fails, back up to Step 4 and then attempt Step 5 again. If they succeed, return to Step 1 and introduce a new stimulus item.

Measuring Response to MIT

The functional goal of MIT is to improve the communication skills of patients with significant expressive impairment. Progress can be measured by using a variety of tools, including: giving a close family member the Communication Questionnaire

(Helm-Estabrooks & Albert, 2004) before and after MIT; standardized aphasia tests that require narrative descriptions of pictures, such as the "Cookie Theft" in the Boston Diagnostic Aphasia Examination (BDAE) and pre- and post-MIT speech samples of the patient.

MossTalk Words (MTW)

The presence of word-finding deficits in patients with aphasia is well documented (Basso, 2003). Such difficulties have been shown to interfere with both daily living and social communication (Lesser & Algar, 1995). MossTalk Words (MTW), developed at Moss Rehab (associated with the Albert Einstein Healthcare Network and Jefferson Health System of Pennsylvania), is a computer-based program focused on word-finding deficits, by training comprehension and production of words at the word, phrase, and sentence levels. MTW is a software program that may be utilized in the clinic with the assistance of a speech-language pathologist or a trained volunteer, or it may be used independently in the patient's own home (Fink, Brecher, Sobel, & Schwartz, 2005). MTW comes equipped with 340 vocabulary words and pictures, which may be presented in both the visual and auditory modalities.

Program Interfaces

There are three separate interfaces within the MTW program. They are as follows:

1. The Standard Interface contains three separate treatment modules. Each module contains an array of exercises that are organized in a hierarchy of easy-to-difficult tasks. For example, a more difficult task might include lower frequency vocabulary words or phonological foils that closely resemble the target production.

2. The Customizing Interface gives clinicians and caregivers the option of "preselecting" the items that will be included in the patient's exercise.

3. The Assigned Exercises Interface allows "patients to access preselected exercises independently" (Fink et al., 2005, p. 947).

Therapy Modules

Fink et al. (2005) describe two general types of therapeutic exercises that they refer to as "therapy modules."

1. Core-Vocabulary Module. Exercises include matching and naming tasks for the more severely impaired patient. This module contains a select group of vocabulary words associated with functional ADLs, such as common objects and the names of foods.
2. Multiple-Choice Matching Module. Includes exercises for strengthening vocabulary and comprehension in both speech and printed formats.
3. Cued-Naming Module. Single-word production is the goal in this module. These exercises contain a cuing hierarchy and 8 possible cues (4 visual and 4 print), which may be used to facilitate word retrieval and production. According to Fink et al., (2005), "The clinician assesses patient deficits and needs, and individualizes this module accordingly. The clinician can select the level of difficulty, the modality, the vocabulary and/or which cues to activate for a given exercise with a particular patient" (Fink et al., 2005, p. 946). The cues are listed below (Ramsberger & Marie, 2007).

Verbal cues:
1) first phoneme
2) sentence completion
3) definition
4) spoken word

Print cues:
1) first letter
2) written sentence completion
3) written definition
4) written word

Fink et al. (2005) instruct the clinician to carefully consider the type of chronic patient before selecting MTW. They advise that MTW is appropriate for patients with primary progressive aphasia, and those who demonstrate semantically based deficits that are moderate in nature. This program is not suited for patients with a Wernicke's type aphasia, cognitive impairments, or patients who perseverate. Both patients and clinicians alike gave high satisfactory remarks regarding MTW, highlighting ease of use and level of enjoyment. Initially, clinicians invested time to learn the software, but the general feeling was that this investment paid off long term, in that MTW saved clinicians time once the program was in use.

The use of computer technology is intimidating to some, especially those patients who are not regularly exposed to computers. Therefore, using a volunteer in the computer lab who is trained and/or supervised by a certified speech-language pathologist may provide an extra level of support (Fink et al., 2005).

Narrative Story Cards

Background

The process of telling and retelling a story involves the interaction of cognitive and linguistic skills. This process includes word-retrieval, correct word morphology, appropriate sentence syntax, narrative cohesion, working memory, pragmatic awareness, and visual perception. Narrative Story Cards as an approach is appropriate for adolescent and adult populations who have brain damage and who may experience deficits in narrative discourse.

Methodology

The Narrative Story Cards include 15 separate stories to facilitate planning, organization, word-retrieval, syntax, topic maintenance, and working memory. The stories contain emotional content, which is thought to stimulate memory function, and each set includes pictures, a text, and titles. The Narrative Story Cards range in order of complexity from 3 to 5 cards each: 6-story sets include 3 cards each; 4-story sets include 4 cards each; and 5-story sets include 5 cards each.

All sets include a story sheet to be used along with the cards for telling and retelling the story. A content unit checklist associated with each story is also included. This is used to record client responses and to determine narrative discourse skills (Helm-Estabrooks & Nicholas, 2002). For example, in the story "Casino Luck," card 3 reads: "It's now four o'clock, and Joe has just a few pennies left. Three hours and no luck!" The following information units are included on the checklist.

1. four
2. o'clock
3. Joe/he
4. has
5. few
6. pennies
7. three
8. hours
9. no luck

If the client mentions any of the above words, a check mark is placed in the column to the right on the score sheet. The final score is calculated by adding the patient's total information units and dividing this number by the total number of possible units. If the total number of possible units was 55, but the patient only expressed 23 units, the final score would be 23/55 or 42%.

List of Tasks

The following list of tasks is suggested for use with Narrative Story Cards (Helm-Estabrooks & Nicholas, 2002).

1. Sequencing the cards.
2. Telling a story once given the cards.
3. Retelling the story and making up a new ending.
4. Giving the story a title.
5. Comprehension for titles read.
6. Comprehension of story read, matched to correct pictures.
7. Writing story given information.
8. Writing story without word prompts.
9. Retelling story in written form.
10. Auditory comprehension of information.

Nonsymbolic Movements for Activation of Intention (NMAI)

Background

The self-initiation of complex behaviors has its origins in the presupplementary motor area, an intentional mechanism center within the brain (Picard & Strick, 1996). Complex behaviors include language tasks such as word generation and hand gesturing, which individuals with nonfluent aphasia have difficulty initiating due to lesions in that area. After a stroke in the left hemisphere, language production mechanisms may move to the right hemisphere, whereas the intention mechanisms remain in the left hemisphere. According to the theory, this may create a disconnection between the two communicating centers. It is this phenomenon that may explain the difficulty of word generation found in nonfluent aphasics.

Previous research has highlighted a successful intervention technique for aphasia, using American Indian Sign Language during verbal naming tasks (Hoodin & Thompson, 1983; Kearns, Simmon, & Sisterhen, 1982; Pashek, 1997; Skelly, Schinsky, Smith, & Fust, 1974). This therapeutic approach required the patient to name objects while simultaneously performing a hand gesture with their nondominant hand. They found that naming accuracy improved using this technique. However, the authors of a more recent pilot study suggested that the complex hand movements actually activated the intentional centers in the right hemisphere, and as a result, helped with word production (Richards, Singletary, Rothi, Koehler, & Crosson, 2002). If these complex hand movements activated intentional centers in the right hemisphere, maybe they could potentially activate the initiation of language. Essentially, switching initiation centers to the same side as the production centers (initiated by complex hand movement in the nondominant hand) would improve naming accuracy.

Treatment

The treatment protocol is described below (Richards et al., 2002), and it can be utilized in the therapy session with a few modifications. In lieu of the computer program, the clinician could provide his or her own black and white line drawings and accompanying words. A stopwatch is also required. The treatment seeks to stimulate right hemisphere initiation centers through the use of complex hand gestures in the nondominant hand. The phases are in succession, beginning with the patient receiving external cues, to the patient receiving no cues and creating their own nonsymbolic hand gesture.

Treatment in the research study consisted of three phases. Each phase included ten 45-minute sessions. During each session, the clinician present-ed and named a set of 50 black and white line drawings, for a total of 150 pictures for all three phases. The 50 words in each phase were broken down into 15 high-frequency, 15 medium-frequency, and 20 low-frequency words. The clinician began each trial by clicking a mouse button, thereby activating a timer. When the black and white line drawing appeared on the computer monitor, the patient was to name the picture as quickly as possible. If the patient was unable to produce the correct name within 20 seconds, the computer program recorded an incorrect response and moved on to the next probe item.

Phase I of Intention Treatment (10 sessions)

The same set of 50 line drawings is trained each day of the treatment phase.

1. The patient sits at a desk. Body and head face straight forward.
2. The computer monitor is positioned in front of the patient.
3. The clinician activates the program by clicking the mouse.
4. An image of a star appears in the center of computer screen along with a 1000-Hz tone.
5. The patient presses a button inside a box to his or her left to make the star and tone go away.
6. After a 2-second delay, a black and white drawing appears, and the timer begins.
7. Correct naming of the object prompts the clinician to click the mouse, which ends the timer and removes the picture from the screen.

8. Incorrect naming of the object prompts the clinician to name a picture while making a circular gesture with the left hand.
9. The patient repeats this word and imitates the hand gesture.

Phase II of Intention Treatment (10 sessions)

A different set of 50 line drawings is introduced.

1. The patient is seated in the same position as in Phase I.
2. The clinician activates the program by clicking the mouse.
3. A star appears in the center of the screen, without tone.
4. The patient presses a button inside a box to his or her left to make the image go away.
5. After a 2-second delay, the black and white drawing appears, and the timer begins.
6. Incorrect responses are corrected in the same way as Phase I.

Phase III of Intention Treatment (10 sessions)

A different set of 50 line drawings is introduced.

1. The patient is seated in the same position as in Phase I.
2. The clinician activates the program by clicking the mouse.
3. A star appears in the center of the screen, without tone.
4. The patient is to produce a meaningless hand gesture with the left hand 3 times.
5. The clinician clicks the mouse button to begin presentation of line drawings.
6. Incorrect responses are corrected in the same way as in Phases I and II.

Results

The authors of the study employed the single subject A-B design. Two tests were administered: the

Rey-Osterrieth Complex Figure Test (Meyers & Meyers, 1995) and the Block Design Subtest of the Wechsler Adult Intelligence Scale-Revised Edition (WAIS-R; Wechsler, 1981). In one subject, gesturing with the left hand appeared to facilitate word generation, aiding in motor production and reducing the patient's groping for words. There was overall improvement in functional communication, as reported by the patient's caretakers. Additionally, there was carryover of the hand gestures to everyday situations. Because there were only three participants in the study, the authors caution against generalizing the findings to the broader population. Additionally, they noted limitations associated with an A-B design. Although results of this study were promising, further investigation is needed. Finally, if this program is utilized as it is described, then it requires at least 30 therapy sessions, which can be an issue with the fiscal constraints imposed by insurers in today's health care environment.

Normal Sentence Production

Despite years of research efforts focused on producing a complete understanding of normal sentence production, that prize has been elusive. More current approaches to understanding the sentence production of aphasic speakers has led to a reconceptualization of not only that process but even the way that process is studied. For many years, the goal of studying sentence production in aphasia was to correlate the findings with anatomic data, so that speakers could be classified according to type, for example, Broca's, Wernicke's, and so forth. However, since the mid-1980s, researchers focused their energy on determining how normal sentence production was disrupted due to aphasia and left the classification issue behind. Borrowing from cognitive neuropsychology, language researchers found that cognitive analyses gave them a method to *interpret* aphasic language rather than *diagnose* it.

Garrett (1988) developed a model of sentence production out of this context. He proposed three levels of cognitive representation used during sentence production: the Message Level Representation, the Functional Level Representation, and the Positional

Level Representation. The Message Level is the level of meaning and intent. It is pre-linguistic and the highest level of sentence production. It is at this level that the speaker decides to "say something." As a consequence, speakers with difficulty at this level are unable to generate neither intent nor meaning rendering them not functionally communicative. Speakers with difficulty at the Functional Level are able to produce grammatical morphemes, but have an impaired ability to express thematic roles, for example, who is doing what to whom. This level specifies word meanings for the content of the sentence, and multiple words are considered as candidates for selection. It also is argued that this level may be implicated in the noun/verb relationship. Thus, the choices made at this level will place some restrictions on the structure of the sentence, although at this level, the sentence contains no formal structure. Finally, there is the Positional Level. It is at this level that the syntactic phrase constituents impose structure on the forming sentence. Phonologically specified words are chosen, and free and bound morphemes are inserted. Impairment at this level produces a person with agrammatic verbal output.

Based on the above description of sentence production, a clinician would view the sentences produced by the aphasic speaker within that context, and their errors also would be viewed from that perspective. The patient's therapy program would be constructed around and within the level the error patterns were found. For example, a patient whose errors were noted to be at the Functional Level would be given tasks to facilitate thematic role production. The clinician would show the patient a picture of a scene, and ask the patient, "Who is doing what to whom?" A patient with difficulty at the Positional Level would be engaged in tasks that focused on argument structure. The fewer the arguments, the easier it is to generate a sentence.

Oral Reading for Language in Aphasia (ORLA) and ORLA with Virtual Therapist (ORLA-VT)

ORLA was developed to help individuals with alexia improve their reading comprehension skills. Early research indicated that patients not only improved reading comprehension but also other language skills such as oral expression and written expression (Cherney, 2004).

ORLA focuses on connected discourse rather than isolated words to support the natural rhythm and intonation of speech. ORLA requires repetition of stimuli with responses that are not forced or corrected. Incorrect responses are followed by additional stimulation. There are four main principles to this program. They are: (1) active participation by the learner, (2) repetitive practice with overlearning, (3) use of meaningful material with graduated difficulty levels, and (4) successful experiences.

ORLA has four levels of treatment based on reading level and length of utterance, making this a program that can be adapted for individuals with a broad range of aphasia. The treatment levels are based on a reading comprehension ability score obtained from a measure such as the Western Aphasia Battery (WAB) or the oral reading fluency portion of the Gray Oral Reading Test.

- Level 1: Simple 3- to 5-word sentences at a first-grade reading level
- Level 2: 8 to 12 words that may be single sentences or two short sentences, at a third-grade reading level
- Level 3: 15 to 30 words, divided into 2 to 3 sentences at a sixth-grade reading level
- Level 4: 50 to 100 words composing 4 to 6 sentences

The ORLA treatment approach has five basic steps. During treatment, the SLP sits across from the patient, providing an opportunity to view oral-motor movements.

Step 1. SLP reads each word to the patient while pointing to it.

Step 2. SLP reads aloud with the patient, pointing to each word as they read it together. The SLP adjusts his or her speaking rate according to the patient's needs.

Step 3. SLP says a word in each line or sentence, and the patient must identify that word by pointing to it.

Step 4. SLP points to a word in a sentence and asks the patient to read the word aloud.

Step 5. The whole sentence is read aloud again in unison by the SLP and the patient. The steps are repeated to further enhance the patient's reading level.

ORLA is an interactive program that is easy to follow. As patients decode words more quickly, they typically begin to comprehend with greater success. Reading comprehension, oral expression, and written expression all improve to benefit those with either fluent or nonfluent aphasia. Rhythm, pacing, and linguistic templates appear to help patients establish their own rhythm, melody, and rate of speech. The ease and repetitive nature of ORLA seems to help patients work independently, with others, or with a computer (Cherney, 2010a). ORLA-VT is the computer-based version of ORLA. It uses a multimodality stimulation approach that includes listening to a sentence, tapping along with a rhythm, and repeating sentences aloud along with the virtual therapist (VT). As in ORLA, with ORLA-VT, responses are not forced or corrected. Instead, correct responses are modeled. When an error is made, additional stimulation is provided.

There are seven steps to ORLA-VT. They are as follows:

Step 1. A sentence or paragraph is shown on the computer screen. The VT reads the sentence to the patient with each word read as it is highlighted on the computer screen.

Step 2. The VT reads aloud again, and the patient points to each highlighted word as it is read.

Step 3. The VT reads the sentence aloud again, and the patient points to each word and reads it aloud in unison with the VT.

Step 4. The VT reads the same sentence again (as in #3 above), but the VT fades the words at the end of the sentence so the patient can read aloud independently.

Step 5. The VT says a word in each sentence that the patient must identify.

Step 6. For each sentence, the VT highlights a word for the patient to read aloud.

Step 7. The patient reads the whole sentence aloud in unison with the VT.

Research has shown that there was no significant difference in outcomes between computer-based ORLA and the traditional SLP-delivered version (Cherney, 2010b). However, one difference was that in using the ORLA-VT program, the patient had to be able to operate a computer, understand directions, and attend to the VT.

Promoting Aphasics' Communicative Effectiveness (PACE)

Background

PACE therapy (Davis, 2007; Wilcox & Davis, 1977) attempts to mimic the natural exchange of conversation between two people. As noted by Wertz (1984), PACE focuses on the *context* of language rather than *content*. In the program, both the clinician and patient assume equal responsibility in communication, much like conversational partners do every day during conversation. Both communicators take turns sending and receiving messages. PACE does not require a specific modality of communication. Instead, the patient is free to communicate through whatever modality he or she chooses. As noted by Peach (2008), PACE falls within the category of Functional Communication Treatment (FCT) and has been used with globally aphasic patients. In this model, improving the patient's ability to communicate individual and daily needs is the central theme.

Methodology

PACE follows a hierarchy, or *phases,* whereby complexity of communication and abstraction of the message increases as therapy continues. Picture cards are used as message-generating stimuli, and the clinician is free to choose the images within a specific phase. The phases are:

1. Phase I uses everyday object picture cards.
2. Phase II uses verb picture cards.
3. Phase III uses story-sequence picture cards.

PACE is composed of the following principles of conversation.

1. New information is exchanged between clinician and patient.
   A stack of picture cards is placed face down between the patient and the clinician. One takes a turn describing the picture and the other deciphering the message. The positive part of both partners assuming equal roles in communication is that the clinician can model appropriate responses for the patient to imitate when it is their turn. Second, the clinician can model communication modalities that the patient may not be using, but is capable of using. Picture cards should follow the aforementioned hierarchy, beginning with everyday object picture cards, moving to verb picture cards, and finally, using story-sequence picture cards. An alternative method is to use a barrier screen between the clinician and patient (Muma, 1978). Through dialogue, each person should end up with identical boards. For example, if the clinician and patient each have a piece of paper with identical objects, both people will communicate the appropriate information in order to end up with identical images or configurations. For more information on this method, refer to Newhoff and Apel (1990).
2. Equal participation of patient and clinician.
   Both people take turns sending and receiving messages. In this way, therapy resembles a natural conversation.
3. The communication mode is chosen by the patient.
   Instead of the clinician training a specific communication modality, the patient chooses their response mode. Drawings, speaking, writing, pantomiming, gesturing, and pointing at objects are all accepted modalities. Leaving options open permits greater chances of patient success.

4. Functional feedback is provided.

The clinician responds to the patient in the same way that a conversational partner would in a typical conversational paradigm. If the clinician successfully understood the patient's message, he or she will respond appropriately. This gets the clinician away from the traditional role of rating a patient's response as either correct or incorrect. If the patient has accurately conveyed the information, the clinician will understand it and give reinforcement in the form of a response.

Response Elaboration Training (RET)

Background

Response Elaboration Training (RET) is a method that attempts to mimic natural communication and promote generalization of responses (Kearns, 1985,1990). RET is different from traditional production methods in that no predetermined set of responses are trained. Instead, the clinician uses patient-initiated responses as the main substance of therapy. These responses are shaped and expanded by the clinician to increase the length and richness of patient utterances. The end goal is to increase a patient's ability to self-initiate responses and become an independent communicator. RET is based on a "loose training" method developed by Stokes and Baer (1977). Loose training procedures create a treatment environment that provides stimuli that are found in the natural environment, allows for response variations that occur in that environment, thus promoting generalization outside the therapy room (Marshall, 2008). The literature does show evidence of generalization with this treatment methodology (Kearns, 1985; Kearns & Potechin, 1988).

Methodology

Action picture cards are the stimuli used in RET, typically consisting of transitive and intransitive verbs.

(The clinician may choose his or her own imagery under these guidelines.) Instead of providing a simple description of the action picture, patients should be encouraged to draw on their world knowledge and personal experience in formulating a response. The clinician follows the steps below for elaborating a patient's self-initiated utterances, as outlined by Kearns (1990):

1. An initial response is elicited to a picture stimulus.
2. This response is modeled and reinforced by the clinician.
3. "Wh" cues are provided to prompt clients to elaborate on their initial responses.
4. The subsequent client-attempted response is reinforced, and then sentences that combine initial and subsequent responses to a given stimulus picture are modeled.
5. A second model of sentences that combine previous responses are modeled, and then the client is instructed to repeat the sentence.
6. Repetitions of combined sentences are reinforced, and a final sentence model is provided.

Table D–1 provides an example of the clinician's and patient's role in RET. The picture stimuli provided to the patient in this example shows a man sweeping the floor.

Schuell's Stimulation Approach

Background

After two decades of working with people with aphasia, Hildred Schuell developed the Stimulation Facilitation Approach, also known as Schuell's Stimulation Approach. She believed that language was neither lost nor destroyed in the patient with aphasia. Rather, she believed that language was no longer easily retrieved due to a damaged, less efficient system. Therefore, her therapy approach does not "reteach" language. Instead, the speech-language pathologist is to "stimulate adequate functioning of disrupted processes" (Schuell, Carroll, & Street, 1955).

Table D–1. RET Steps and Responses

Ret Steps	Clinician's Stimulus	Patient's Response	Clinician's Feedback
1. Elicit initial verbal response to picture.	Line drawing of simple event (man with a broom). "Tell me what's happening in this picture."	"Man . . . sweeping."	
2. Reinforce, model, and shape initial response.			"Great. The man is sweeping."
3. "Wh"-cue to elicit elaboration of initial response	"Why is he sweeping?"	"Wife . . . mad."	
4. Reinforce, model, and shape the two patient responses combined.			"Way to go! The man is sweeping the floor because his wife is mad."
5. Second model and request repetition.	"Try and say the whole thing after me. Say, 'The man is sweeping the floor because his wife is mad.'"	"Man . . . sweeping . . . wife . . . mad."	"Good job."
6. After reinforcement, elicit a delayed imitation of the combined response.	"Now, try to say it one more time."	"The man . . . sweeping because his wife . . . mad."	

Sources: Kearns & Potechin, 1988; Kearns & Yedor, 1991.

Coelho, Sinotte, and Duffy (2008) state that Schuell's approach to aphasia is one "that places its primary emphasis on the stimulation presented to the patient" (p. 403). The goal is to help maximize the patient's reorganization of language. It is generally understood that a majority of patients with aphasia demonstrate weaknesses in the auditory modality (Duffy & Ulrich; 1976; Schuell, Jenkins, & Jiménez-Pabón, 1964; Smith, 1971). Schuell's stimulation approach encourages speech-language pathologists to strengthen language input and output. The intensive stimulation involved in this approach is thought to strengthen the disrupted neural pathways important to language processing.

Schuell did not classify aphasic patients into the orderly and traditional paradigms, such as expressive aphasia, receptive aphasia, and so forth. Instead, the aphasias were classified according to three other criteria: the severity of the language impairment, the presence of sensory or motor deficits, and the patient's prognosis (Duffy & Coelho, 2001).

System of Classification

Schuell's system of categorizing aphasia included the following (Jenkins, Jiménez-Pabón, Shaw, & Sefer, 1975):

- Simple aphasia
- Aphasia with visual involvement
- Aphasia with persisting dysfluency
- Aphasia with scattered findings
- Aphasia with sensorimotor involvement
- Aphasia with intermittent auditory imperception
- Irreversible aphasia syndrome

The stimulation approach to aphasia has general principles that will facilitate success with the patient (Brookshire, 1992; Schuell, 1974; Schuell et al., 1964). They are:

1. Use intensive auditory stimulation.
2. Pair visual and auditory modalities together.
3. Stimulation should be sufficient enough to reach the brain.
4. Sensory stimulation should be repetitive.
5. Stimuli provided to the patient should evoke a response.
6. Try for a maximum number of responses from the patient.
7. Provide feedback to the patient about his or her progress.
8. Treatment should be systematic and often.
9. Each session should follow a hierarchy from easy to more difficult tasks.
10. The clinician should have a variety of materials on hand to help ward off boredom if using drill-style formats.

Where to Begin Therapy (Brookshire, 1992)

1. The clinician should begin at a level where the patient is demonstrating only minor deficiencies.
2. Begin with tasks in which the patient's responses are correct about 60% to 80% of the time.
3. Increase the level of difficulty when performance reaches 90%.

The use of standardized assessments can measure baseline performance and pinpoint an appropriate starting point. For instance, if a patient is incorrect 50% of the time during a two-step direction task on a standardized test, use that as the therapeutic starting point.

Tasks

Tasks Highlighting the Patient's Auditory Capabilities

1. Point-to tasks
2. Following directions of varied length and complexity

3. Answering yes-or-no questions and verify sentences
4. Response switching (rapidly changing directions to follow, questions to answer)

Tasks Highlighting the Patient's Verbal and Auditory Capabilities

1. Repetition tasks
2. Sentence or phrase completion
3. Verbal association
4. Answering "wh"-questions
5. Connected utterances in response to single words (define words and complete phrases)
6. Retelling paragraphs and stories
7. "Self-initiated" or conversational verbal tasks (name pictures, describe function of objects, describe activities, etc.).

Tasks Targeting the Patient's Reading and Writing Abilities

1. Reading (match written words and sentences to pictures, identify letters named, read in unison, fill in missing words in sentences, read aloud and retell, etc.).
2. Writing (copy forms, letters, words, write letters to dictation, write known information, fill in missing words in sentences, write down essential information told, etc.).

Semantic Feature Analysis (SFA)

The underlying premise of Semantic Feature Analysis (SFA; Boyle & Coelho, 1995) is that by accessing the semantic network of a target word, the patient will be more likely to retrieve it because all like concepts are linked. The closer the concepts are, the stronger the link. Therefore, patients are encouraged to produce words that are semantically related to the target word. Strongly associated words activate phonological information, and the likelihood of target word production increases. One of the techniques used in the approach is the semantic feature diagram (Figure D–2). Another important aspect of

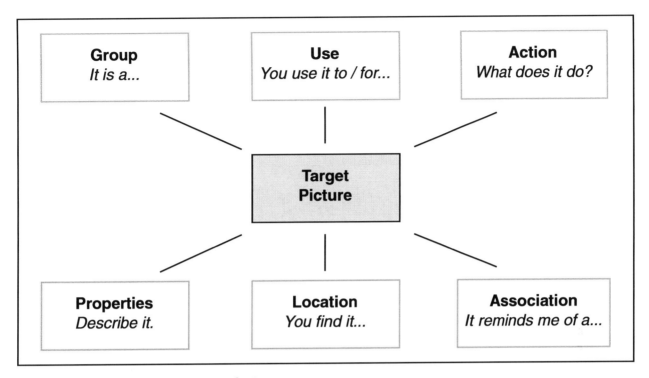

Figure D–2. Semantic Feature Analysis.

this approach is that the patient must produce all of the semantic features of the target work, even if it is named successfully. The intent is to strengthen the semantic network associated with that word.

Sentence Production Program for Aphasia (SPPA)

Background

According to Helm-Estabrooks and Nicholas (2000), sentence-level deficits are a diagnostic indicator for nonfluent aphasia. In a previous study, Gleason, Goodglass, Green, Ackerman, and Hyde (1975), using story-completion tasks with patients who displayed Broca's Aphasia and agrammatism, concluded that the patients were not lacking in *knowledge* of syntax, but *access* to that knowledge (Davis, 2000). This study was the inspiration behind training a hierarchy of syntactic structures in Sentence Production Program for Aphasia (SPPA), beginning with easy-to-produce structures and ending with

more complex ones. Results of the study indicated that patients had the ability to produce a wide variety of syntactically correct utterances (Helm-Estabrooks & Albert, 2004).

The overarching goal of SPPA is to improve functional communication skills in the patient's daily interactions, such as making requests, conversing socially with others, and asking questions. Potential candidates for SPPA include patients who are nonfluent with agrammatic speech patterns and who have relatively spared auditory comprehension. SPPA seeks to reduce the impact of agrammatism on spoken communication by improving the patient's ability to speak in increasingly longer and more complex sentences.

Program Overview

SPPA contains 8 sentence types that are presented in a hierarchy of increasing difficulty, with 15 target sentences each and two separate levels of difficulty (Helm-Estabrooks & Nicholas, 2000). A spiral-bound booklet contains all materials needed for the SPPA program. This includes stories, pictures, and target stimuli. In addition to the published version (Helm-Estabrooks & Nicholas, 2000), clinicians may use their own target stimuli, pictures, and stories, as long as they follow the sentence-type hierarchy. The 8 sentence types are:

1. Imperative intransitive   "Wake up."
2. Imperative transitive   "Drink your milk."
3. Wh-interrogative (what and who)   "What are you watching?"; "Who is coming?"
4. Wh-interrogative (where and when)   "Where is the hospital?"; "When are we landing?"
5. Declarative transitive   "I teach school."
6. Declarative intransitive   "He swims."
7. Comparative   "She's taller."
8. Yes/No questions   "Is it sad?"

Picture Stimuli

Pictorial representations include three different families of various ethnic backgrounds engaged in verbal interactions during everyday situations. For example, to functionally demonstrate what to do in an emergency, an illustration of a family is shown responding to an accident, reaching for the phone. The target phrase is, "Call 911."

Difficulty Levels. There are two difficulty levels for each picture. One provides a clinician model, and the other one does not provide a model.

Level A: Clinician model provided Patient repeats a modeled sentence in response to a question.

Level B: No clinician model provided Patient completes the story with the target sentence, without requiring the use of a clinician model.

Example of Level A and Level B Sentence Type 1: Imperative Intransitive Sample Target:

Phrase: "Wake up."

Level A: Nick's school bus arrives in 15 minutes, and Nick is still asleep. So his mother tells him, "Wake up!" What does his mother say?

Level B: Nick's school bus arrives in 15 minutes, and he is still asleep. So what does his mother tell him to do?

Presentation Suggestions

1. Speak in a natural voice.
2. Use a slow, natural rhythm with appropriate pauses and intonation.
3. Level A probe: Pause right before saying the target stimuli, so the patient is attuned to it, therefore enhancing his or her ability to repeat it.
4. Level B probe: Use rising intonation at the end of reading, so the patient is clued in to when it's time to complete the story.
5. If the patient fails to respond, one repetition only is granted at each level.
6. Upon successful response to Level A, immediately administer Level B to the patient.
7. Once an 85% accuracy level is achieved with Level B, present the 15 items for each sentence type using only Level B.
8. Progress to next sentence type in hierarchy.

Scoring

Patients may receive a score of 0, .5, or 1. The manual includes specific instructions, as well as scoring sheets that may be reproduced. For more information, refer to Helm-Estabrooks and Albert (2004).

Measuring Progress

The functional goal of SPPA is to reduce the patient's agrammatism and to improve the ability to communicate using more syntactically complex sentences. To assess progress, formal measures such as the Communicative Effectiveness Profile (CEP) (Menn, Ramsberger, & Helm-Estabrooks, 1994) may be used. It also is important to obtain feedback from caregivers who interact with the patient in everyday situations. To assess carryover, ask the caregiver to keep a journal of the patient's functional use of conversations in activities of daily living for your review.

SentenceShaper

SentenceShaper is a software program that helps individuals with aphasia communicate systematically by creating sentences and narratives from words. The program has more than 800 different therapeutic exercises organized in workbooks to elicit different grammatical structures. It is based on the premise that people with aphasia have delays in processing, experience word-finding problems, and have difficulty formulating sentences (Linebarger, Romania, Fink, Bartlett, & Schwartz, 2008). Accordingly, these authors stated that the program "is based on evidence that words are retrieved more slowly and may decay more quickly in persons with aphasia, causing them to have difficulty assembling all the elements of a sentence in memory simultaneously" (Linebarger et al., 2008, p. 1403). As a result, SentenceShaper makes it possible for patients to record words and phrases, and build them into sentences. Once they build the sentence, they can hear it by clicking on a series of icons that are replayed on the computer. The steps in SentenceShaper are:

1. Record speech by touching the microphone button. Once recorded, an icon will appear. Clicking on it will allow the patient to hear the recording or snippet just said.
2. Drag the recording or snippet up to the sentence row and place it in the first of two designated spots.
3. Press the play button above the snippets to play them in the order they were created.
4. Continue building the sentence by recording another word or phrase and adding it to the sequence.
5. Play the entire sequence forming the sentence.
6. Click the button on the upper right of the sentence and words or phrases will be added to a story row where it will be represented by a single icon such as a purple oval.
7. Hear the sentence by clicking the purple oval. By dragging the oval back to the sentence row, it will once again separate the snippets.
8. By recording a snippet, arranging it in the sentence row, and then adding it to the story row, one can continue to build and separate sentences and stories.

Treatment with SentenceShaper has assisted with carryover of sentences into spontaneous speech and stories (narratives). Studies have shown that continual use of SentenceShaper may lead to improved generalization and spontaneous speech. This program has been found helpful for individuals with agrammatic aphasia. The program has been found to be most appropriate for individuals with aphasia who have the ability to produce some speech and who also have sufficient working memory to manipulate the program (Linebarger, Schwartz, & Kohn, 2001; McCall, Virata, Linebarger, & Berndt, 2009). According to Fink, Bartlett, Lowery, Linebarger and Schwartz (2008), narratives produced with SentenceShaper contained a higher percentage of information (more than 90% correct informational units) than those not using the program. Results also found that patients had greater ability to generate sentences that carried over to unaided speech (Linebarger, McCall, Virata, & Berndt, 2007).

Speech Entrainment

People with Broca's aphasia tend to speak telegraphically, that is, in two- to three-word phrases, and occasionally, one to two words depending on the level of severity of the disorder. However, some patients can mimic the audiovisual stimuli of a fluent, nonaphasic speaker, enabling them to produce fluent speech. This effect is referred to as "speech entrainment" (Fridriksson et al., 2012). Fridriksson et al. (2012) conducted three experiments to examine the possible neural mechanism for the effect as well as its possible therapeutic value.

The results of the first experiment involving 13 patients with Broca's aphasia revealed that they produced a greater variety of words using an audiovisual feedback model (modeling speech while listening and watching another speak) versus audio-only feedback (modeling speech while listening to another speak), and spontaneous speech (speaking without listening or hearing another speak). Experiment 2 used 12 of the 13 aphasic patients and 20 normal controls, and asked questions regarding underlying neural mechanisms for the speech entrainment effect. Those results showed that during entrainment, there was bilateral cortical activation at the juncture of the anterior insula and Brodmann areas 47, 37, and in the left middle temporal gyrus unilaterally.

Experiment 3 was a treatment program in which all of the patients from Experiment 1 participated in 6 weeks of speech entrainment therapy. At the end of the treatment phase and for 1 to 6 weeks afterward, the aphasic patients were able to increase their speech output by a factor of >2, producing a greater variety of words with and without entrainment. The authors felt that these preliminary results suggest that using speech entrainment therapeutically can improve speech production in people with a nonfluent, Broca's type aphasia. The authors believe that speech entrainment is effective because it provides an external mechanism via the visual modality, that is, watching the other speaker model the word, and that compensates for the damage to Broca's area. They do caution, however, that speech entrainment was not effective in all cases, which implied that motor programming still needs to be partially preserved for it to have an effect because they feel that Broca's area is responsible for "uniting language and articulatory processing for speech production" (p. 3827).

This study lends support to the use of articulatory cueing in people with aphasia and helps explain why it can be so effective with certain patients. However, adding the audio (speaking the word aloud) to the visual (just the articulatory cue) improved speech fluency and variety. As noted above, this suggests that the motor plans remain intact in these patients; another helpful insight for planning treatment.

Treatment of Underlying Forms (TUF)

This therapeutic approach was developed to treat people with poor sentence comprehension and production, that is, agrammatism commonly associated with the nonfluent, Broca's type aphasia. Individuals with agrammatism have a degraded grammatical structure, based on the type of sentences that they produce. They produce short Subject-Verb-Object (SVO) sentences with misordered or absent verb forms. They also have difficulty comprehending and producing non-canonical sentences, that is, sentences in which the Noun Phrases (NP) have been moved out of their canonical order, as they are in passives. Treatment of Underlying Forms (TUF) (Thompson, 2001) is a linguistic approach that focuses on training complex, noncanonical sentences. The training hierarchy proceeds from complex to simpler sentence structures. The example below illustrates how the clinician facilitates simpler sentence construction from a more complex form. The stimulus is the sentence, "It was the artist who the thief chased."

1. Present cards (read aloud and repeat): [the thief] [chased] [the artist] [it was] [who]
2. Point to the verb, "This is *chase,* it is the action." Point to the theme, "This is the *thief,* the person doing the chasing." "This is the *artist,* the artist is the person who is chased."
3. The <u>who</u> card is placed next to the theme card (the artist). Say, "To make a sentence, *who* is added next to the artist because the artist is the person who was chased." [the thief] [chased] [the artist] [who]
4. The theme (<u>the artist</u>) and the <u>who</u> cards are moved to the sentence initial position. "To make the correct sentence, these words are moved to the beginning of the sentence." [the artist] [who] [the thief] [chased]
5. The *it was* card is added to the beginning of the sentence. The examiner states: "*It was* is added to the sentence because it was the artist who the thief chased." The client reads and repeats: [it was] [the artist] [who] [the thief] [chased]
6. Sentence parts are rearranged in active sentence form together with the *it was* and *who* cards, and the steps are repeated with the cards moving to form the target sentence.

Visual Action Therapy (VAT)

Background

Visual Action Therapy (VAT) is a nonverbal therapeutic approach to aphasia, which is appropriate for patients with severe impairment (i.e., global aphasia). Patients are trained to generate and produce hand/arm gestures that represent objects. The intent is to ultimately improve the patient's functional communication. (Helm-Estabrooks & Albert, 2004). For example, if a patient is thirsty, he or she will produce a gesture that represents drinking from a cup. VAT takes advantage of preserved skills, such as nonlinguistic, visuospatial, and memory skills, and the ability to spontaneously use overlearned gestures. The patient's motivation and ability to attend to tasks will assist in a successful response to intervention.

This particular treatment program utilizes "alternate symbol systems" (Helm-Estabrooks & Albert, 2004). Researchers discovered that patients with global aphasia still had intact abilities to conceptualize (Gardner, Zurif, Berry, & Baker, 1976). For some of these patients, they had the cognitive abilities needed to produce language that led Helm and Benson (1978) to create the initial VAT program. Helm-Estabrooks, Ramsberger, Brownell, and Albert (1989) found that it was easier for patients to produce proximal gestures (hand and arm movements) prior to distal gestures (hand-finger movements). The initial program was thereby revised to include a new hierarchy of phases, which are discussed in the following.

Treatment Phases

There are three phases to the VAT treatment program: proximal limb VAT (hand-arm movements, such as motor activity of sawing), distal limb VAT (hand-finger movements, such as turning a screwdriver), and oral VAT such as blowing. The stimuli used for all three phases include real objects, line drawings, and action pictures of a figure using the object. The patient moves sequentially through a hierarchy of nine steps that progress from simple (matching objects to pictures) to complex (using gestures to represent hidden objects). The clinician tracks ongoing progress to determine if the patient is ready to progress to the next level or phase (Helm-Estabrooks & Albert, 2004). The 9 steps are as follows and proceed in a hierarchical progression from 1 to 9: (1) matching pictures and objects; (2) object use

training; (3) action picture demonstration; (4) following action picture commands; (5) pantomimed gesture demonstration; (6) pantomimed gesture recognition; (7) pantomimed gesture production; (8) representation of hidden objects demonstration; and (9) production of gestures for hidden objects.

Preparation for Training

Clinicians will need:

1. 15 real objects (toys do not count)
2. Shaded line drawings of those objects
3. Action pictures of a simple figure using those objects

Suggestions for proximal limb gestures may include motions used to represent paint stick, gavel, saw, and iron. Distal limb gestures may include motions using a screwdriver, teaspoon, telephone, artist's fine paintbrush, and tea bag, and so forth. For oral gestures, motions may involve postures to indicate a whistle, flower, lollipop, and straw, plus others. For a complete overview of the 9 steps of VAT, see Helm-Estabrooks and Albert (2004).

Measuring Outcomes

Pre and post-VAT measurements are suggested. The Boston Assessment of Severe Aphasia (Helm-Estabrooks, Ramsberger, Nicholas, & Morgan, 1989); and the Nonvocal Communication Scale (NCS) (Borod, Fitzpatrick, Helm-Estabrooks, & Goodglass, 1989) have been used pre- and post-VAT. The clinician can also use the Communication Questionnaire, which has two components, Expressing Self and Understanding Information (Helm-Estabrooks, 1996).

VAT Follow-Up Treatment

Helm-Estabrooks and Albert (2004) suggest several steps following successful outcome of VAT:

1. The Amer-Ind Code program, which has been modified by Skelly (1979) for patients with aphasia is based on Native American hand signals. Thirty additional gestures are taught. Such gestures may be used to communicate functional

needs, such as "bathroom" and "sleep." Refer to Rao (1994) for a recent review of this method.

2. PACE (Davis & Wilcox, 1981; Helm-Estabrooks & Albert, 2004) suggest using the PACE photo cards to teach two-gesture combinations, such as "man drinking."

3. To ease some of the patient's burden of communication, a family member or other communication partner may be brought into the therapy sessions. The patient is first shown an illustration of an object or concept that is new. They are then asked to use a gesture to communicate the illustration that the family member must identify. The clinician's job is to monitor and review progress, so the patient and their communication partner are able to identify areas of weakness that still need improvement. This can be accomplished by carefully charting data or videotaping sessions and reviewing them with both communication partners.

References

Basso, A. (2003). *Aphasia and its therapy*. New York, NY: Oxford University Press.

Beeson, P. M. (1999). Treating acquired writing impairment: Strengthening grapheme representations. *Aphasiologoy, 13*, 767–785.

Beeson, P. M., Hirsch, F. M., & Rewega, M. A. (2002). Successful single-word writing treatment: Experimental analyses of fours cases. *Aphasiology, 16*, 473–491.

Beeson, P. M., Rising, K., Kim, E. S., & Rapcsak, S. Z. (2010). A treatment sequence for phonological alexia/agraphia. *Journal of Speech, Language, and Hearing Research, 53*, 450–468.

Beeson, P. M., Rising, K., & Volk, J. (2003). Writing treatment for severe aphasia: Who benefits. *Journal of Speech, Language and Hearing Research, 46*, 1038–1060.

Benson, D. F., & Ardilia, A. (1996). *Aphasia: A clinical perspective*. New York, NY: Oxford University Press.

Boles, L. (1998). Conducting conversation: A case study using the spouse in aphasia treatment. *ASHA SID 2 Newsletter. Neurophysiology and Neurogenic Speech and Language Disorders*, 24–31.

Borod, J., Fitzpatrick, R., Helm-Estabrooks, N., & Goodglass, H. (1989). The relationship between limb apraxia and the spontaneous use of communicative gesture in aphasia. *Brain and Cognition, 10*, 121–131.

Boyle, M., & Coelho, C. A. (1995). Application of semantic feature analysis as a treatment for aphasic dysnomia. *American Journal of Speech-Language Pathology, 4*, 94–98.

Brookshire, R. H. (1992). *An introduction to neurogenic communication disorders* (4th ed.). St. Louis, MO: Mosby Year Book.

Chapey, R. (1994). *Language intervention strategies in adult aphasia* (3rd ed.). Baltimore, MD: Lippincott Williams & Wilkins.

Chapey, R. (2001). *Language intervention strategies in aphasia and related neurogenic communication disorders* (4th ed.). Philadelphia, PA: Lippincott Williams & Wilkins.

Chapey, R., Duchan, J. F., Elman, R. J., Garcia, L. J., Kagan, A., Lyon, J. G., & Simmons-Mackie, N. (2008). Life-participation approach to aphasia: A statement of values for the future. In R. Chapey (Ed.), *Language intervention strategies in aphasia and related neurogenic communication disorders* (5th ed.). Philadelphia, PA: Lippincott Williams & Wilkins.

Chapey, R., Rigrodsky, S., & Morrison, E. B. (1997). Aphasia: A divergent semantic interpretation. *Journal of Speech and Hearing Disorders, 42*, 287–295.

Cherney, L. R. (2004). Aphasia, alexia, and oral reading. *Topics in Stroke Rehabilitation, 11*(1), 22–36.

Cherney, L. R. (2010a). Oral reading for language in aphasia: Impact of aphasia severity on cross-modal outcomes in chronic nonfluent aphasia. *Seminars in Speech and Language, 31*, 42–51.

Cherney, L. R. (2010b). Oral reading for language in aphasia: Evaluating the efficacy of computer-delivered therapy in chronic nonfluent aphasia. *Topics in Stroke Rehabilitation, 17*, 423–431.

Cherney, L. R., Patterson, J. P., Raymer, A., Frymark, T., & Schooling, T. (2008). Evidence-based systematic review: Effects of intensity of treatment and constraint-induced language therapy for individuals with stroke-induce aphasia. *Journal of Speech, Language, and Hearing Research, 51*, 2282–2299.

Coelho, C. A., Sinotte, M. P., & Duffy, J. R. (2008). Schuell's stimulation approach to rehabilitation. In R. Chapey (Ed.), *Language intervention strategies in aphasia and related neurogenic communication disorders* (5th ed.). Philadelphia, PA: Lippincott Williams & Wilkins.

Davis, G. A. (2000). *Aphasiology: Disorders and clinical practice*. Needham Heights, MA: Allyn & Bacon.

Davis, G. A. (2007). *Aphasiology: Disorders and clinical practice* (2nd ed.). Boston, MA: Allyn & Bacon.

Davis, G. A., & Wilcox, M. J. (1981). Incorporating parameters of natural conversation in aphasia treatment. In R. Chapey (Ed.), *Language intervention strategies in adult aphasia*. Baltimore, MD: Lippincott Williams & Wilkins.

Duffy, J. R., & Coelho, C. A. (2001). Schuell's stimulation approach to rehabilitation. In R. Chapey (Ed.), *Language intervention strategies in aphasia and related neurogenic communication disorders* (4th ed.). Philadelphia, PA: Lippincott Williams & Wilkins.

Duffy, R. J., & Ulrich, S. R. (1976). A comparison of impairments in verbal comprehension, speech, reading, and writing in adult aphasics. *Journal of Speech and Hearing Disorders, 41*, 110–119.

Elman, R. J. (2000, November). *Language disorders in adults grand rounds: Life participation approaches to aphasia*. Presented to the American Speech-Language-Hearing Association Convention.

Fink, R. B. , Bartlett, M. R., Lowery, J. S., Linebarger, M. C., Schwartz, M. F. (2008). Aphasic speech with and without SentenceShaper: Two methods for assessing informativeness. *Aphasiology, 22*(7–8), 679–690.

Fink, R. B., Brecher, A., Sobel, P., & Schwartz, M. F. (2005). Computer-assisted treatment of word retrieval deficits in aphasia. *Aphasiology, 19*, 943–954.

Fridriksson, J., Hubbard, H., Hudspeth, I., Grace, S., Holland, A. L., Bonhila, L., . . . Rorden, C. (2012). Speech entrainment enables patients with Broca's aphasia to produce fluent speech. *Brain, 135*, 3815–3829.

Gardner, H., Zurif, E. B., Berry, T., & Baker, E. H. (1976).Visual communication in aphasia. *Neuropsychologia, 14*, 275–292.

Garrett, M. F. (1988). Processes in language production. In F. J. Newmeyer (Ed.), *Lingusitics: The Cambridge Survey: 111. Language: Psychological and biological aspects*. Cambridge, UK: Cambridge University Press.

Gleason, J. B., Goodglass, H., Green, E., Ackerman, N., & Hyde, M. R. (1975). The retrieval of syntax in Broca's aphasia. *Brain and Language, 2*, 451–471.

Goldstein, K. (1942). *After effects of brain-injuries in war: Their evaluation and treatment*. New York, NY: Grune & Stratton.

Goodglass, H., & Kaplan, E. (1983). *Boston Diagnostic Aphasia Examination*. Hagerstown, MD: Lippincott Williams & Wilkins.

Grossman, M. (1981). A bird is a bird is a bird: Making reference within and without superordinate categories. *Brain and Language, 12*, 313–331.

Guilford, J. P. (1967). *The nature of human intelligence*. New York, NY: McGraw-Hill.

Helm, N. A., & Benson, D. F. (1978). *Visual Action Therapy for global aphasia*. Paper presented at the annual meeting of the Academy of Aphasia, Chicago, IL.

Helm-Estabrooks, N.(1996). Communication Questionnaire. In N. Helm-Estabrooks and M. Albert, *Manual of aphasia and aphasia therapy* (pp.188–189). Austin, TX: Pro-Ed.

Helm-Estabrooks, N. (2001). *Cognitive Linguistic Quick Test*. San Antonio, TX: Psychological Corp.

Helm-Estabrooks, N., & Albert, M. (2004). *Manual of aphasia and aphasia therapy* (2nd ed.). Austin, TX: Pro-Ed.

Helm-Estabrooks, N., & Nicholas, M. (2000). *Sentence production program for aphasia*. Austin, TX: Pro-Ed.

Helm-Estabrooks, N., & Nicholas, M. (2002). *Narrative story cards*. Austin, TX: Pro-Ed.

Helm-Estabrooks, N., Ramsberger, G., Brownell, H., & Albert, M. (1989). Distal versus proximal movement in limb apraxia [Abstract]. *Journal of Clinical and Experimental Neuropsychology, 7*, 608.

Helm-Estabrooks, N., Ramsberger, G., Nicholas, M., & Morgan, A. (1989). *Boston Assessment of Severe Aphasia*. Austin, TX: Pro-Ed.

Holland, A. (1999). *Counseling adults with neurogenic communication disorders* [Videotape]. Rockville, MD: American Speech-Language-Hearing Association.

Hoodin, R. B., & Thompson, C. K. (1983). Facilitation of verbal labeling in adult aphasia by gestural, verbal, or verbal plus gestural training. *Clinical Aphasiology, 13*, 62–64.

Ireland, C., & Wootten, G. (1996). Time to talk: Counseling for people with dysphasia. *Disability and Rehabilitation, 18*(11), 585–591.

Jenkins, J., Jimnez-Pabn, E., Shaw, R., & Sefer, J. (1975). *Schuell's aphasia in adults* (2nd ed.). New York, NY: Harper & Row.

Kagan, A., & Gailey, G. (1993). Functional is not enough: Training conversation partners in aphasia. In A. Holland & M. Forbes (Eds.), *Aphasia treatment: World perspectives* (pp. 199–226). San Diego, CA: Singular.

Kaplan, E., Goodglass, H., & Weintraub, S. (2000). *Boston Naming Test*. Philadelphia, PA: Lea & Febiger.

Kearns, K. P. (1985). Response elaboration training for patient initiated utterances. In R. H. Brookshire (Ed.), *Clinical aphasiology conference proceedings* (pp. 196–204). Minneapolis, MN: BRK.

Kearns, K. P. (1990). Broca's aphasia. In L. L. LaPointe (Ed.), *Aphasia and related neurogenic language disorders*. New York, NY: Thieme Medical.

Kearns, K. P., & Potechin, G. (1988). The generalization of response elaboration training effects. In T.

Prescott (Ed.), *Clinical aphasiology* (pp. 223–246). Boston, MA: College-Hill Press.

Kearns, K. P., Simmon, N. N., & Sisterhen, C. (1982). Gestural sign (Amer-Ind) as a facilitator of verbalization in patients with aphasia. *Clinical Aphasiology, 12*, 183–191.

Kearns, K. P., & Yedor, K. (1991). An alternating treatments comparison of loose training and a convergent treatment strategy. In T. E. Prescott (Ed.), *Clinical aphasiology* (Vol. 20, pp. 223–238). Austin, TX: Pro-Ed.

Kirmess, M., & Lind, M. (2011). Spoken language production as outcome measurement following constraint induced language therapy. *Aphasiology, 25*, 1207–1238.

Kirmess, M., & Maher, L. M. (2010). Constraint induced language therapy in early aphasia rehabilitation. *Aphasiology, 24*, 725–736.

Lesser, R., & Algar, L. (1995). Towards combing the cognitive neuropsychological and the pragmatic in aphasia therapy. *Neuropsychological Rehabilitation, 5*, 67–92.

Lindfors, J. W. (1987 [1980]). *Children's language and learning*. Englewood Cliffs, NJ: Prentice-Hall.

Linebarger, M. C., McCall, D., Virata, T., & Berndt, R. S. (2007). Widening the temporal window: Processing support in the treatment of aphasic language production. *Brain and Language, 100*, 53–68.

Linebarger, M. C., Romania, J. R., Fink, R. B., Bartlett, M. R., & Schwartz, M. F. (2008). Building on residual speech: A portable processing prosthesis for aphasia. *Journal of Rehabilitation Research and Development, 45*, 1401–1414.

Linebarger, M. C., Schwartz, M. F., & Kohn, S. E. (2001). Computer-based training of language production: An exploratory study. *Neuropsychological Rehabilitation, 11*, 57–96.

Linebaugh, C., & Lehner, L. (1977). Cuing hierarchies and word retrieval: A treatment program. In R. H. Brookshire (Ed.), *Clinical aphasiology: Conferences proceedings*. Minneapolis, MN: BRK.

Linebaugh, C. W., Pryor, A. P., & Margulies, C. P. (1983). A comparison of picture descriptions by family members of aphasic patients to aphasic and non-aphasic listeners. In R. H. Brookshire (Ed.), *Clinical aphasiology conference proceedings*. Minneapolis, MN: BRK.

Lyon, J. G., Cariski, D., Keisler, L., Rosenbek, J., Levine, R., Kumpula, J., Ryff, C., Coyne, S., & Blanc, M. (1997) Communication partners: Enhancing participation in life and communication for adults with aphasia in natural settings. *Aphasiology, 11*(7), 693–708.

Marshall, R. C. (2008). Early management of Wernicke's aphasia: A context-based approach. In R. Chapey (Ed.), *Language intervention strategies in aphasia and related neurogenic communication disorders* (5th ed.). Philadelphia, PA: Lippincott Williams & Wilkins.

McCall, D., Virata, T., Linebarger, M. D., & Berndt, R. S. (2009). Integrating technology and targeted treatment to improve narrative production in aphasia: A case study. *Aphasiology, 23*, 438–461.

Meinzer, M., Djundja, D., Barthel, G., Elbert, T., & Rockstroh, B. (2005). Long-term stability of improved language functions in chronic aphasia after constraint-induced aphasia therapy. *Stroke: Journal of American Heart Association, 36*, 1462–1466.

Menn, L., Ramsberger, G., & Helm-Estabrooks, N. (1994). A linguistic communication measure for aphasic narratives. *Aphasiology, 8*, 343–359.

Meyers, J. E., & Meyers, K. R. (1995). *Rey complex figure test and recognition trial*. Lutz, FL: Psychological Assessment Resources.

Muma, J. R. (1978). *Language handbook: Concepts, assessment and intervention*. Englewood Cliffs, NJ: Prentice-Hall.

Newhoff, M., & Apel, K. (1990). Impairments in pragmatics. In L. L. LaPointe (Ed.), *Aphasia and related neurogenic language disorders* (pp. 221–233). New York, NY: Thieme Medical.

Orjada, S. A., & Beeson, P. M. (2005). Concurrent treatment for reading and spelling in aphasia. *Aphasiology, 19*, 341–351.

Pashek, G. (1997). A case study of gesturally cued naming in aphasia: Dominant versus non-dominant hand training. *Journal of Communication Disorders, 30*, 349–366.

Peach, R. K. (2008). Global aphasia: Identification and management. In R. Chapey (Ed.), *Language intervention strategies in aphasia and related neurogenic communication disorders* (5th ed.). Philadelphia, PA: Lippincott Williams & Wilkins.

Picard, N., & Strick, P. L. (1996). Motor areas of the medial wall: A review of their location and functional activation. *Cerebral Cortex, 6*, 342–353.

Pulvermuller, F., Neininger, B., Elbert, T., Mohr, B., Rockstroh, B., Koebbel, P., & Taub, E., . . . (2001). Constraint-induced therapy of chronic aphasia after stroke. *Stroke, 32*, 1621–1626.

Ramsberger, G., & Marie, B. (2007). Self-administered cued naming therapy: A single- participant investigation of a computer-based therapy program replicated in four cases. *American Journal of Speech-Language Pathology, 16*, 343–358.

Rao, P. R. (1994). Use of Amer-Ind code by persons with aphasia. In R. Chapey (Ed.), *Language intervention strategies in adult aphasia* (pp. 359–367). Baltimore, MD: Lippincott Williams & Wilkins.

Richards, K., Singletary, F., Gonzalez Rothi, L. J., & Koehler, S., & Crosson, B. (2002). Activation of intentional mechanisms through utilization of nonsymbolic movements in aphasia rehabilitation. *Journal of Rehabilitation Research and Development, 39*, 445–454.

Schuell, H. (1974). The treatment of aphasia. In L. F. Sies (Ed.), *Aphasia theory and therapy: Selected lectures and papers of Hildred Schuell*. Baltimore, MD: University Park Press.

Schuell, H., Carroll, V., & Street, B. S. (1955). Clinical treatment of aphasia. *Journal of Speech and Hearing Disorders, 20*, 43–53.

Schuell, H., Jenkins, J., & Jiménez-Pabón, E. (1964). *Aphasia in adults: Diagnosis, prognosis and treatment*. New York, NY: Harper & Row.

Shelton, J. R., Weinrich, M., McCall, D., & Cox, D. M. (1996). Differentiating globally aphasic patients: Data from in-depth language assessments and production training using C-ViC. *Aphasiology, 10*, 319–342.

Skelly, M. (1979). *Amer-Ind gestural code based on universal American Indian hand talk*. New York, NY: Elsevier.

Skelly, M., Schinsky, L., Smith, R., & Fust, R. S. (1974). American Indian (AmerInd) Sign as a facilitation of verbalization for the oral verbal apraxic. *Journal of Speech and Hearing Disorders, 39*, 445–456.

Smith, A. (1971). Objective indices of severity of chronic aphasia in stroke patients. *Journal of Speech and Hearing Disorders, 36*, 167–207.

Steele, R. D., Kleczewska, M. K., Carlson, G. S., & Weinrich, M. (1992). Computers in the rehabilitation of chronic, severe aphasia: C-ViC 2.0 cross-modal studies. *Aphasiology, 6*, 185–194.

Steele, R. D., Weinrich, M., Wertz, R. T., Kleczewska, M. K., & Carlson, G. S. (1989). Computer-based visual communication in aphasia. *Neuropsychologia, 27*, 409–426.

Stokes, T., & Baer, D. M. (1977). An implicit technology of generalization. *Journal of Applied Behavior Analysis, 10*, 349–367.

Thompson, C. K. (2001). Treatment of underlying forms: A linguistic specific approach for sentence production deficits in agrammatic aphasia. In R. Chapey (Ed.), *Language intervention strategies in aphasia and related neurogenic communication disorders* (4th ed., pp. 605–628). Philadelphia, PA: Lippincott Williams & Wilkins.

Wechsler, D. (1981). *The Wechsler Adult Intelligence Scale*. New York, NY: The Psychological Corporation.

Wechsler, D. (1997). *Wechsler Memory Scale* (3rd ed.). San Antonio, TX: Psychological Corp.

Weinrich, M., Steele, R. D., Carlson, G. S., Kleczewska, M. K., Wertz, R. T., & Baker, E. (1989). Processing of visual syntax in a globally aphasic patient. *Brain and Language, 36*, 391–405.

Weinrich, M., Steele, R. D., Kleczewska, M. K., Carlson, G. S., Baker, E., & Wertz, R. T. (1989). Representation of "verbs" in a computerized visual communication system. *Aphasiology, 3*, 501–512.

Wepman, J. (1972). Aphasia therapy: A new look. *Journal of Speech and Hearing Disorders, 37*, 203–214.

Wepman, J. (1976). Aphasia: Language without thought or thought without language. *ASHA, 18*, 131–136.

Wertz, R. T. (1984). Language disorders in adults: State of the clinical art. In A. Holland (Ed.), *Language disorders in adults*. San Diego, CA: College-Hill Press.

Wilcox, M. H., & Davis, G. (1977). Speech act analysis of aphasic communication in individual and group settings. In R. H. Brookshire (Ed.), *Clinical aphasiology conference proceedings* (pp. 166–174). Minneapolis, MN: BRK.

Appendix E

THE WORLD HEALTH ORGANIZATION AND THE INTERNATIONAL CLASSIFICATION OF FUNCTIONING, DISABILITY, AND HEALTH

The International Classification of Functioning, Disability, and Health (ICF) shifts from a medical model to a more integrated bio-psychosocial model for analyzing human functioning and disability. The ICF is important to the definitions, measurement practices, and policies of the health and disability of people around the world. Furthermore, it provides individuals with a common language and a framework to describe issues of health. It provides a classification of health-related domains used to describe body structure and function, and what an individual with a specific health condition can do in their environment based on their capacity level and performance ability. The ICF shifts the focus from cause to the impact health conditions can place on one's functioning in the world. The ICF is a tool that allows individuals to compare information about health and disability. It provides the general basis for the World Health Organization's overall approach to health. Service provision using the ICF is geared to answer such individualized questions as:

- What is the individual's level of functioning?
- What treatments or interventions can maximize functioning?

- What are the outcomes of the treatment, and how useful were the interventions?
- How would I rate my capacity in mobility or communication?

The underlying principle of the ICF is that anyone can have a disability, and that disease/disorder is multidimensional. Disease is not culturally, geographically, or gender-specific; it can occur at any time across the lifetime; and there are barriers and facilitators—personal and environmental—that can affect a person's rehabilitation. The person with a disability is viewed as a whole person in this model and not as a medical condition. For example, *context-inclusive* addressees the need to consider the social network and resources of the person with the disorder, not only the disorder itself. The outcomes of a rehabilitation program should be functional and ultimately facilitating the person's return to the social fabric. The foundations of the ICF can be summarized by the following schema:

Human Functioning	—*not merely disability*
Universal Model	—*not a minority model*
Integrative Model	—*not merely medical or social*

Interactive Model   —*not linear progressive*

Parity   —*not etiological causality*

Context-Inclusive   —*not person alone*

Cultural Applicability —*not western concepts*

Operational   —*not theory driven alone*

Life Span Coverage   —*not adult driven*

The original system, instituted in 1980, used the categories of *Disorder, Impairment, Disability,* and *Handicap.* Graphically, this can be represented as:

Disorder→Impairment→Disability→Handicap

The interpretation for a particular disorder or disease could be explained as a disease/disorder leads to an impairment, which creates a disability, and has handicapping consequences. This was an important first step because it captured the condition of the whole person within one framework. This was refined further with the ICF of 2001 and 2007 (Table E–1, Comparison Chart). The change involved a redefinition of the impact of the disease on the patient and added barriers and facilitators impacting rehabilitation.

This familiar graphic in Figure E–1, illustrates the current ICF conceptualization of disease/disorder. The interactive aspect of this model is readily visible.

Table E–1. A Comparison of ICIDH 1980 with the Most Current Model

Handicap	Impairment		Disability
ICIDH 1980 (Noninteractive)	Deviation from the norm	Functional consequences of impairment	A social consequence of the impairment or disability; defined by social attitudes and responses.
ICF 2007 (Interactive)	Body Structure/ Functions	Activities	Participation
	Functions Structures	*Capacity Performance*	*Barriers Facilitators*

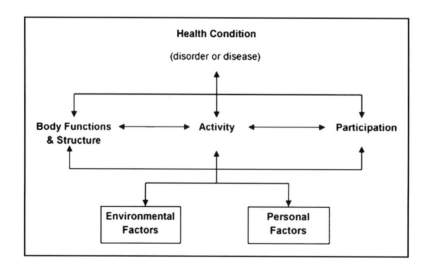

Figure E–1. World Health Organization (2002) ICF Model.

Body Functions and Structures

The ICF (2001) has systematized body functions and structures, and placed them in relational pairs. For example, *Mental Functions* is paired with *Structures of the Nervous System*, and *Voice and Speech Functions* is paired with *Structures Involved in Voice and Speech*. It is notable that there is no pair such as "Language Functions/Structures Related to Language Production and Comprehension" to characterize the aphasias, for example. However, there is a classification under *Specific Mental Functions* (b140–b189), which is *Mental Functions of Language* (b1670), and that covers the aphasias. (See http://apps.who.int/classifications/icfbrowser/

Activities and Participation

This element of the model addresses the functional effects of the disease or disorder. A list of the *Activities* and *Participation* component is below:

- Learning and applying knowledge
- General tasks and demands
- Communication
- Movement
- Self-care
- Domestic life areas
- Interpersonal interactions
- Major life areas
- Community, social, and civic life.

Contextual Factors (Environmental Factors and Personal Factors)

The environmental factors and personal factors affecting rehabilitation are jointly referred to as *Contextual Factors* in the ICF (2007) model. The model recognizes the impact that context can have on a patient's recovery, and the context within which each individual operates in the world is unique to that individual. Therefore, a clinician must consider these factors so that the whole person is considered during treatment planning.

There are many environmental factors and personal factors that can affect a person's rehabilitation, and as a consequence, their ability to be a participant in social interactions and activities. The current ICF model asks the provider to take those factors into consideration during the rehabilitation process. The *Environmental Factors* are divided into barriers and facilitators. A particular factor can be either a barrier or a facilitator, because the model requires that the patient be considered as a unique individual, with unique life circumstances. For example, for one patient, their natural environment may act as a facilitator in the rehabilitation, yet for another it may be a barrier. The *Environmental Factors* are listed below:

- Natural environment and human-made changes to the environment
- Products and technology
- Support and relationships
- Attitudes
- Services, systems, and policies.

The ICF and the Rehabilitation of the Person with an Acquired Language Disorder

As rehabilitation professionals, the value of this model cannot be overstated. If the goal of treatment is to restore the individual to the social fabric —the context—of his or her life, then treating the whole person makes eminent sense. This model is also consistent with the ASHA Code of Ethics that mandates individualized treatment while holding the "welfare of the patient paramount." Any of the disorders discussed in this book can be interpreted and addressed using the current ICF model, and a wise clinician will find great benefit in doing so. We provide an example of how to use the ICF model with a person with aphasia in Table E–2.

The follow categories complete the list of primary considerations within the ICF.

Table E–2. How to Use the ICF Model with a Person with Aphasia

Disease/ Disorder	Body Structure/ Function	Activity	Participation	Barriers	Facilitators
CVA	Neurological structures and functions; Mental functions for language	Communication	Interpersonal interactions; movement; learning and applying new knowledge	No caregiver support; depression; low socioeconomic status	Nephew nearby willing to visit; social worker assigned; in-home aide 3 times per week for 4 hours

Body

Function

Mental Functions

Sensory Functions and Pain

Voice and Speech Functions

Functions of the Cardiovascular, Hematological, Immunological, and Respiratory Systems

Functions of the Digestive, Metabolic, Endocrine Systems

Genitourinary and Reproductive Functions

Neuromusculoskeletal and Movement-Related Functions

Functions of the Skin and Related Structures

Structure

Structure of the Nervous System

The Eye, Ear, and Related Structures

Structures Involved in Voice and Speech

Structure of the Cardiovascular, Immunological, and Respiratory Systems

Structures Related to the Digestive, Metabolic, and Endocrine Systems

Structure Related to Genitourinary and Reproductive Systems

Structure Related to Movement

Skin and Related Structures

Activities and Participation

Learning and Applying Knowledge

General Tasks and Demands

Communication

Mobility

Self-Care

Domestic Life

Interpersonal Interactions and Relationships

Major Life Areas

Community, Social, and Civic Life

Environmental Factors

Products and Technology

Natural Environment and Human-Made Changes to Environment

Support and Relationships

Attitudes

Services, Systems, and Policies

Reference

World Health Organization. (2002). *Towards a common language for functioning, disability and health: International classification of functioning, disability and health.* Geneva, Switzerland. Retrieved from http://www.who.int/classifications/icf/training/icf beginnersguide.pdf

Appendix F

THE OCTAGON WORKSHEET FOR FUNCTIONAL COMMUNICATION

FUNCTIONAL COMMUNICATION CONNECTIONS

VISUALLY MEDIATED

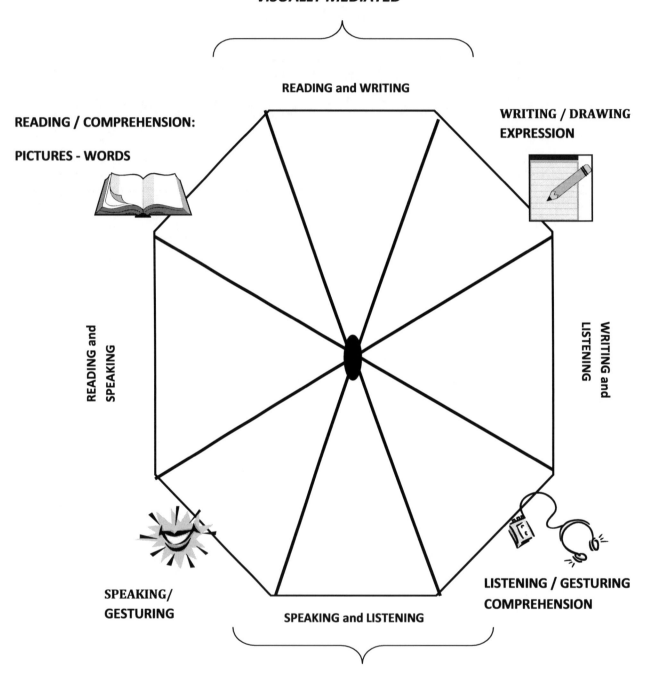

READING and WRITING

READING / COMPREHENSION:

PICTURES - WORDS

WRITING / DRAWING
EXPRESSION

READING and SPEAKING

WRITING and LISTENING

SPEAKING/
GESTURING

LISTENING / GESTURING
COMPREHENSION

SPEAKING and LISTENING

VERBALLY MEDIATED

Appendix G

TEST YOUR KNOWLEDGE

■ This examination focuses on *critical thinking,* given detailed clinical information.

■ There are 50 questions on this examination, based on seven case scenarios. Read the case scenarios very carefully. This is a skill that you must master in this discipline.

■ Choose the one best response and circle your response on the answer sheet below and darken the appropriate corresponding responses.

Case #1

This patient is a 60-year-old WM found down by his son in the living room of a house that they share. The patient was not breathing and had no pulse. The patient's son started CPR after calling 911, and he continued with CPR until EMS arrived, 10 minutes later. EMS found the patient to be unconscious, not breathing, and pulseless. They implemented the cardiac arrest protocol. A respiration and a pulse were restored. The son told EMS that the patient must have been down "for at least 10 minutes" before he called 911. The patient was transferred to the EMS vehicle and taken to the local hospital.

The patient was stabilized in the emergency department and transferred to the cardiac care unit. Two weeks post-event, the critical care attending consulted speech-language pathology to assess the patient's cognitive-linguistic status in preparation for eventual transfer to the next level of care. The chart review indicated that the patient had variable levels of alertness; mumbles "occasionally"; is totally dependent on nursing for his activities of daily living. Nursing reports that he "just lays there most of the day." His family is present in the afternoon hours, and they are asking for "rehab."

1. Based on the history above, it is most likely that this patient is presenting with:
   a. Lewy body dementia
   b. PPA
   c. Anoxic encephalopathy
   d. RHD

2. As the family is asking for "rehab," is it reasonable to assume that the DRS would be the appropriate rating scale for this patient as part of your assessment?
   a. Yes, because the DRS is a scale related to functioning post-hospitalization and therefore describes the patient from a rehab potential perspective.
   b. Yes, because the DRS assesses brain injury.
   c. Yes, because the DRS is the best and most efficacious assessment instrument for all anoxic patients.
   d. No, I would still use the Rancho rating system for this patient.

3. This family is asking for inpatient rehab services at a free-standing rehabilitation hospital 2 weeks post event. This may pose a counseling and education problem for you. How would you handle this?
   a. I would refer to social work and step aside.
   b. I would notify the resident and tell her that this family is irate and unrealistic and demand a social work consult from her.

c. I would ask for a family meeting and explain the goals and procedures of my treatment plan while the patient is at this level of care. Then I would take their questions.

d. I would advocate for the patient and family and start an intense rehabilitation treatment plan immediately.

4. Once you complete the assessment on this patient while he is in acute care, which approach would you use at the outset of therapy?

a. I would start immediately with ORLA.

b. I would address his poor attentional skills, gradually increasing his ability to attend to me for longer periods of time.

c. I would start with a verbal expression goal, so that he can communicate his basic needs.

d. I would start developing a writing treatment plan as he is nonverbal.

5. The patient is transferred to a rehab facility. He stays there for 8 weeks. He then comes back to your hospital for continued OP therapy because it is closer to his home than going back to the rehab facility. He is now verbal, and still mildly lethargic although attentive, and with a mild auditory processing deficit. What would you do first?

a. I would conduct my own formal assessment in order to delineate his current strengths and weaknesses.

b. I would use the rehab therapist's notes and continue with his treatment.

c. I would refer the patient to a community reentry program in order to prepare him for his eventual return to work.

d. I would not treat this patient as this is as good as he will get, based on his initial clinical presentation.

Case #2

The patient is a 24-year-old WM who sustained a TBI as an unrestrained passenger in a motor vehicle accident. He was unresponsive at the scene of the accident. He was taken to an acute care hospital where a CAT scan revealed cerebral edema, left tha-lamic bleed, and an intraventricular bleed. He was transferred to another acute care hospital, where he underwent a left ventriculostomy. He also suffered a left tibia fracture that was repaired by open reduction internal fixation (ORIF), a left ulna fracture that was casted, and a left clavicle fracture. Thirteen days later, the patient went into respiratory failure that required a tracheostomy. He was placed on 28% oxygen. A G-tube was also placed at this time for nutritional needs and provision of medication.

The patient was transferred to a rehabilitation center approximately 4 weeks post-injury, at a Rancho Level 2. He was making generalized responses to auditory stimuli but was unresponsive to both visual and tactile stimuli. He was unable to follow commands and dependent in all self-care, communication, and mobility. He continued to receive all nutrition through the G-tube and still required the tracheostomy with room air. At this time in his rehabilitation stay, he was receiving physical, occupational, and speech-language pathology services. As noted above, the patient was transferred to rehab when he was 4 weeks out from the injury, and he began receiving therapeutic services from PT, OT, and speech. He arrived as a Rancho Level 2 patient. He is now 8 weeks out from the injury, and he is able to participate in 3 hours of treatment per day—one hour in each therapy. He is now at Rancho Level 6. They are weaning him from the G-tube feedings, and he is starting to meet his nutritional goals via PO feeds (PO = eating by mouth). His current cognitive/communication profile is as follows:

- LOA: Usually awake and alert in the morning. Needs more attentional cues in the afternoon to attend to tasks.
- Receptive language: 1-step commands, 2-step simple commands with objects: 100%;
- Confrontation naming: moderate impairment, improved from baseline 4 weeks ago;
- Expressive language: Semantic paraphasias persist; syntax WFL at sentence level for short declarative sentences, more paraphasic at conversational level.
- Speech Production: flat intonation, slow rate, but 100% intelligible in known

and unknown contexts despite mild consonantal distortions.

- Memory: Declarative memory is impaired; procedural memory for activities of daily living needs is mildly impaired.
- Behavior: Emerging awareness of deficits; still asks to "leave to go to work," but can be redirected; emotional lability noted, but decreasing.

6. According to the admission record, this patient was diagnosed with cerebral edema. To monitor the pressure on his brain, the neurosurgeons will need to insert:
   a. A craniotomy
   b. an IV
   c. an intraventricular shunt
   d. an ICP bolt

7. The initial imaging studies revealed a "left thalamic bleed." As this patient has sustained a TBI, it is unlikely that he will also present with a subcortical aphasia.
   a. TRUE
   b. FALSE

8. The GCS on this patient was:
   a. Not reported
   b. 3/15
   c. 15/15
   d. 0/15

9. According to the patient's record, he was at Rancho Level 2 four weeks out from his injury. At that level, therapeutic intervention is focused on intense rehabilitation efforts.
   a. TRUE
   b. FALSE

10. This patient is presenting with clinical symptomatology consistent with aphasia secondary to a TBI.
    a. TRUE
    b. FALSE

11. Once this patient was ready to participate in treatment, I would focus my goals on optimizing his functional communication with others by addressing which of the following:
    a. Speech production
    b. Sentence building
    c. Developing his awareness of his paraphasic errors
    d. Writing

12. The patient is now in rehab at your facility. As noted above, he has intelligible speech, despite mild distortions and a flat intonation contour. What would you do in this case?
    a. Initiate an intense oromotor program since this would eliminate his muscle weakness and make his speech more articulate.
    b. Take stimulability data on his ability to benefit from contrastive stress drills, which teaches him to vary the intonation based on meaning.
    c. I would use MIT and start at the sound segment level.
    d. I would not address the speech impairment since he is functional in the social context.

13. Every time the patient sees his parents, he begins to cry and asks if he can "go to work today." His parents are aware that this is organic; however, it is beginning to affect them, and one morning, the nurse found all of them crying together. However, when she asked, "Why are you crying?" the patient responded, "I don't know, I just do." If this happens during a therapeutic session with you, it is your responsibility to:
    a. Leave the room and allow them to be alone.
    b. Stay in the room with them, ask them how you can help, and then follow their lead.
    c. Leave the room and immediately call social work.
    d. Explain to the parents and the patient that this will not improve, and that they must adjust, that is, using a "tough love" approach to counseling them.

14. At Level 6, this patient is characterized as:
    a. Localized responses: total assistance
    b. Confused-agitated: Max assist
    c. Appropriate: Min assist for activities of daily living
    d. Confused-appropriate: Mod assist

15. This patient, like all TBI patients, has memory impairment. His declarative memory is worse than his procedural memory. OT has asked that you cotreat with them during his morning activities of daily living. Since OT focuses on the *acts* of shaving, bathing, dressing, and so forth, your primary role in this cotreatment scenario is to:
    a. Monitor his language use during these activities.
    b. Provide memory strategies so that he can remember the names of the items being used.
    c. Provide a script so that he can communicate during the activity(ies).
    d. Provide memory strategies, cue him during processing as needed, and provide strategies that he can use to self-cue during these activities.

Case #3

This is a case of a 60-year-old male, with a history of HTN and Type I diabetes for the past 15 years. He presented at the emergency department with complaints of mild left upper limb weakness and slurred speech, which started simultaneously half an hour earlier. His PMH included stroke in 2001 as well as a CABG (coronary artery bypass and graft) done in 1996. He was admitted to rule out stroke. On day 2 of the admission, he complained of severe weakness of the left upper extremity with no sensory changes. The following morning his left upper extremity was flaccid, and his speech abnormality worsened. The nursing assessment from that morning reported the following:

- He was conscious and oriented to person, time, and place.
- He stood with assistance, and his gait was normal walking to the bathroom.
- Vital signs were stable (BP; heart rate/rhythm; respiratory rate; afebrile)
- The CNS examination revealed the following:
- Mild dysarthria; no hypernasality, with pitch breaks.

- Left facial weakness; tongue was deviated to the left on protrusion; palate was normal; uvula central and gag reflex present.

16. Based on the case history information above, this patient is presenting with:
    a. A right CVA with speech impairment and buccofacial weakness.
    b. A right CVA with anoxia.
    c. A left CVA with dysarthria and aphasia
    d. A right CVA with no buccofacial involvement.

17. Once stabilized, this patient may present with cognitive-linguistic impairment. The following would be true in this case:
    a. He may be aphasic, and as I do not know if he is left-handed, I would administer a test for aphasia.
    b. He will resolve into a TBI-type patient.
    c. Paralinguistic and extralinguistic deficits would predominate.
    d. There would be syntactic, morphologic, and phonologic deficits in this patient.

18. In order to evaluate this patient, I would use:
    a. The MIRBI
    b. The SCATBI
    c. The WAB-R
    d. The ABCD

19. Based on the case history as reported above, this patient appears to be a high *cardiac* risk. Therefore, the case history supports the probability that the etiology of this stroke is most likely:
    a. Thrombotic or embolic
    b. Hemorrhagic
    c. Intraventricular
    d. Subdural hematoma

20. Based on the information that you have about this patient, it is also possible that he may present with:
    a. Behavioral abnormalities, language issues, emotional lability
    b. Prosopagnosia, anosagnosia, tangential output

c. Attentional problems, apraxia of speech, and dysgraphia without alexia

d. Personality changes exacerbated by the intracerebral pressure

Case #4

This patient is a 14-year-old male who had a skateboard accident at the skateboard park. This was witnessed by his friends. According to their report, the patient attempted a trick that involved a maneuver that he hadn't perfected, and he fell backward and hit his head on the concrete. They described him as sitting up briefly, but then he passed out. They called 911.

EMS arrived, and the patient was breathing with a strong pulse, but had his eyes closed and was very lethargic. His GCS was as follows: Eye Opening: 3; Verbal Response: 4; Motor Response: 5. He was transferred to the local hospital, admitted to neurosurgery service, and was placed under observation in the neuro-intensive care unit. His parents, who were both in health care, were notified, and they arrived promptly.

Once the CT of the head and the MRI was read, neurosurgery determined that he did not have a subdural, subarachnoid, or an epidural hemorrhage. He was described as "out-of-the-woods," and they wanted to release him the next day. However, the parents said that, "He's not sharp. He is a very bright boy, and he doesn't know the state capital or our home state." They wanted a rehab consult to assess his cognition. Neurosurgery stated that there is no medical reason for him to be in the hospital, so they will still discharge him. However, they will write for an OP evaluation and treatment by speech, PT, and OT. The patient was discharged the next day at 11 AM.

21. This patient presents with a case history consistent with:
   a. PPA
   b. PCS
   c. SDAT
   d. TBI with anosagnosia

22. According to the report of the patient's friends at the scene of the event, this patient fell backward and hit his head on the concrete. Most likely, this caused:
   a. Occipital involvement due to a coup injury from the fall
   b. Temporal involvement due to a contrecoup injury from the fall
   c. Parieto-occipital hemorrhage
   d. An occipital skull fracture

23. The patient did lose consciousness at the scene, but only briefly. As a consequence, he is not considered a patient with a TBI.
   a. TRUE
   b. FALSE

24. This young man and his parents arrived on time for the OP evaluation 2 weeks post-discharge. They were pleasant, cooperative, and obviously very informed about their son's status and health care issues in general. You decide to administer which test?
   a. WAB-2
   b. MTDDA
   c. Revised Token Test
   d. SCATBI

25. The results of the assessment revealed the following deficit areas: memory, attention, information processing, and concrete thinking. You inform the parents that you will be recommending treatment to focus on these deficit areas. You discover that this patient cannot attend for 15 minutes without asking for a "walk outside." The mother reports that he is not doing well in class and is getting up to go to the bathroom very often. She thinks that he is taking these breaks because he cannot manage the classroom context. She asks you if this "makes any sense based on your experience." You state:
   a. No, it does not. He had no identifiable injury on the MRI, so this is probably laziness.
   b. Yes it does. He had a severe brain injury, and this is always expected.
   c. Yes, it does. His testing revealed attentional problems, and these types of injuries have very subtle symptoms after the fact.
   d. Yes it does. He's 14 and hates school!

Case #5

A 36-year-old WF was shopping at the local super-market. A witness reported that the patient "wobbled to the right, and then fell down." The witness alerted the store manager who immediately called 911. EMS arrived in 6 minutes. The patient was breathing nor-mally, eyes open, moaning, and conscious.

The patient was an accounts manager for a pub-lic relations firm and is at her desk at least 12 hours per day. Her family reported that her firm downsized and that she was "furloughed." As a consequence, she has been feeling very stressed. She often reported to her friends and family that her heart "feels funny sometimes." The patient smokes cigarettes 1 ppd, drinks socially, and "loves her coffee." Her family reported that she has gained at least 50 lbs. recently, causing great embarrassment. She does not partici-pate in a fitness program of any sort. Her sleep has been negatively affected by her life circumstances.

When EMS arrived on the scene, their assess-ment included the following data:

- Nonverbal; not following commands; eyes open; paretic (paretic = weak) right arm; right facial droop
- Slightly irregular heart rate
- Pulse 80, BP 160/85, respiratory rate 20, afebrile

EMS called the patient in as a "probable stroke." She was transferred to the local hospital and admitted to the critical care unit for monitoring. The patient was stabilized in the critical care unit and transferred to a telemetry floor.

26. You were consulted on day 5 of this admission. The medical diagnosis on your *Request for Con-sultation* print out was L CVA. You have 30 to 40 minutes to evaluate this patient due to a depart-mental staff meeting on the hour. You decide to use which assessment tool to evaluate this patient?
    a. MIRBI
    b. CADL
    c. WAB-R
    d. BDAE

27. When you enter the patient's room, she is sitting up in bed. You notice that her head is turned to the left. You stand at the foot of the bed and call her name, and she responds but does not turn toward the sound of your voice. Which of the following disorders must be ruled out?
    a. Simultagnosia
    b. Prosopagnosia
    c. Auditory agnosia
    d. Visual neglect due to hemianopsia

28. The patient is awake, alert, and cooperative with no complaint of pain. You administer the selected test instrument. Selected findings indicate: sig-nificant logorrhea and neologistic output; mod-erate-severe auditory comprehension deficit. This suggests that this patient is presenting with:
    a. A posterior aphasia, probably of the Wer-nicke's type
    b. An anterior aphasia, more consistent with a Broca's type
    c. A mixed aphasia due to the occluded territory
    d. A subcortical aphasia due to the visual involvement

29. The etiology of this stroke is most likely from a:
    a. Subdural hemorrhage
    b. Cardiac source
    c. Blood disorder
    d. Eating disorder

30. When reviewing this patient's chart before you enter to begin the evaluation, the most relevant information in the history taken by EMS, for your purposes, is:
    a. Pulmonary and social histories
    b. Neuro, vitals taken in the field, and CV status
    c. Neuro, social, and pulmonary
    d. CV only

31. On day 6 of the admission, you enter the room to begin treatment with this patient. It makes the most sense to:
    a. Place sequencing cards in front of her and ask her to "tell the story."
    b. Begin a word-finding task.
    c. Stand midline and have her locate you, and then explain why.

d. Explain the phonological elements of her neologisms in order to heighten her awareness of them.

32. The reading subtest of the test instrument indicated that this patient had a reading disorder. As a consequence, you decide to administer the Reading Comprehension Battery for Aphasia (RCBA). You find the following:
    a. Unable to sound out words
    b. There is a sound-symbol disassociation
    c. Uses word shape to facilitate meaning
    d. Uses memory as a strategy to facilitate reading

33. This patient is presenting with an alexia with the characteristics of:
    a. A peripheral type with global characteristics
    b. A central type with surface alexia characteristics
    c. A central type with phonological alexia characteristics
    d. A peripheral type with pure characteristics

34. This patient is presenting with a dysarthria.
    a. TRUE
    b. FALSE

35. One of the packaged programs that can be useful for a patient with this type of aphasia is:
    a. MIT
    b. PACE
    c. SPPA
    d. NMAI

36. In the acute care setting, your goals for this patient will include:
    a. Optimizing her auditory comprehension; addressing the logorrhea; and providing her with a functional means of communication for her immediate needs.
    b. Developing her repetition skills; facilitating her writing skills; aggressively addressing the alexia.
    c. Addressing lexical retrieval functions; optimizing her narrative discourse; addressing auditory processing
    d. Encouraging more conversational speech with family and friends; do not address the logorrhea as this is a sign of recovery; optimize attentional skills.

Case #6

A 57-year-old female retired business owner began having difficulty finding words. Over time, she found it more difficult to express her thoughts and started become socially withdrawn and was characterized by family as "a quiet little mouse." She used mostly nouns and struggled with connected speech. There was no family history of stroke or dementia. The case history described her pleasant, well-groomed, cooperative, and courteous. Her neurological examination was WNL.

The neurologist's report indicated that her MMSE (Mini Mental State Exam) was 29/30, missing only a repetition item. Her speech was nonfluent, agrammatic, with struggle behavior noted. Her auditory comprehension was WNL. Working memory was mildly impaired. She generated 17 animals in 1 minute but only 8 "d" words. She correctly named 57 of 60 words on the Boston Naming Test (BNT). Recognizing facial emotions was normal.

The patient's MRI revealed asymmetric atrophy of the left frontal lobes. EMG was normal. The neurologist reported that he tested for tau protein in the blood, but it was absent. Unfortunately, this patient had a significant decline within 2 years. She became mute and developed a moderate dysphagia. The neurologist diagnosed this patient with dementia, most likely of the FTP type.

37. This patient is presenting with Alzheimer's Disease.
    a. TRUE
    b. FALSE

38. From the choices below, which is the linguistic symptom that *most* indicates frontal lobe involvement?
    a. Agraphia
    b. Visual perceptual deficits
    c. Agrammatism
    d. Lexical retrieval problems

39. Based on the case history above, the evaluator noted that the patient had no problem recognizing faces. The technical name for the inability to recognize faces is:

    a. Visual agnosia
    b. Simultagnosia
    c. Prosopagnosia
    d. Incomplete gestalt phenomenon

40. Is it atypical to read that lexical retrieval issues are an early symptom in a case history of a patient with dementia?
    a. YES
    b. NO

41. The physician requested that a test for "tau" be included in the patient's bloodwork profile. This is because:
    a. The tau protein is the marker for all dementias.
    b. Tau accumulation in the CSF indicates a FTP-type dementia.
    c. It has been shown that an accumulation of the tau protein in the CSF is indicative of SDAT. He wanted to make a differential.
    d. The tau protein breaks down cells in the language area of the cortex.

42. You are consulted at the 2-year mark in this patient's process. The role of the speech-language pathologist in this case at that time is:
    a. To work with the family, providing counseling and education around the issues of the patient's cognitive-linguistic decline.
    b. To begin training the patient in compensatory strategies for her activities of daily living needs.
    c. OP treatment 2 times per week for 8 weeks in order to establish a baseline for her cognitive-linguistic functions.
    d. Aggressive cognitive-linguistic treatment to restore communicative functions.

43. When working with this patient, it is wise to redirect her gently if she is caught up in an obsessive, unrealistic thought pattern.
    a. TRUE—Because they are unable to reason clearly, so challenging them to alter that pattern will be futile.
    b. FALSE—You must challenge their irrational thoughts, so that they can learn to break the cycle.

44. The patient was able to name 17 animals in 1 minute but only 8 words with initial /d/ in the phonological configuration. This shows that:
    a. Lexical retrieval is still intact.
    b. Retrieving nouns is easier than retrieving verbs.
    c. Lexical retrieval is not yet an issue.
    d. The sound-symbol relationship is beginning to fracture.

45. Agrammatic productions were noted in this patient's output. She also presented with "articulatory groping" and "a stuttering output." Therefore, this patient's symptoms are consistent with which type of aphasia?
    a. Conduction aphasia
    b. Anomic aphasia
    c. Jargon aphasia
    d. Nonfluent aphasia

46. The patient is described as "mute" at the 2-year mark. This is when you meet her. Although her auditory comprehension is still functional, though mildly impaired, which of the options below would you choose to pursue?
    a. I would take baseline data on her ability to use an AAC system, from the most simple to the most complex available in our hospital at that time.
    b. I would use CILT to facilitate verbal expression.
    c. I would teach the patient a simple gestural language for use in the home.
    d. a and c

Case #7

This patient is a 60-year-old, right-handed WM with h/o HTN, and recent MI (myocardial infarction), who had a sudden onset of right central facial paralysis, right upper and lower extremity hemiparesis, and the inability to speak. The patient was sitting in his car, waiting to pull out of his driveway. His neighbor came by approximately 15 minutes later and found him slumped against the window on the driver's side. He was awake but unable to speak. The neighbor called 911. They arrived within 6 minutes. The patient was stabilized by EMS and transferred to the local hospital, called in as a "stroke in progress."

The patient's PMH included: morbid obesity, HTN, MI, ASCVD (atherosclerotic cardiovascular disease), and hypercholesterolemia. The patient is a 2 ppd smoker. No ETOH.

Both the CT scan and MRI supported a diagnosis of left MCA branch infarct. The areas infarcted included the pre-Rolandic region (specifically Brodmann's 44 and 45), the motor strip, with some involvement of the inferior frontal region. Radiology also noted that there was "some question about white matter involvement" but his may have been old. Radiology and neurology agreed that the probable etiology was cardioembolic.

47. The clinical presentation of this patient in the field raised the question of etiology. Why did radiology believe that his stroke was "cardioembolic"?
    a. The patient was obese and a smoker.
    b. A history of MI, HTN and ASCVD, and hypercholesterolemia support the diagnosis.
    c. The patient already sustained one MI, and this stroke was likely caused by a second one.
    d. The facial paralysis always indicates a cardioembolic event.

48. Upon reviewing the chart, and reading the imaging studies, which type of aphasia are you anticipating?
    a. An anterior aphasia
    b. A mixed aphasia
    c. A posterior aphasia

d. A subcortical aphasia

49. This patient was transferred to a free-standing rehab facility after 8 days in acute care. You are consulted to evaluate the patient. You choose the WAB-R and the BNT. You chose these two instruments because:
    a. They are reimbursable.
    b. The WAB-R gives an aphasia quotient and is brief; and the BNT can give a detailed picture of the word-finding deficit that you expect to find.
    c. The WAB-R gives an aphasia quotient and the BNT assesses naming and auditory comprehension.
    d. The family insisted on these two tests.

50. The patient does present with a mild dysarthria, although his speech intelligibility is 100% in known and unknown contexts. Why would you choose *not* to include speech articulation as a goal in his therapy plan?
    a. I would still choose to work on articulation because it would get him even closer to normal, premorbid levels.
    b. I would choose not to work on his speech articulation because it would only make him more frustrated to correct something that is functional.
    c. I would choose not to work on his speech articulation because he is 100% intelligible, and there are other deficit areas requiring more intense focus.
    d. I would not choose to work on his speech articulation because he is depressed and unwilling to participate in treatment anyway.

Answer Key

1. c	11. c	21. b	31. c	41. c
2. a	12. b	22. a	32. c	42. a
3. c	13. b	23. b	33. b	43. a
4. b	14. d	24. d	34. b	44. d
5. a	15. d	25. c	35. b	45. d
6. d	16. a	26. c	36. a	46. d
7. b	17. c	27. d	37. b	47. b
8. a	18. a	28. a	38. c	48. a
9. b	19. a	29. b	39. c	49. b
10. a	20. b	30. b	40. a	50. c

INDEX

Note: Page numbers in **bold** reference non-text material.